THE ENGLISH–CHINESE ENCYCLOPEDIA OF PRACTICAL TRADITIONAL CHINESE MEDICINE

Chief Editor   Xu Xiangcai

Assistants   You Ke   Kang Kai

                  Bao Xuequan   Lu Yubin

英汉实用中医药大全

主　编　　徐象才

主编助理　尤　可　　康　凯

　　　　　鲍学全　　路玉滨

D1670502

Higher Education Press

高等教育出版社

Preface

I am delighted to learn that THE ENGLISH−CHINESE ENCYCLOPEDIA OF PRACTICAL TRADITIONAL CHINESE MEDICINE will soon come into the world.

TCM has experienced many vicissitudes of times but has remained evergreen. It has made great contributions not only to the power and prosperity of our Chinese nation but to the enrichment and improvement of world medicine. Unfortunately, differences in nations, states and languages have slowed down its spreading and flowing outside China. At present, however, an upsurge in learning, researching and applying Traditional Chinese Medicine (TCM) is unfolding. In order to maximize the effect of this upsurge and to lead TCM, one of the brilliant cultural heritages of the Chinese nation, to the world for it to expand and bring benefit to the people of all nations, Mr. Xu Xiangcai called intellectuals of noble aspirations and high intelligence together from Shandong and many other provinces in China and took charge of the work of both compilation and translation of THE ENGLISH−CHINESE ENCYCLOPEDIA OF PRACTICAL TRADITIONAL CHINESE MEDICINE. With great pleasure, the medical staff both at home and abroad will hail the appearance of this encyclopedia.

I believe that the day when the world's medicine is fully

developed will be the day when TCM has spread throughout the world.

I am pleased to give it my preface.

Prof. Dr. Hu Ximing

    Deputy Ministerof the Ministry of Public Health of the People's Republic of China,

    Director General of the State Administrative Bureau of Traditional Chinese Medicine and Pharmacology,

    President of the World Federation of Acupuncture—Moxibustion Societies,

    Member of China Association of Science & Technology,

    Deputy President of All—China Association of Traditional Chinese Medicine,

    President of China Acupuncture & Moxibustion Society.

December, 1989

Preface

The Chinese nation has been through a long, arduous course of struggling against diseases and has developed its own traditional medicine—Traditional Chinese Medicine and Pharmacology (TCMP). TCMP has a unique, comprehensive, scientific system including both theories and clinical practice. Some thousand years since it(its)beginnings,not only has it been well preserved but also continuously developed. It has special advantages, such as remarkable curative effects and few side effects. Hence it is an effective means by which people prevent and treat diseases and keep themselves strong and healthy.

All achievements attained by any nation in the development of medicine are the public wealth of all mankind. They should not be confined within a single country. What is more, the need to set them free to flow throughout the world as quickly and precisely as possible is greater than that of any other kind of science. During my more than thirty years of being engaged in Traditional Chinese Medicine(TCM), I have been looking forward to the day when TCMP will have spread all over the world and made its contributions to the elimination of diseases of all mankind. However it is to be deeply regretted that the pace of TCMP in extending outside China has been unsatisfactory due to the major difficulties in expressing its concepts in foreign languages.

Mr. Xu Xiangcai, a teacher of Shandong College of TCM, has sponsored and taken charge of the work of compilation and translation of The English—Chinese Encyclopedia of Practical Traditional Chinese Medicine—an extensive series. This work is a great project, a large—scale scientific research, a courageous effort and a novel creation. I deeply esteem Mr. Xu Xiangcai and his compilers and translators, who have been working day and night for such a long time, for their hard labor and for their firm and indomitable will displayed in overcoming one difficulty after another, and for their great success achieved in this way. As a leader in the circles of TCM, I am duty—bound to do my best to support them.

I believe this encyclopedia will be certain to find its position both in the history of Chinese medicine and in the history of world science and technology.

Mr. Zhang Qiwen
Member of the Standing Committee of
All—China Association of TCM,
Deputy Head of the Health Department
of Shandong Province.
March, 1990

Publisher's Preface

Traditional Chinese Medicine(TCM) is one of China's great cultural heritages. Since the founding of the People's Republic of China in 1949, guided by the farsighted TCM policy of the Chinese Communist Party and the Chinese government, the treasure house of the theories of TCM has been continuously explored and the plentiful literature researched and compiled. As a result, great success has been achieved. Today there has appeared a world—wide upsurge in the studying and researching of TCM. To promote even more vigorous development of this trend in order that TCM may better serve all mankind, efforts are required to further it throughout the world. To bring this about, the language barriers must be overcome as soon as possible in order that TCM can be accurately expressed in foreign languages.

Thus the compilation and translation of a series of English—Chinese books of basic knowledge of TCM has become of great urgency to serve the needs of medical and educational circles both inside and outside China.

In recent years, at the request of the health departments, satisfactory achievements have been made in researching the expression of TCM in English. Based on the investigation into the history and current state of the research work mentioned above, the English—Chinese Encyclopedia of Practical TCM has been published to meet the needs of extending the knowledge of TCM around the world.

The encyclopedia consists of twenty—one volumes, each dealing with a particular branch of TCM. In the process of compilation, the distinguishing features of TCM have been given close attention and great efforts have been made to ensure that the content is scientific, practical, comprehensive and concise. The chief writers of the Chinese manuscripts include professors or associate professors with at least twenty years of practical clinical and / or teaching experience in TCM. The Chinese manuscript of each volume has been checked and approved by a specialist of the relevant branch of TCM. The team of the translators and revisers of the English versions consists of TCM specialists with a good command of English professional medical translators, and teachers of English from TCM colleges or universities. At a symposium to standardize the English versions, scholars from twenty—two colleges or universities, research institutes of TCM or other health institutes probed the question of how to express TCM in English more comprehensively, systematically and accurately, and discussed and deliberated in detail the English versions of some volumes in order to upgrade the English versions of the whole series. The English version of each volume has been re—examined and then given a final checking.

Obviously this encyclopedia will provide extensive reading material of TCM English for senior students in colleges of TCM in China and will also greatly benefit foreigners studying TCM.

The assiduous efforts of compiling and translating this encyclopedia have been supported by the responsible leaders of the State Education Commission of the People's Republic of China, the State Administrative Bureau of TCM and Pharmacy, and the Education Commission and Health Department of Shandong

Province. Under the direction of the Higher Education Department of the State Education Commission, the leading board of compilation and translation of this encyclopedia was set up. The leaders of many colleges of TCM and pharmaceutical factories of TCM have also given assistance.

We hope that this encyclopedia will bring about a good effect on enhancing the teaching of TCM English at the colleges of TCM in China, on cultivating skills in medical circles in exchanging ideas of TCM with patients in English, and on giving an impetus to the study of TCM outside China.

Higher Education Press
March, 1990

Foreword

The English—Chinese Encyclopedia of Practical Traditional Chinese Medicine is an extensive series of twenty—one volumes. Based on the fundamental theories of traditional Chinese medicine(TCM) and with emphasis on the clinical practice of TCM, it is a semi—advanced English—Chinese academic works which is quite comprehensive, systematic, concise, practical and easy to read. It caters mainly to the following readers: senior students of colleges of TCM, young and middle—aged teachers of colleges of TCM, young and middle—aged physicians of hospitals of TCM, personnel of scientific research institutions of TCM, teachers giving correspondence courses in TCM to foreigners, TCM personnel going abroad in the capacity of lecturers or physicians, those trained in Western medicine but wishing to study TCM, and foreigners coming to China to learn TCM or to take refresher courses in TCM.

Because Traditional Chinese Medicine and Pharmacology is unique to our Chinese nation, putting TCM into English has been the crux of the compilation and translation of this encyclopedia. Owing to the fact that no one can be proficient both in the theories of Traditional Chinese Medicine and Pharmacology and the clinical practice of every branch of TCM, as well as in English, to ensure that the English versions express accurately the inherent meanings of TCM, collective translation measures have been taken. That is, teachers of English familiar with TCM, professional medical translators, teachers or physicians of TCM and even teachers of palaeography with a strong command of English were all invited together to co−translate the Chinese manuscripts and, then, to co−deliberate and discuss the English versions. Finally English−speaking foreigners studying TCM or teaching English in China were asked to polish the English versions. In this way, the skills of the above translators and foreigners were merged to ensure the quality of the English versions. However, even using this method, the uncertainty that the English versions will be wholly accepted still remains. As for the Chinese manuscripts, they do reflect the essence, and give a general picture, of traditional Chinese medicine and pharmacology. It is not asserted, though, that they are perfect, I whole−heartedly look forward to any criticisms or opinions from readers in order to make improvements to future editions.

More than 200 people have taken part in the activities of compiling, translating and revising this encyclopedia. They come from twenty−eight institutions in all parts of China. Among these institutions, there are fifteen colleges of TCM:Shandong, Beijing, Shanghai, Tianjin, Nanjing, Zhejiang, Anhui, Henan, Hubei, Guangxi, Guiyang, Gansu, Chengdu, Shanxi and Changchun, and scientific research centers of TCM such as China Academy of TCM and Shandong Scientific Research Institute of TCM.

The Education Commission of Shandong province has included the compilation and translation of this encyclopedia in its scientific research projects and allocated funds accordingly. The Health Department of Shandong Province has also given financial aid together with a number of pharmaceutical factories of TCM. The subsidization from Jinan Pharmaceutical Factory of

TCM provided the impetus for the work of compilation and translation to get under way.

The success of compiling and translating this encyclopedia is not only the fruit of the collective labor of all the compilers, translators and revisers but also the result of the support of the responsible leaders of the relevant leading institutions. As the encyclopedia is going to be published, I express my heartfelt thanks to all the compilers. translators and revisers for their sincere cooperation, and to the specialists, professors, leaders at all levels and pharmaceutical factories of TCM for their warm support.

It is my most profound wish that the publication of this encyclopedia will take its role in cultivating talented persons of TCM having a very good command of TCM English and in extending, rapidly, comprehensive knowledge of TCM to all corners of the globe.

Chief Editor   Xu Xiangcai
Shandong College of TCM
March, 1990

Contents

3　Drugs for Acting on the Respiratory System ·········· 46

15 Drugs Used in the Departments of Eye, Ear, Nose and Throat ································· 339

Notes

"Commonly Used Chinese Patent Medicines" is the 5th volume of "THE ENGLISH-CHINESE ENCYCLOPEDIA OF PRACTICAL TRADITIONAL CHINESE MEDICINE".

This volume consists of 18 chapters and deals with 449 Chinese patent medicines. In it, the medicines are classified as modern ones with their indications pointed out clearly and definitely in the terms of western medicine. Besides, two indexes are attached for the readers', convenience.

As an important component of traditional Chinese medicine and pharmacy, Chinese patent medicines are preparations made with Chinese medicinal herbs.With sure curative effects and without sideones, they are easy to use.This volume will help them fly out of China to serve overseas people, and that is our purpose. But compiling and translating a book of this kind is making a completely new effort for the first time. So, shortcomings and even mistakes are hardly avoided. We hope eagerly to be corrected by the readers both in and outside China.

In order to make the English Version come up to the desirable standards, a comprehensive re-translation has been undertaken on the basis of the original version. There are also other ladies and gentlemen who once made certain contributions towards the translation work. Among them are Sun Xiangxie, Xun Jianying, Li Junlin, Chen Qing and Guo Hongzhu. Here, we express our thanks to them.

The Editors

1 Drugs For Acting on Central Nervous System

1.1 Antiepileptics

Baijin Wan

Ingredients:

Radix Curcumae	70%	*Yujin*
Alumen	30%	*Baifan*

Actions: Relieving stagnation–syndrome and elimin–ating phlegm for resuscitation, tranquilizing the mind and relieving convulsion.

Indications: Stagnation of phlegm in the interior, epilepsy induced by terror, mania and unconsciousness.

Administration and Dosage: Taken orally, 0.3 g each time, once a day.

Preparation Form: Water–paste pill.

Package: Every 150 Pills weighs 3 g.

Notes: The prescription originates from the book *Wai Ke Zheng Zhi Quan Sheng Ji* compiled by Wang Hongxu in the Qing Dynasty.

This drug has the effects of regulating the function of central nervous system, tranquilizing the mind, relieving restlessness and resisting epilepsy. It is clinically indicated for epilepsy, convulsion, mania and unconsciousness.

Yangxianfeng Wan

Ingredients:

Radix Curcumae	*Yujin*
Alumen	*Baifan*
Semen Sinapis	*Jiezi*
Exocarpium Citri Reticulatae	*Juhong*
Radix et Rhizoma Rhei	*Dahuang*
Radix Scutellariae	*Huangqin*
Rhizoma Coptidis	*Huanglian*
Cortex Phellodendri	*Huangbai*
Fructus Gardeniae	*Zhizi*
Massa Fermentata Medicinalis	*Shenqu*
magnetitum	*Cishi*
Lignum Aquilariae Resinatum	*Chenxiang*

Actions: Removing heat—phlehm, tranquilizing the mind and relieving convulsion.

Indications: Abundant sputum, unconsciousness opisthotonos.

Administration and Dosage: Taken orally once a day, 1.5g each time for children of 1—4 years old, 3g each time for children of 5—7 years old, 9g each time for adults.

Preparation Form: Water—paste pill.

Package: Every 50 pills weighs 3g.

Notes: This drug has the effects of relieving fever, tranquilizing the mind, relieving convulsion and resisting epilepsy. It is clinically indicated for epilepsy, etc.

It is contraindicated for pregnant women and those who are weak due to prolonged illness.

Yixian Wan

Ingredients:

Rhizoma Typhonii	4.3%	*Baifuzi*
Rhizoma Arisaematis	8.6%	*Tiannanxing*
Rhizoma Pinelliae	8.6%	*Banxia*
Fructus Gleditsiae Abnormalis	43.2%	*Zhuyazao*
Alumen	13.0%	*Baifan*
Bombyx Batryticatus	8.6%	*Jiangcan*
Scolopendra	0.2%	*Wugong*
Scorpio	1.7%	*Quanxie*
Zaocys	8.6%	*Wushaoshe*
Realgar	1.3%	*Xionghuong*
Cinnabaris	1.7%	*Zhusha*

Actions: Expelling wind and removing phlegm, relieving epilepsy and stopping clonic convulsion.

Indications: Clonic convulsion due to epilepsy occuring now and then.

Administration and Dosage: Taken orally 3g each time, twice a day.

Preparation Form: Water—paste pill.

Package: 3g in per bag.

Notes: The pill can tranquilize the mind, relax muscular spasm and resist epilepsy. It is clinically indicated for epilepsy and convulsion.

Compared with *Yangxianfeng wan*, the pill is better in relaxing muscular spasm and fighting against convulsion, but poorer in preventing coma.

It is contraindicated for pregnant women

1.2　Antipsychotics

Mengshi Guntan Wan

Ingredients:

Lapis Micae Aureus	10%	*Jinmengshi*
Lignum Aquilariae Resinatum	5%	*Chenxiang*
Radix Scutellariae	42.5%	*Huangqin*
Radix et Rhizoma Rhei	42.5%	*Dahuang*

Actions: Promoting diuresis and removing phlegm.

Indications: Stubborn phlegm due to sthenic heat resulting in manic—depressive psychosis and palpitation due to fright, or cough, dyspnea and thick sputum, and constipation.

Administration and Dosage: Taken orally 6—12g each time, once a day.

Preparation Form: Water—paste pill.

Package: Every 20 pills weighs 1g.

Notes: The pill can eliminate phlegm and fight against psychosis. It is clinically indicated for schizophrenia due to stubborn phlegm caused by sthenic heat, chronic bronchitis, pulmonary emphysema with infection, and epilepsy.

It is contraindicated for pregnant women.

Zhuli Datan Wan

Ingredients:

Bamboo Juice	*Zhuli*
Lapis Chloriti	*Qingmengshi*
Exocarpium Citri Rubrum	*Juhong*
Rhizoma Pinelliae	*Banxia*

Radix et Rhizoma Rhei	*Dahuang*
Radix Scutellariae	*Huangqin*
Lignum Aquilariae Resinatum	*Chenxiang*
Rhizoma Zingiberis Recens	*Shengjiang*
Radix Glycyrrhizae	*Gancao*

Actions: Clearing away fire and eliminating phlegm for resuscitation, facilitating the flow of the lung—Qi *to relieve asthma.*

Indications: Heart disturbed by phlegm—fire, rapid respiration and coma, accumulation of stubborn phlegm, restless and oppressed feelings, insanity abundant expectoration, etc.

Administration and Dosage: Taken orally 6—9g each time, 1—2 times a day.

Preparation Form: Water—paste pill.

Package: 18g in per bag.

Notes: The pill can eliminate phlegm and struggle against psychosis due to sthenic heat and stubborn phlegm.

1.3 Sedative—hypnoticcs (drugs for Regulating Nervous System)

Tianwang Buxin Dan

Ingredients:
Radix Salviae Miltiorrhizae	3.4%	*Danshen*
Radix Angelicae Sinenisis	.7%	*Danggui*
Rhizoma Acori Graminei	3.5%	*Shi chang Pu*
Radix Codonopsis Pilosulae	3.5%	*Dang shen*
Poria	3.5%	*Fuling*
Fructus Schisandrae	7%	*Wu Weizi*
Radix Ophiopogonis	7%	*Mei Dong*

Radix Asparagi	7%	*Tian Dong*
Radix Rehmanniae	28.2%	*Dihuang*
Radix Scrophulariae	3.5%	*Xuanshen*
Radix Polygalae	3.5%	*Yuanzhi*
Semen Ziziphi Spinosae	7%	*Suan zaoren*
Semen Biotae	7%	*Baiziren*
Radix Platycodi	3.5%	*Jiegeng*
Radix Glycyrrhizae	3.5%	*Gancao*
Cinnabaris	1.4%	*Zhusha*

Actions: Nourishing *Yin*, supplementing blood and enhancing the heart to calm the mind.

Indications: Deficiency of the heart—*Yin*, palpitation. amnesia, insomnia, dreaminess and constipation.

Administration and Dosage: Taken orally 1 bolus each time, twice a day.

Preparation Form: Honeyed bolus.

Package: Each bolus weighs 9g.

Notes: The prescription originates from the book *Shi Yi De Xiao Fang* compiled by Wei Yili in the Yuan Dynasty.

Having tranquilizing, nourishing and strengthening actions, this bolus can regulate the functions of the central nervous system and other organs. It is clinically indicated for neurasthenia, rheumatic heart disease, heyperthyrcidism, climacteric syndrome due to insufficiency of blood and hyperactivity of fire due to deficiency of *Yin*, palpitation, insomnia, dreaminess, amnesia, and aphthae.

Zhusha Anshen Wan

Ingredients:

Cinnabaris	21.4%	*ZhuSha*
Rhizoma Coptidis	32.2%	*Huanglian*
Radix Angelicae Sinensis	21.4%	*Danggui*
Radix Rehmanniae	21.4%	*ShengDi*
Radix Glycyrrhizae	3.6%	*Gancao*

Actions: Relieving convulsion, tranquillizing the mind, clearing away heart—fire and nourishing blood.

Indications: Irritability due to flaring heart—fire and damage of the heart, blood fidgetiness, sleeplessness, dysphoria with smothery sensation in the chest, dreaminess in the night, etc.

Administration and Dosage: Taken orally, 1 bolus each time, 1—2 times a day.

Preparation Form: Honeyed bolus.

Package: Each bolus weighs 9g

Notes: The prescription is recorded in the book *Shou Shi Bao Yuan*, written by Gong Tingxian in the Ming Dynasty.

This kind of bolus has the action of relieving restlessness and regulating the central nervous system. It is clinically indicated for fidgetiness due to excessive heart—fire or deficiency of heart—blood, palpitation, insomnia, neurasthenia, mental depression and epilepsy.

It is not allowed to be administered together with potassium bromide, sodium bromide, and sodium iodide.

Zhenzhong Dan

Ingredients:

Plastrum Testudinis	25%	*Guiban*
Os Draconis Fossilia Ossis Mastodi	25%	*Longgu*

Rhizoma Acori Graminei	25%	ShiChangpu
Radix Polygalae	25%	Yuanzhi

Actions: Nourishing *Yin* to reduce pathogenic fire, relieving palpitation to tranquilize the mind.

Indications: Deficiency of heart—blood, excessive consideration, hyperactivity of fire due to *Yin* deficiency, severe palpitation, dizziness, insomnia, emission and night sweat.

Administration and Dosage: Taken orally, 1 bolus each time, 1—2 times a day.

Preparation Form: Honeyed bolus.

Package: Each bolus weighs 9g.

Notes: The prescription is recorded in the book *Qian Jin Yao Fang*, written by Sun Simiao in the Tang Dynasty.

The bolus of this kind can tranquilize the mind, regulate the central nervous system and the vegetative nervous system. It can be clinically used for neurasthenia, palpitation, insomnia, poor memory, emission and night sweat.

Baizi Yangxin Wan

Ingredients:

Semen Biotae	3.2%	Baiziren
Radix Codonopsis Pilosulae	3.2%	Dangshen
Radix Astragali	12.8%	Huangqi
Rhizoma Chuanxiong	12.8%	Chuanxiong
Radix Angelicae Sinensis	12.8%	Danggui
Poria	25.6%	Fuling
Radix Polygalae	3.2%	Yuanzhi
Semen Ziziphi Spinosae	3.2%	Suan zaoren
Cortex Cinnamomi	3.2%	Rougui

Radix Glycyrrhizae	1.3%	*Gancao*
Leaven of Rhizoma pinelliae	12.8%	*Banxiaqu*
Fructus Schisandrae	3.2%	*Wuweizi*
Cinnabaris	2.8%	*Zhusha*

Actions: Invigorating *Qi*, nourishing blood, benefiting intelligence and calming the mind.

Indications:Palpitation and shortness of breath, insomnia, amnesia, lassitude, spontaneous perspiration, night sweet, etc, all of which are due to deficiency of heart—blood, flaring—up fire of deficiency type.

Administration and Dosage: Taken orally, 1 bolus each time, twice a day.

Preparation Form: Honeyed bolus.

Package: 9 g in Each bolus

Notes: The prescription is recorded in the book *Zheng Zhi Zhun Sheng* written by wang Kentang in the Ming Dynasty.

The bolus of this kind can be clinically used for palpitation and shortness of breath due to neuraschenia, insomnia, amnesia, lassitude, spontaneous perspiration and night sweat.

Anshen Buxin Wan

Ingredients:

Radix Salviae Miltiorrhizae	27%	*Danshen*
Fructus Schisandrae	13.5%	*Wuweizi*
Rhizoma Acori Graminei	9%	*ShiChangPu*
Anshen Gao	50.5%	*Anshengao*

Actions: Nourishing the heart to calm the mind.

Indications: Palpitation, insomnia, amnesia, dizziness and tinnitus.

Administration and Dosage: Taken orally, 15 pills each time, three times a day.

Preparation Form: Water—paste pill.

Package: 2g in Every 15 pills

Notes: The pill of this kind has the action of tranquilizing the mind, regulating the central nervous system and enriching the blood.It can be clinically used for neurasthenia due to deficiency of heart—blood, nearosis, insomnia, amnesia, restlessness and dizziness.

Naolingsu Pian

Ingredients:

Rhizoma Polygonati	*Huangjing*
Herba Epimedii	*Yinyanghuo*
Fructus Xanthii	*Cangerzi*
Radix Ophiopogonis	*Maidong*
Radix Polygalae	*Yuan zhi*
Radix Ginseng Rubra	*Hong shen*
Semen Ziziphi Spinosae	*Suanzaoren*
Fructus Schisandrae	*Wu wei zi*
Plastrum Testudinis	*Guiban*
Fructus Lycii	*Gouqizi*
Cornu Cervi Pantotrichum	*Lurong*
Poria	*FuLing*
Fructus Ziziphi Jujubae	*Dazaorou*
Radix Rehmanniae Praeparata	*Shudihuang*
Colla Cornus Cervi	*Lujiaojiao*

Actions: Invigorating *Qi*, enriching blood, nourishing the heart, supplementing the kidney, strengthening the brain and calming the mind.

Indications: Amnesia, sleeplessness, dizziness, palpitation, tiredness and spontaneous perspiration due to general debility, impotence, seminal emission and abalienation.

Administration and Dosage: Taken orally, 2—3 tablets each time, 2—3 times a day.

Preparation Form: Sugar—coated tablet.

Package: 3 g in Each tablet.

Notes: Possessig nourishing action, this medicine can regulate the function of the boly organs, especially that of the central nervous system. It can be clinically used for neurasthenia, psychosis, chronic nephritis, anemia, chronic hepatitis, diabetes, etc.

Wuweizi Chongji

Ingredients:

Fructus Schisandrae 100% *Wuweizi*

Actions: Invigorating *Qi* to tonify the kidney and tranquilizing the mind to treat insomnia.

Indications: Deficiency of the kidney—*Qi*, vexation, insomnia and tiredness.

Administration and Dosage: Infused with boiling water and taken, 10g each time, three times a day.

Preparation Form: Granule or powder preparation dissolvable in water.

Package: 10g in each bag.

Notes: This medicine is clinically indicated for neurasthenia, heart musclestrain, excessive tiredness, insomnia, etc.

Niuhuang Qingnao Pian

Ingredients:

Radix Scrophulariae	6.6%	Xuanshen
Radix Scutellariae	6.6%	Huangqin
Flos Lonicerae	2.8%	Jinyinhua
Herba Taraxaci	9.5%	Pugongying
Radix Glycyrrhizae	6.6%	Gancao
Radix Isatidis	6.5%	Ban Langen
Radix Trichosanthis	6.6%	Tianhuafen
Radix et Rhizoma Rhei	4.8%	Dahuang
Fructus Forsythiae	3.9%	Lianqiao
Concha Haliotidis	1.4%	Shijueming
Gypsum Fibrosum	6.6%	Shigao
Realgar	7.3%	Xionghuang
Haematitum	6.6%	Zheshi
Borneolum Syntheticum	0.7%	Bingpian
Cinnabaris	0.2%	Zhusha
Radix Ophiopogonis	6.6%	Maidong
Fructus Gardeniae	3.9%	Zhizi
Radix Rehmanniae	4.8%	Shengdi huang
Radix Puerariae	3.9%	Gegen
concentrated pig bile	0.3%	Kudangao
Rhizoma Coptidis	0.7%	Huanglian
Margarita	0.3%	Zhenzhu
Magnetitum calcined	2.8%	Cishi

Actions: Clearing away heat and toxic material, removing heat from the brain and tranquillizing the mind.

Indications: High fever, dizziness, distension in the head

mania, dry tongue, dim eyesight, swelling and pain in the throat, interior heat and infuntile convulsion.

Administration and Dosage: Taken orally, 2—4 tablets each time, three times a day.

Preparation Form: Sugar—coated tablet.

Package: Each tablet weighs 0.34 g.

Notes: Maybe served as a tranquilizer and antibiotic, this medicine can relax spasm, relieve pain, fight against shock and reduce blood pressure. It is clinically indicated for hypertension, neurosis, nruralgic headache, insomnia, dizziness due to high fever, fidgetiness, fever and convulsion.

This medicine should be cautiously used for children who are weak or those with lower blood pressure.It is contraindicated for pregnant women.

Jiannao Bushen Wan

Ingredients:

Radix Ginseng	3.5%	Renshen
Cornu Cervi Pantotrichum	0.8%	Lurong
Dog's Testis	1.6%	Goushen
Coptex Cinnamomi	3.5%	Rougui
Herba Lysimachiae	1.4%	Jinqiancao
Fructus Arctii	2.0%	Niubangzi
Fructus Rosae Laevigatae	1.4%	Jinyinzi
Cortex Eucommiae	4.2%	Duzhong
Ramulus Cyathulae	4.2%	Chuang xiteng
Flos Lonicerae	3.0%	Jinyenhua
Fructus Forsythiae	2.8%	Lianqiao
Periostracum Cicadae	2.8%	Chantui

Rhizoma Dioscoreae	5.6%	Shanyao
Radix Polygalae	4.9%	Yuanzhi
Semen Ziziphi Spinosae	4.2%	Suanzaorei
Fructus Amomi	4.9%	Sharei
Radix Angelicae Sinensis	4.2%	Danggui
Dragon's Bone	4.1%	Longgu
Oyster Shell	4.9%	Muli
Poria	9.7%	Fuling
Rhizoma Atractylodis Macrocephalae	4.9%	Baizhu
Ramulus Cinnamomi	4.1%	Guizhi
Radix Paeoniae Alba	4.1%	Baishuo
Cinnabaris	5.2%	Zhusha
Fructus Amomi Rotundus	4.1%	Doukou
Radix Glycyrrhizae	3.2%	Gancao

Actions: Strengthening the brain and supplementing Qi, tonifying the kidney to replenish essence.

Indications: Amnesia, sleeplessness, dizziness, tinnitus palpitation, lassitude in the loins and and knees, emission due to the kidney deficiency.

Administration and Dosage: Taken orally, 15 pills each time, twice a day.

Preparation Form: Water—paste pill.

Package: 1 g in every 20 pills.

Notes: This pill can improve the function of the brain, reduce blood pressure and tranquilize the mind. It can be clinically used for neurasthenia, chronic hepatitis, anemia and neurosis.

Jiannao Wan

Ingredients:

Semen Ziziphi Spinosae	19.4%	*Suanzaoren*
Herba Cistanchis	9.7%	*Roucongrong*
Fructus lycii	9.7%	*Gouqizi*
Semen Alpiniae Oxyphllae	9.7%	*Yizhiren*
Fructus Schisandrae	7.3%	*Wuweizi*
Semen Biotae	7.3%	*Baiziren*
Arisaema Cum Blle	4.8%	*Dan nanxing*
Radix Polygalae	4.8%	*Yuanzhi*
Concretio Silicea Bambusae	4.8%	*Tian zhuhuang*
Rhizoma Acori Gramineis		
(Rhizoma Anemoni)	4.8%	*Jiujie changpu*
Radix Angelicae Sinensis	3.6%	*Danggui*
Cinnabaris	4.8%	*Zhusha*
Dragon's Teeth	4.8%	*Longgu*
Succinum	4.8%	*Hubo*

Actions: Nourishing the brain, calming the mind to benefit wisdom and relieving mental stress.

Indications: Severe palpitation and amnesia, dizziness, palpitation, dysphoria and sleeplessness.

Administration and Dosage: Taken orally, 20 pills each time, twice a day.

Preparetion Form: Water—paste pill.

Package: 200 pills in each bottle.

Notes: The pill of this kind can tranquilize the mind, regulate the central nervous system and blood pressure as well. It can be clinically used for execssive tiredness of brain, neurasthenia, insomnia and amnesia, dizziness, palpitation and fidgetiness.

Lingzhi Tangjiang

Ingredients:

Dried Fructification of the Fungus Ganoderma Lucidum	42.6%	*Lingzhi zishiti*
Mycelium of the Fungus Ganoderma Lucidum	38.5%	*Ling zhiguensiti*
Folium Eriobotryae	7.7%	*Pibaye*
Mentholum	0.008%	*Behenao*
Rdaix Platycodi	7.7%	*Jiegeng*

Actions: Protecting the liver, invigorating the spleen, supplementing *Qi*, relieving asthma and convulsion, and lowering blood pressure.

Indications: Acute icterohepatitis, Ke—shan disease, hypertension, neurasthenia and asthmatic trachitis.

Administration and Dosage: Taken orally, 15—20ml each time, three times a day.

Preparation Form: Sirupus.

Package: 500ml in each bottle.

Notes: This medicine can increase the immune and disease—resistant ability of the organism, reduce blood—fat, regulate blood pressure and the function of central nervous system as well, and relieve fidgetiness, allergy and asthma. It is clinically indicated for acute icterohepatitis, Ke—Shan disease, hypertensi, neurasthenia and asthmatic trachitis.

Cizhu Wan

Ingredients:

Magnetitum	28.6%	*Cishi*
Cinnabaris	14.3%	*Zhusha*
Medicinalis	57.1%	*Liushenqu*

Actions: Relieving palpitation, tranquilizing the mind and improving vision.

Indications: *Yin* deficiency of the heart and kidney, hyperfunction of the heart—*Yang*, palpitation, insomnia, tinnitus, deafness, poor vision and dysphoria.

Administration and Dosage: Taken orally, 3g each time, twice a day.

Preparation form: Water—paste pill.

Package: 18g in each bag.

Notes: The pill of this kind can regulate the function of the central nervous system, improve cerebral blood circulation and relive fidgtiness. It can be clinically used for neurasthenia, palpitation, insomnia, tinnitus, deafness, epilepsy, anxiety, etc.

2 Drugs for Acting on Cardiovascular System

2.1 Drugs for Treating Coronary heart Disease and Angina Pectoris

Huoxin Wan

Main Ingredients:

Radix Ginseng   *Ren shen*

Calcullus Bovis   *Niuhuang*

Actions: Clearing away heart—fire, calming the mind and inducing resuscitation.

Indications: Obstruction of *Qi* in the chest, angina pectoris, chest tightness, shortness of breath and palpitation.

Administration and Dosage: Taken orally, 1—2 pills each time, three times a day.

Preparation Form: Small water—paste pill.

Package: 20mg included in each pill.

Notes: The pill of this kind can regulate heart rate.improve the function of the heart and blood microcirculation, expand the coronary arteries and cerebral blood vessels, excert actions against myocardial ischemia, relieve angina pectoris and increase cerebral blood flow. Clinically it can be used to treat coronary heart diseases, angina pectoris caused by various heart diseases, myocardial ischemia and chronic heart function insufficiency and cerebral ischemia syndrome due to cerebral arteriosclerosis.

Caution is needed when it is administrated to treat pregnant women or women in the period.

Yixin Wan

Main Ingredients:

Radix Ginseng	*Ren shen*
Calculus Bovis	*Niuhuang*
Venenum Bufonis	*Chansu*
Margarita	*Zhenzhu*
Borncolum Snytheticum	*Bingpian*
Radix Notoginseng	*Tiansanqi*

Actions: Supplementing *Qi*, reinforcing heart, inducing resuscitation by means of aromatics and promoting blood circulation by removing blood stasis.

Indications: Angina pectoris, precordial pain with cold limbs, chest tightness, shortness of breath and palpitation.

Administration and Dosage: It is sucked sublingually, 1−2 pills each time, 1−2 times a day.

Preparation Form: Water−paste pill.

Package: 20 pills in each bottle.

Notes: The pill of this kind can expand the coronary arteries, regulate heart rate, increase the ability of cardiac muscle against oxygen deficit, strengthen the systolic force of the heart muscles. Clinically it can be used to treat coronary heart diseases, angina pectoris, arrhythmia and heart function insufficiency.

After 332 cases were clinically observed, the total effective rate reached 85.4% in patients with angina pectoris and 82.7% in patients with chronic coronary ischemia whose ECG is of a little change.

It is contraindicated for pregnant women and suggested with caution to women in menstrual period.

Huanxin Dan

Main Ingredients:

Radix Notoginseng	*Sanqi*
Radix Ginseng	*Renshen*
Margarita	*Zhenzhu*

Actions: Promoting blood circulation by removing blood stasis, invigorating pulse—beat and activating the collaterals.

Indications: Angina pectoris, chest tightness, shortness of breath, and palpitation.

Administration and Dosage: Taken orally, 2 pills each time, 1—3 times a day.

3—4 pills may be chewed and sucked when sudden attack of the disease occurs.

Preparation Form: Semiconcentrated pill.

Package: 0.25g in every 10 pills.

Notes: The pill of this kind can expand the coronary arteries, increase coronary arterial blood flow, improve microcirculation, reduce oxygen consumption in the cardiac muscles, regulate heart rate, increase the ability of the heart muscles against ischemia and oxygen deficit and relieve angina pectoris. It can be clinically used to treat coronary heart disease, angina pectoris, arrhythmia and myocardiac infarction.

It is contraindicated for fever, attack of asthma, haemorrhage and pregnanty women.

Shengmaiyin Koufuye

Ingredients:

Radix Ginseng	25%	*Renshen*
Radix Ophiopogonis	50%	*Maidong*
Fructus Schisandrae	25%	*Wuweizi*

Actions: Supplementing *Qi* to recover pulse, nourishing *Yin* to promote the production of body fluid.

Indications: Deficiency of both *Qi* and *Yin*, palpitation, shortness of breath, faint pulse and sweating due to debility, and weak body resulting from prolonged illness.

Administration and Dosage: Taken orally, 10ml each time, three times a day.

Preparation Form: Oral sterile—liquid.

Package: 10ml in each bottle.

Notes: The prescription is recorded in the book *Nei Wai Shang Bian Huo Lun* written by Li Gao in the Jin Dynasty.

This medicine can regulate heart rate and the functions of the organs, increase heart output and the ability of the body against diseases, strengthen cardiac contractility, reduce oxygen consumption in the heart muscles, adjust blood pressure, excert actions against shock, expand the coronary arteries and increase coronary arterial blood flow. It can be clinically used to treat coronary heart disease, pulmonary diseases, rheumatic heart disease, arrhythmia, heart neurosis, hypotension, sunstroke, chronic bronchitis and tuberculosis.

Baoxin Wan

Main Ingredients:

Styrax Liquidus	*Suhexiangzhi*
Venenum Bufonis	*Chansu*
Cortex Cinnamomi	*Rougui*
Calculus Bovis	*Niuhuang*
Borneolum	*Bing Pian*
Radix Ginseng	*Renshen*

Actions: Inducing resuscitation by means of aromatics, regulating the flow of *Qi* to alleviate pain, and promoting blood circulation by removing blood stasis.

Indications: Angina pectoris, precordial pain with cold limbs, chest tightness, shortness of breath, palpitation, etc.

Administration and Dosage: Taken orally, 1−2 pills each time, three times a day.

Preparation Form: Minipill.

Package: 1g in every 300 pills.

Notes: The pill of this kind can expand coronary arteries, improve myocardial blood supply, reduce oxygen consumption in the cardiac muscles, increase the ability of the heart muscles to endure oxygen deficit, and relieve angina pectoris. It can be clinically used to treat coronary heart diseases, various angina pectoris and oppressed feeling in the chest.

It is reported that this drug comes into its effect 50 seconds after its administration and plays its full part within five minutes. Its action can generally continue for eleven hours with the longest for twenty−four hours and the shortest for thirty minutes.

Dryness of the mouth, distension in the head, or slight

numbness of the lips and tongue may happen to some individuals after this drug is taken. It is contraindicated for pregnant women and used cautiously for those who will be ill with urticaria after it is taken.

Suxiao Jiuxin Wan

Main Ingredients:

Rhizoma Chuanxiong   *Chuanxiong*

Borneolum   *Bingpian*

Actions: Promoting blood circulation by removing blood stasis, inducing resuscitation by means of aromatics, and regulating the flow of *Qi* to alleviate pain.

Indications: Angina pectoris, chest tightness, shortness of breath and palpitation.

Administration and Dosage: Sucked, 4—6 pills each time, three times a day. While the disease is in acute stage, 10—15 pills is to be sucked.

Preparation Form: Drip—pill.

Package: 40 pills in each bottle.

Notes: This pill can expand the coronary arteries, increase coronary arterial blood flow, slow down heart rate, reduce oxygen consumption of cardiac muscles and improve microcirculation. It can be clinically used to treat coronary heart disease, angina pectoris and oppressed feeling in the chest. It can be served both as first—aid and routine medicine for the coronary disease.

Mai luotong Pian

Main Ingredients:

Radix Salviae Miltiorrhizae	*Danshen*
Radix Ophiopogonis	*Maidong*
Radix Notoginseng	*Sanqi*
Radix Curcumae	*Yujin*
Radix Scutellariae	*Huangqin*
Ramulus Uncariae Cum Uncis	*Gouteng*
Spica Prunellae	*Xiakucao*
Radix Aucklandiae	*Muxiang*
Lignum Dalbergiae Odoriferae	*Jiangxiang*
Flos Sophorae Immaturus	*Huaimi*
Radix Ginseng	*Renshen*
Succinum	*Hubo*
Rhizoma Nardostachydis	*Gansong*
Ochra Haematitum	*Daizheshi*
Rhizoma Coptidis	*Huanglian*
Rhizoma Acori Graminei	*Shichangpu*
Calculus Bovis	*Niuhuang*
Radix Glycyrrhizae	*Gancao*
Lignum Santali	*Tanxiang*
Borneolum	*Bingpian*
Margarita	*Zhenzhu*

Actions: Promoting circulation of *Qi*, through the channels and collaterals, removing blood stasis, and invigorating pulse—beat.

Indications: Obstruction of *Qi* in the chest, chest tightness, shortness of breath, and draging pain in the chest and back.

Administration and Dosage: Taken orally, 4 tablets each time, 2—3 times a day.

Preparation Form: Tablet.

Package: Each tablet weighs 0.4g.

Notes: The tablet of this kind can expand the coronary arteries, increase coronary arterial blood flow, improve microcirculation, reduce blood grease and its mucosity. It can be clinically employed to treat coronary heart diseases, angina pectoris, hypertension, cerebral embolism, myocardiac infarction and atheroscleorsis.

Guanxin Suhe Wan

Ingredients:

Styrax Liquidus	7.4%	*Suhexiang*
Borneolum	15.4%	*Bingpian*
Resina Olibani	15.4%	*Zhruxiang*
Lignum Santali	30.9%	*Tanxiang*
Radix Aristolochiae	30.9%	*Qingmuxiang*

Actions: Inducing resuscitation by means of aromatics, soothing chest oppression, regulating the flow of *Qi* and alleviating pain.

Indications: Obstruction of *Qi* in the chest, angina pectoris, palpitation and shortness of breath.

Administration and Dosage: It is sucked or swallowed after chewed, 1 pill each time, three times a day. It may be taken at the onset of the disease.

Preparation Form: Honeyed bolus.

Package: Each bolus includes 3g.

Notes: This bolus can expand the coronary arteries, increase coronary arterial blood flow and reduce myocardial oxygen consumption. It can be clinically used to treat coronary heart diseases due to stagnation of *Qi* and cold, angina pectoris and oppressed feeling in the chest. Compared with *Suhexiang Wan*, this medicine is better in expanding the coronary arteries and reducing oxygen consumption, but not as good as *Suhexiang Wan* in fighting against coma.

This bolus should not be administered along with potassium bromide, sodium bromide and sodium iodide.

Yufeng Ningxin Pian

Ingredient:

Radix Puerariar   100%   *Gegen*

Actions:Dispelling pathogenic factors from the superficial muscles, reducing heat, promoting the production of body fluid, inducing eruption and elevating the spleen *Yang* to stop diarrhea.

Indications: Angina pectoris, precordial pain with cold limbs, obstruction of *Qi* in the chest and vertigo due to hyperactivity of the liver *Yang*.

Administration and Dosage: Taken orally, 5 tablets each time, three times a day.

Preparation Form: Tablet.

Package: 0.25 g in each tablet.

Notes: This tablet is made of the alcoholic extract of Gegen Radix Puerariar, whose main effective ingredient is the flavonoid of kudzuvine root.

Pharmacological experiments have showed that the flavone can expand the coronary arteries and cerebral blood vessels, increase coronary and cerebral blood flow, reduce the resistance in blood vessels and myocardial oxygen consumption, excert the actions against coronary blood vessel spasm caused by pituitrin, improve metabolism of the cardiac muscles and lower blood pressure. It can be clinically used to treat coronary heart diseases, hypertensim, dizziness and deafness due to Meniere's syndrome.

Jiexintong Pian

Ingredients:

Rhizom Cyperi	25%	*Xiangfu*
Fructus Trichosanthis	50%	*Gualou*
Herba Epimedii	25%	*Yinyanghuo*

Actions: Soothing chest oppression, regulating the flow of *Qi*, invigorating pulse—beat and relieving pain.

Indications: Angina pectoris, precordial pain with cold limbs, obstruction of *Qi* and tightness in the chest.

Administration and Dosage: Taken orally, 6—8 tablets each time, three times a day.

Preparation Form: Sugar—coated tablet.

Package: 0.28g in each tablet.

Notes: This tablet can increase coronary arterial blood flow, fight against adrenaline arrhythmia, reduce myocardial oxygen consumption, strengthen the ability of ECG. Served as sedative and hypnotic.it can be clinically used to treat coronary heart diseases, angina pectoris and arrhythemia.

Fufang Danshen Pian

Ingredients:

Radix Salviae Miltiorrhizae	22.5%	*Danshen*
Radix Notoginseng	75%	*Sanqi*
Borneolum	2.5%	*Bingpian*

Actions: Promoting blood circulation by removing blood stasis, inducing resuscitation by means of aromatics, and regulating the flow of *Qi* to alleviate pain.

Indications: Angina pectoris, precordial pain with cold limbs, chest tightness, palpitation and shortness of breath.

Administration and Dosage: Taken orally, 3 tablets each time, three times a day.

Preparation Form: Tablet.

Package: 0.25g in each tablet.

Notes: The drug of this kind can dilate the coronary artery to increase the blood volume of it, decrease myocardial oxygen consumption, lighten angina pectoris, decrease blood lipid level etc. It can be clinically used to treat coronary heart disease and angina pectoris, both due to stagnancy of *Qi* and blood.

It has reported that 85.6% of 377 patients with angina pectoris treated with this drug have enjoyed its curative effect.

This drug shouldn't be taken with gastropine.

Xinkeshu Pian

Ingredients:

Fructus Crataegi	31.9%	*Shanzha*
Radix Salviae Miltiorrhizae	31.9%	*Danshen*
Radix Puerariae	31.9%	*Gegen*
Radix Notoginseng	2.2%	*Sanqi*
Radix Aucklandiae	2.1%	*Muxiang*

Actions: Promoting blood circulation to remove blood stasis, benefiting the heart and lowering blood pressure.

Indications: Angina pectoris, precordial pain with cold limbs, chest tightness, shortness of breath and palpitation.

Administration and Dosage: Taken orally, 4 tablets each time, three times a day.

Preparation Form: Sugar—coated tablet.

Package: 0.25g in each tablet.

Notes: This drug can dilate the coronary artery, improve cardiac function and microcir culation, decrease the concentration of trigly—ceride and cholesterol, lower down blood viscosity, and change blood stream denature, Clinically, it is suitable for chronic coronary blood insufficiency, cardica insufficiency, etc.

Subing Diwan

Ingredients:

Styrax Liquidus	33.3%	*Suhexiangzhi*
Borneolum Syntheticum	66.7%	*Bing pian*

Actions: Inducing resuscitation by means of aromatics, and regulating the flow of *Qi* to alleviate pain.

Indications: Angina pectoris, precordial pain with cold limbs, chest tightness, etc.

Administration and Dosage: Taken orally, 2—4 pills each time, three times a day; or swallowed, or sucked immediately at the onset of the disease.

Preparation Form: Drop pills.

Package: 50mg in each pill.

Notes: This drug is characterized by the effect of dilating coronary artery and resisting angina pectoris. It is derived from *Suhexiang Wan* with the effect of resisting coronary heart disease, myocardiac infarction and shock strengthened.

This drug has a powerful ability to dilate the coronary

artery, to increase the volume of coronary arterial blood, to reduce myocardial oxygen consumption to enrich cerebral blood flow, and to resist shock. In clinical practice it can be used to treat angina pectoris due to coronary heart disease.

Those with stomach disease should take it with caution, for this drug is irrtant.

Guanxin Tongmailing Pian

Ingredients:

Radix Angelicae Sinensis	5.9%	*Danggui*
Radix Salviae Miltiorrhizae	14.7%	*Danshen*
Radix Polygoni Multiflori	9.8%	*Heshouwu*
Semen Persicae	3.9%	*Taoren*
Flos Carthami	3.9%	Honghua
Radix Curcumae	5.9%	*Yujin*
Rhizoma Polygonati	9.8%	*Huangjing*
Radix Puerariae	14.7%	*Gegen*
Resina Draconis	3.3%	*Xuejie*
Myrrha	3.3%	*Moyao*
Rhizoma Corydalis	5.9%	*Yuanhu*
Borneolum	0.6%	*Bingpian*
Resina Olibani	3.3%	*Ru xiang*
Caulis Spatholobi	14.7%	*Ji xueteng*

Actions: Promoting blood circulation by removing blood stasis.

Indications: Angina pectoris, chest tightness shortness of breath and palpitation.

Administration and Dosage: Taken orally, 5 tablets each time, three times a day.

Preparation Form: Sugar–coated tablet.

Package: 0.3g in each tablet.

Notes: This drug can help to dilate the coronary arterial blood vessels, improve heart, blood supply, decrease myocardial oxygen consumption, decrease blood lipid and blood viscosity, dilate cerebral arteries and improve cerebral blood flow.It is clinically used to treat coronary insufficiency angina pectoris, brain thrombus, etc.

Fufang Danshen Zhusheye

Ingredients:

Radix Salviae Miltiorrhizae　　90.9%　　Danshen

Lignum Dalbergiae Odoriferae　9.1%　　Jiangxiang

Actions: Promoting blood circulation to remove obstruction in the channels and activating the circulation of Qi to relieve pain.

Indications: Angina pectoris, precordial pain with cold limbs, chest tightness, etc.

Administration and Dosage: Given by intramuscular injection, 2ml each time, twice a day, or intravenous–drip according to the order of a doctor.

Preparation Form: Injection.

Package: 2ml in each ampoule.

Notes: Pharmacological experiments show that Danshen Radix Salviae Miltiorrhizae and Jiangxiang Lignum Dalbergiae Odoriferae both have the effects of improving the contraction of the cardial muscle, dilating the coronary artery, increasing coronary blood flow, decreasing heart rate and apparently improving heart function. Besides, Danshan can also reduce blood viscosity and improve microcirculation. This product is clinically indicated for coronary heart disease, myocardiac infarction, etc.

The effects of *Danshen Zhusheye* is similar to this product but its effect of improving microcirculation and decreasing myocardial oxygen consumption is lower.

2.2 Antihypertensives

Niuhuang Jiangya Wan

Main Ingredients:

Calculus Bovis and others   *Niuhuang*

Actions: Clearing away heart—fire, resolving phlegm, tranquilizing the mind and reducing hypertension.

Indications: Hyperactivity of the liver—*Yang*, vertigo, abundant phlegm—fire, coma, lockjaw, numbness of the limbs, hemiplegia and deviation of the eye and mouth.

Administration and Dosage: Taken orally, 1—2 boluses each time, twice a day.

Preparation Form: Honeyed bolus.

Package: 1.6g in each bolus.

Notes: This product can decrease blood pressure, adjust the central nervous system and calm the mind. It can be clinically used to treat hypertension due to hyperactivity of the liver—*Yang*, accumulation of phlegm—fire and cerebrovascular accident.

It is contraindicated for diarrhea.

Naoliqing Wan

Ingredients:

Haematitum   18.4%   *Zheshi*

Magnetitum	10.5%	*Cishi*
Rhizoma Pinelliae	10.5%	*Zhibanxia*
Distiller's Yeast	10.5%	*Jiuqu*
Cooked Distiller's Yeast	10.5%	*Shujiuqu*
Radix Achyranthis Bidentatae	10.5%	*Niuxi*
Concha Margaritifera Usta	5.3%	*Zhenzhumu*
Mentholum	2.6%	*Behenao*
Borneolum	2.6%	*Bing pian*
Fresh Pig's Bile	18.4%	*Xianzhudanzhi*

Actions: Checking exuberance of Yang with its heavy materials, restoring consciousness and tranquilizing the mind.

Indications: Hyperactivity of *Yang* due to *Yin* deficiency, vertigo, apoplexy, and deviation of eyes and mouth.

Administration and Dosage: Taken orally, 10 pills each time twice a day.

Preparation Form: Water—paste pill.

Package: 1g in every 10 pills.

Notes: This product can dilate the peripheral cappillaries, decrease blood pressure and relieve fever and pain. It is clinically indicated for I or II type of hypertension resulting from hyperactivity of *Yang* due to *Yin* deficiency, and spasm of blood vessels of brain.

Shuxin Jiangya Pian

Ingredients:

Radix Salviae Miltiorrhizae	11.8%	*Danshen*
Radix Curcumae	5.9%	*Yujin*
Flos Chrysanthemi	7.8%	*Juhua*
Flos Carthami	5.9%	*Honghua*

· 33 ·

Flos Sophorae Immaturus	7.8%	*Huaimi*
Rhizoma Acori Graminei	5.9%	*Shichangpu*
Ramulus Visci	9.8%	*Huojisheng*
Radix Puerariae	11.8%	*Gegen*
Semen Persicae	7.8%	*Taoren*
Semen Biotae	7.8%	*Baiziren*
Ramulus Uncariae cum Uncis	11.8%	*Gouteng*
Radix Achyranthis Bidentatae	5.9%	*Niuxi*

Actions: Promoting blood circulation to remove blood stasis, relaxing the heart and reducing hypertension.

Indications: Vertigo, headache, distension in the brain, angina pectoris and precordial pain with cold limbs.

Administration and Dosage: Taken orally, 6—8 tablets each time, three times a day.

Preparation Form: Tablet.

Package: 0.3g in each tablet.

Notes: This product can dilate the coronary artery and peripheral blood vessels, decrease the blood pressure and blood—lipid concentration, ruduce the blood viscosity, and prolong the time of pleteletes coagulation, It is clinically indicated for primary hypertension, coronary heart disease, arteriosclerosis, etc.

Fufang Luobuma Pian

Main Ingredients:

Folium Apocini Veneti	*Luobuma*
Radix Stephaniae Tetrandrae	*Fangji*
Flos Chrysanthemi Indici	*Yejuhua*

Actions: Clearing away heat, inducing diuresis, calming

the liver and tranquilizing the mind.

Indications: Hyperactivity of the liver—*Yang*, vertigo, headache and distension in the brain.

Administration and Dosage: Taken orally, 2 tablets each time, three times a day.

Preparation Form: Tablet.

Package: 0.1g in each tablet.

Notes: This product can decrease blood pressure, dilate the periphercal capillaries and induce diuresis. It can be clinically applied to mild and moderate hypentention.to relieve headache, dizziness and sleeplessness.

Hypentention with gastric ulcer, chronic rhinitis, depression, etc.may be treated with it.

Duzhong Jiangya Pian

Ingredients:

Cortex Eucommiae	*Duzhong*
Radix Scutellariae	*Huangqin*
Ramulus Uncariae cum Uncis	*Gou teng*
Spica Prunellae	*Xiakucao*
Herba Leonuri	*Yimucao*

Actions: Calming the liver to stop the wind.

Indications: Hyperactivity of the liver—*Yang*, vertigo, headache and distension in the brain.

Administration and Dosage: Taken orally, 5 tablets each time, three times a day.

Preparation Form: tablet.

Package: 0.3g in each Tablet.

Notes: This product can dilate the capillaries, induce

diuresis and decrease blood pressure. It can be clinically applied to mild and moderate hypertention.

It is forbidden for pregnant women.

Jiangyaping Pian

Ingredients:

Spica Prunellae	10.5%	*Xiakucao*
Radix Scutellariae	10.5%	*Huangqin*
Herba Visci	10.5%	*Huojisheng*
Radix Puerariae	10.5%	*Gegen*
Concha Margaritifera Usta	10.5%	*Zhenzhumu*
Flos sophorae	10.5%	*Huaihua*
Radix Rehmanniae	5.4%	*Shengdi*
Flos Chrysanthemi	10.5%	*Juhua*
Herba Lophatheri	10.5%	*Danzhuye*
Mentholum	0.01%	*Bing pian*
Lumbrieus	10.5%	*Dilong*

Actions: Calming the liver to stop the wind.

Indications: Hyperactivity of the liver−*Yang*, dizziness, and vertigo.

Administration and Dosage: Taken orally, 4 tablets each time, three times a day.

Preparation Form: Sugar−coated tablet.

Package: 0.3g in each tablet.

Notes: This product can decrease blood−lipid concentration and blood viscosity, dilate the peripheral capillaries, and decrease blood pressure. It can be clinically applied to treat hypertention and prevent arteriosclerosis.

Luobuma Jiangya Pian

Ingredients:

Folium Apocyni Veneti   *Luobuma*

Rhizoma Alismatis   *Zexie*

Spica Prunellae   *Xiakucao*

Concha Margaritifera Usta   *Zhenzhumu*

Actions: Calming the liver, reducing hypertension, tranquilizing and allaying excitement, strengthening the heart and inducing diuresis.

Indications: Hyperactivity of the liver—*Yang*, and dizziness.

Administration and Dosage: Taken orally, 2—4 tablets each time, three times a day.

Preparation Form: Tablet.

Package: 0.3g in each tablet.

Notes: This drug is clinically indicated for mild and moderate hypertension.

2.3 Drugs for Decreasing Blood—lipid

Jiangzhiling Jiaowan

Ingredients:

Pollen Typhae   *Puhuang*

Oleum Vegetable Seeds   *Caiziyou*

Actions: Reducing serum cholesterol and triglyceride.

Indication: Hyperlipemia.

Administration and Dosage: Taken orally, 5 pills each time, three times a day.

Preparation Form: Glue—pill.

Package: 0.25g in each pill.

Notes: This drug is clinically indicated not only for the treatment of hyperlipemia but for the prevention of coronary heart disease.

Xiaoshuan Tongluo Pian

Ingredients:

Radix Notoginseng	8%	*Sanqi*
Rhizoma Chuanxiong	15.9%	*Chuanxiong*
Radix Astragali	23.9%	*Huangqi*
Radix Curcumae	8%	*Yujin*
Ramulus Cinnamomi	8%	*Guizhi*
Fructus Crataegi	8%	*Shanzha*
Radix Aucklandiae	4%	*Muxiang*
Rhizoma Alismatis	8%	*Zexie*
Flos Sophorae	4%	*Huaimi*
Radix Salviae Miltiorrhizae	12.0%	*Danshen*
Borneolum	0.3%	*Bing pian*

Actions: Promoting blood circulation to remove blood stasis and warming the channel, to activate the flow of *Qi*

Indications: Apoplexy, unconsciousness, listlessness, stiff tongue, dysphasia, unclear speaking, cool hands and feet.

Administration and Dosage: Taken orally, 8 tablets each time, three times a day.

Preparation Form: Sugar—coated tablet.

Package: 0.4g in each tablet.

Notes: This drug can reduce serum cholesterol, triglyceride, β—lipoprotein, blood viscosity and aggregation of platelets. It can also dilate the blood vesseles of brain and heart to provide blood for the brains of patients with cerebrovascular sclerosis, and has certain effect of reducing blood pressure. It is clinically indicated for hyponoia caused by cerebrovascular sclerosis, cerebral thrombosis and hyperlipoidemia.

Maian Chongji

Ingredients:

Fructus Crataegi	50%	Shanzha
Fructus Hordei Germinatus	50%	Maiya

Actions: Reducing blood lipid and guarding against atheroscleorsis.

Indications: Hyperlipoidemia.

Administration and Dosage: Taken orally, 20g each time, twice a day.

Preparation Form: Granule or powder dissolvable in water.

Package: 20g in each bag.

Notes: This product has the effects of reducing blood lipid, triglyceride, cholesterol, B—lipoprotein and blood viscosity, dilating coronary arteries, strengthening the heart and brain, decreasing myocardial oxygen consumption, regulating blood pressure and promoting diuresis.

It is clinically used for hyperlipoidemia.

2.4　Drugs for Treating Cerebrovasular Disease

Zaizao Wan

Main Ingredients:

Agkistrodon	Qisharou

Scorpio	*Quanxie*
Lumbricus	*Dilong*
Bombyx Batryticatus	*Jiongchan*
Calculus Bovis	*N iuhuang*

Action: Expelling wind to resolve phlegm, promoting blood circulation to remove obstruction in the channels.

Indications: Apoplexy, facial hemiparalysis, hemiplegia, numbness of hands and fee with spasm and pain, and language—clog.

Administration and Dosage: Honeyed bolus.

Package: 9g in each blous.

Notes: This product can regulate metabolism body, improve physiological functions, promote microcirculation, and nourish the nerves. Clinically indicated for sequela of cerebrovascular accident, it can prevent hypertension and cerebrovascular accident.

It is forbidden for pregnant women.

Renshen Zaizao Wan

Main Ingredients:

Zaocys	*Wuqiaoshe*
Herba Visci	*Huojisheng*
Radix Clematidis	*Weilingxian*
Scorpio	*Quanxie*
Radix Puerariae	*Gegen*
Herba Ephedrae	*Mahuang*
Radix Angelicae Dahuricae	*Baizhi*
Radix et Rhizoma Rhai	*Dahuang*
Radix Ginseng	*Renshen*

Actions: Relaxing muscles and tendons to promote blood circulation, expelling wind to resolve phlegm.

Indications: Apoplexy, facicl hemiparalysis, slurred speech, spasm of hands and feelt and hemiplegia.

Administration and Dosage: Taken orally, 1 bolus each time, twice a day.

Preparation Form: 10g in each bolus.

Notes: This product can improve microcirculation, regulate physiological function and promote body metabolism. With the effect of nourishing and strengthening the body, it is clinically used in the convalescence of cerebrovascular accident sequela.

Compared with *Zaizao Wan*, it has the stronger effect of nourishing the body and improving microcirculation. Therefore it is more suitable for patients with prolonged illness and weakness.

It is forbidden for pregnant women.

Xiaoshuan Zaizao Wan

Main Ingredients:

Rhizoma Chuanxiong   *Chuanxiong*
Radix Salviae Miltiorrhizae   *Danshen*
Radix Notoginseng   *Sanqi*
Rhizoma Gastrodiae   *Tianma*
Bungarus Parvus   *Baihuasha*
Benzoinum   *Anxixiang*
Styrax   *Suhexiang*
Radix Ginseng   *Renshen*
Ligunum Aqui lariae Resinatum *Chenxiang*

Actions: Promoting blood circulation to remove blood

stasis, dispelling wind to remove obstruction in the channels, invigorating *Qi* and enriching blood.

Indications: Apoplexy, facial hemiparalysis and hemiplegia.

Administration and Dosage: Taken orally, 1–2 pill boluses each time, twice a day.

Preparation: 9g in each bolus.

Notes: This product has the effect of reducing blood lipid and blood viscosity, improving microcirculation and cranovessel blood supply, guarding against agulation of platelets and removing coagulated platelets. It is clinically indicated for cerebral thrombosis, cerebral embolism and hyperlipemia.

Honghua Zhusheye

Ingredient:

Flos Carthami   100%   *Honghua*

Actions: Promoting blood circulation to remove blood stasis.

Indications: Apoplexy, facial hemiparalysis, hemiplegia, obstruction of *Qi* in the chest and angina pectoris.

Administration and Dosage: Given through Intravenous drip, 15ml each time which is diluted with 250–500ml of 10% glucose injection, 15–20 days being a course; 5–20ml each time for coronary heart disease.

Intramuscular injection for angiitis, 2.5–5ml each time, 1–2 times a day.

Preparation Form: Injection.

Package: 5ml in each ampule.

Notes: This product has the effect of dilating the coronary

artery, increasing artery coronary flow, decreasing blood viscosity, improving microcirculation, etc. It is clinically indicated for closed cerebrovascular disease, coronary heart disease, myocardiac infarction, angiitis, etc.

Jufang Niuhuang Qingxin Wan

Main Ingredients:

Calculus Bovis	*Niuhuang*
Cornu Saigae Tataricae	*Lingyangjiao*
Borneolum	*Bing pian*
Radix Scutellariae	*Huangqin*
Radix Ampelopsis	*Bailian*
Realgar	*Xonghuang*
Radix Bupleuri	*Chaihu*
Radix Ophiopogonis	*Maidong*
Radix Paeoniae	*Baishao*
Radix Angelicae Sinensis	*Danggui*
Cortex Cinnamomi	*Rougui*
Rhizoma Zingiberis	*Ganjiang*
Radix Ledebouriellae	*Fangfeng*
Radix Platycodi	*Jiegeng*
Massa Fermentata Madicinalis	*Shenqu*
Semen Armeniacae Amarum	*Xingren*

Actions: Clearing away heart fire to resolve phlegm, and expelling wind to relieve convulsion.

Indications: Abundant phlegm and expectoration, unconsciousness, vertigo, epilepsy, infantile convulsion and mental confusion due to phlegm.

Administration and Dosage: Taken orally, 1 bolus each

time, once a day.

Preparation Form: Honeyed bolus.

Package: 3g in each bolus.

Notes: The prescription is recorded in the bood *Tai Ping Hui Min He Ji Ju Fang* written by Chen Shiwen in the Song Dynasty.

This product has the effect of tranqui lizing to relieve muscle spasm, lowering fever, improving microcirculation and decreasing blood pressure. It is clinically indicated for cerebrovessel spasm, sequelae of cerebral hemorrhage encephalorrhagia and epilepsy.

It's forbidden for pregnant women.

Huatuo Zaizao Wan

Ingredients: (Omission)

Actions: Relaxing muscles and tendons, activating the flow of *Qi* and blood in the channels and collaterals, expelling wind and norishing blood.

Indications: Apoplexy, hemiplegia, facicl hemiparalysis, muscular spasm of hands and feet, slurred speech, and obstruction of *Qi in the chest*.

Administration and Dosage: Taken orally, 1—2 boluses each time, 1—2 times a day.

Preparation Form: Honeyed bolus.

Package: 3g in each bolus.

Notes: This product can adjust the function of each organ, improve microcirculation, dilate the coronary arteries to increase the blood flow through them, raise the ability of the heart against oxygen deficit, nourish the body, decrease blood cholesterol, triglyceride and blood viscosity as well, and improve cerebral circulation. It is clinically indicated for cerebrovasular diseases such as cerebral hemorrhage encephalorrhagia, cerebral embolism, cerebral vasospasm, etc, for angiocardiopathy such as coronary heart disease, angina pectoris, cardiac insufficiency, etc.

It is reported that the curative effect, of this product has reached 94.2% when used to treat cerbrovasular diseases and 93.2% when used to treat angiocardiopathy.

3　Drugs for Acting on Respiratory System

3.1　Drugs for Removing the Phlegm and Cough

Fuling Wan

Ingredients:

Poria	33.3%	*Fuling*
Rhizoma Pinelliae	16.7%	*Banxia*
Fructus Aurantii	8.3%	*Zhiqiao*
Mirabilitum	41.7%	*Fenghuaxiao*

Actions: Eliminating dampness, resolving phlegm, and removing obstruction in the channels to relieve pain.

Indications: Weakness of the spleen and stomach, spasm of muscles, numbness and pain of limbs.

Administration and Dosage: Taken orally, 5—9g each time, twice daily.

Preparation Form: Concentrated pills

Package: 18g in each bag

Notes: The prescription is quoted from the book *Zheng Zhi Zhun Sheng* compiled by Wang Kentang in the Ming Dynasty.

This drug is clinically efficacious for chronic bronchitis, asthma, rheumatic muscle fibrositis, neuritis, etc.

It is contraindicated for patients with loose stools.

Ermu Ningsou Wan

Ingredients:

Gypsum Fibrosum	16.0%	Shengshigao
Fructus Gardeniae	9.6%	Zhi zi
Poria	8.0%	Fuling
Fructus Aurantii Immaturus	5.6%	Zhishi
Rhizoma Anemarrhenae	12.0%	Zhimu
Cortex Mori Radicis	8.0%	Sangbaipi
Radix Scutellariae	9.6%	Huangqin
Semen Trichosanthis	8.0%	Gualouzi
Radix Glycyrrhizae	1.6%	Gancao
Bulbus Fritillariae Thunbergii	12.0%	Beimu
Pericarpium Citri Reticulatae	8.0%	Chenpi
Fructus Schisandrae	1.6%	Wuweizi

Actions: Removing heat—phlegm, checking upward adverse flow of the lung—Qi and relieving cough.

Indications: Cough due to lung—heat, short and rapid breathing due to excessive phlegm.

Administration and Dosage: Taken orally, 2 boluses each time, twice daily.

Preparation Form: Honeyed holus

Package: 9 g in each bolus.

Notes: The prescription is quoted from the book Gu Jin Yi Jian compiled by Gong Xin in the Ming Dynasty.

This drug has the effects of bacteriostasis and anti—inflammation. It is clinically efficacious for chronic bronchitis, pulmonary abscess, etc.

It is contraindicated for patients with pulmonary tuberculosis.

Baihe Gujin Wan

Ingredients:

Bulbus lilii	7.6%	*Baihe*
Radix Rehmanniae Praeparata	22.9%	*Shudihuang*
Radix Ophiopogonis	11.5%	*Maimendong*
Bulbus Fritillariae Cirrhosae	7.6%	*Chuanbeimu*
Radix Scrophulariae	6.1%	*Xuanshen*
Radix Rehmanniae	15.3%	*Dihuang*
Radix Angelicae Sinensis	7.6%	*Danggui*
Radix Paeoniae Alba	7.6%	*Baishao*
Radix Platycodi	6.2%	*Jiegeng*
Radix Glycyrrhizae	7.6%	*Gancao*

Actions: Nourishing the lung to moisten dryness and relieving cough.

Indications: Cough with dyspnea, pharyngodynia, blood loss, hectic fever due to consumptive disease, tidal fever in the afternoon, dry mouth and dark urine, all of which are caused by *Yin* deficiency of both the lung and kidney.

Administration and Dosage: Taken orally, 1 bolus each time, once or twice daily.

Preparation Form: Honeyed bolus.

Package: 9 g in each bolus.

Notes: The prescription originates from the book *Yi Fang Ji Jie* compiled by Wang Ang in the Qing Dynasty.

This drug has the effects of bacteriostasis, anti-inflammatory, antipyresis, relieving cough, hemostasis, nourishing and sthenia. It is clinically efficacious for pulmonary tuberculosis, pneumonia, pharyngitis, whooping cough, hemoptysis, etc.

Zhisou Qingguo Wan

Ingredients:

Bulbus Fritillariae Cirrhosae	3.4%	*Chuanbeimu*
Bulbus lilii	4.5%	*Baihe*
Radix Scutellariae	8.9%	*Huangqin*
Gypsum Fibrosum	3.4%	*Shigao*
Fructus Canarii	5.6%	*Qingguo*
Cortex Mori	8.9%	*Sangbaipi*
Semen Ginkgo	22.3%	*Baiguo*
Herba Ephedrae	17.9%	*Mahuang*
Semen Pruni Armeniacae	1.7%	*Xingren*
Flos Farfarae	8.9%	*Kuandonghua*
Rhizoma Pinelliae	8.9%	*Banxia*
Fructus Aristolochiae	2.2%	*Madouling*
Radix Glycyrrhizae	3.4%	*Gancao*

Actions: Removing heat-phlegm, and relieving cough and asthma.

Indications: Cough with phlegm and dyspnea, dry throat with bitter taste, and senile asthma.

Administration and Dosage: Taken orally, 1 bolus each time, twice daily.

Preparation Form: Honeyed bolus.

Package: 9 g in each bolus.

Notes: The drug has the effects of relieving cough and asthma, and removing phlegm. It is clinically suitable for chronic bronchitis, bronchial asthma, etc.

It is contraindicated for those with dyspnea due to plenty of phlegm or with pulmonary tuberculosis.

Qingfei Yihuo Wan

Ingredients:

Radix Scutellariae	20%	*Huangqin*
Fructus Gardeniae	14.1%	*Zhizi*
Radix et Rhizoma Rhei	17.1%	*Dahuang*
Cortex Phellodendri	5.7%	*Huangbai*
Radix Sophorae Flavescentis	8.3%	*Kushen*
Radix Trichosanthis	10.4%	*Tianhuafen*
Rhizoma Anemarrhenae	8.3%	*Zhimu*
Radix Platycodi	10.4%	*Jiegeng*
Radix Peucedani	5.7%	*Qianhu*

Actions: Clearing away heat, relaxing the bowels, relieving cough and eliminating phlegm.

Indications: Cough with profuse sputum, swollen and sore throat, dry mouth and tongue, and constipation.

Administration and Dosage: Taken orally, 1 bolus each time, twice a day.

Preparation Form: Honeyed bolus.

Package: 9 g in each bolus.

Notes: The prescription comes from the book *Shou Shi Bao Yuan* compiled by Gong Tingxian in the Ming Dynasty.

This drug has the effects of removing phlegm, relieving cough and asthma, restraining bacteria and resisting inflammation. It is clinically good for chronic bronchitis, bronchiectasis, pulmonary tuberculosis, pulmonary abscess, parasitosis of lung, tumor of bronchus, etc.

It should be administrated with caution when used to treat cough due to cold.

This bolus has other dosage forms with the same name, ingredients and actions, such as tablet, water–paste pill and liquid extract.

Erchen Wan

Ingredients:

Rhizoma Pinelliae	34.5%	*Banxia*
Pericarpium Citri Reticulatae	34.5%	*Chenpi*
Poria	20.7%	*Fuling*
Radix Glycyrrhizae	10.3%	*Gancao*

Actions: Eliminating phlegm, removing dampness, and regulating the stomach and *Qi*.

Indications: Cough with profuse and mucous sputum, fullness in the chest and abdomen, nausea, vomiting, dizziness and palpitation.

Administration and Dosage: Taken orally, 1 bolus each time, twice daily.

Preparation Form: Honeyed bolus.

Package: 6 g in each bolus.

Notes: The prescription is quoted from the book, *Tai Ping Hui Min He Ji Ju Fang* compiled by Chen Shiwen in the Song Dynasty.

This drug has the effects of restraining bacteria, resisting inflammation, relieving cough, strengthening the stomach to benefit digestion, promoting secretion of the respiratory tract and eliminating sputum. It is clinically effective not only for chronic bronchitis with such gastrointestinal symptoms as anorexia, acid regurgitation and heart–burn, but also for chronic gastroenteritis with productive cough.

Juhong Wan

Ingredients:

Exocorpium Citri Reticulatae	11.1%	*Juhong*
Pericarpium Citri Reticulatae	7.4%	*Chenpi*
Rhizoma Pinelliae Praeparata	5.6%	*Fabanxia*
Gypsum Fibrosum	7.4%	*Shigao*
Bulbus Fritillariae Thunbergii	7.4%	*Zhebeimu*
Pericarpium Trichosanthis	7.4%	*Gualoupi*
Radix Asteris	5.6%	*Ziyuan*
Flos Farfarae	3.7%	*Kuandonghua*
Semen Armeniacae Amarum	7.4%	*Kuxingren*
Fructus Perillae	5.6%	*Zisuzi*
Radix Platycodi	5.6%	*Jiegeng*
Radix Ophiopogonis	7.4%	*Maimendong*
Radix Rehmanniae	7.4%	*Dihuang*
Poria	7.4%	*Fuling*
Radix Glycyrrhizae	3.6%	*Gancao*

Actions: Clearing away lung—heat, eliminating dampness, relieving cough and resolving phlegm.

Indications: Cough with profuse sputum rapid breathing, dry throat with a bitter taste, stuffiness in the chest, and inappetence.

Administration and Dosage: Taken orally, 2 boluses each time, twice a day.

Preparation Form: Honeyed bolus.

Package: 6 g in each bolus.

Notes: The prescription is quoted from the book *Gu Jin Yi Jian* compiled by Gong Xin in the Ming Dynasty.

This drug has the actions of restraining bacteria, resisting inflammation, removing phlegm, dilating bronchial smooth muscles, etc. It is clinically beneficial to acute or chronic bronchitis with productive cough, rapid breathing, dry mouth, anorexia, etc.

It is contraindicated for common cold with fever.

This drug also has a granule or powder preparation with the same name, ingredients and actions, which is to be dissolved in boiling water before taken.

Qingqi Huatan Wan

Ingredients:

Arisaemacum Bile	16.7%	*Dannanxing*
Radix Scutellariae	11.1%	*Huangqin*
Semen Trichosanthis	11.1%	*Gualouren*
Fructus Aurantii Immaturus	11.1%	*Zhishi*
Exocarpium Citri Reticulatae	11.1%	*Juhong*
Rhizoma Pinelliae	16.7%	*Jiangbanxia*
Semen Armeniacae Amarum	11.1%	*Xingren*
Poria	11.1%	*Fuling*

Actions: Removing heat from the lung to relieve cough, checking upward adverse flow of *Qi* and resolving phlegm.

Indications: cough with dyspnea, stuffiness in the chest, nausea and vomiting.

Administration and Dosage: Taken orally, 6 to 9g each time, twice daily.

Preparation Form: Water—paste pill.

Package: 18g in each bag.

Notes: The prescription is recorded in the book *Jing Yue*

Quan Shu written by Zhang Jiebin in the Ming Dynasty.

This drug has the effects of restraining bacteria, resisting inflammation, dilating the bronchial smooth muscles to relax bronchial spasm, and enhancing secretion of the respiratory tract to eliminate sputum. It is clinically suitable for chronic bronchitis, abundant expectoration, constipation, yellowish urine.

It is not to be used for those with cough due to wind–cold or those having dry cough without sputum.

Kongxian Wan

Ingredients:

Semen Sinapis	33.3%	*Baijiezi*
Radix Kansui	33.3%	*Gansui*
Radix Knoxiae	33.3%	*Hongdaji*

Actions: Eliminating stagnated phlegm and water by purgation and removing toxic substances.

Indications: Cough with dyspnea, hypochondriac pain due to retention of phlegm, and hydrothorax.

Administration and Dosage: Taken orally, 1 to 3g each time, once or twice a day.

Preparation Form: Water–paste pill.

Package: 6g in each bag.

Notes: The prescription comes from the book *San Yin Ji Yi Bing Zheng Fang Lun* written by Chen Yan in the Song Dynasty.

This pill acts as a bacteriostatic, an antiphlogistic, an expectorant and a more potent diuretic. It is clinically efficacious for bronchitis, pneumonia, chronic lymphnoditis, tuberculosis of lymph nodes in the neck, bone tuberculosis, ascites due to cirrhosis, wet pleurisy, ascites due to late schistosomiasis, etc.

It is contraindicated for pregnant women and weak patients. This pill has other dosage form with the same name, ingredients and actions, such as paste pill and honeyed pill.

Tongxuan Lifei Wan

Ingredients:

Herba Ephedrae	9.2%	Mahuang
Folium Perillae	14%	Zisuye
Radix Peucedani	9.3%	Qianhu
Semen Armeniacae Amarum	7%	Xingren
Radix Platycodi	9.3%	Jiegeng
Pericarpium Citri Reticulatae	9.3%	Chenpi
Rhizoma Pinelliae	7%	Banxia
Poria	9.3%	Fuling
Fructus Aurantii	9.3%	Zhique
Radix Scutellariae	9.3%	Huangqin
Radix Glycyrrhizae	7%	Gancao

Actions: Ventilating the lung to relieve cough.

Indications: Cough, fever with chills, headache, anhidrosis and arthrodynia of the extremities due to pathogenic wind—cold.

Administration and Dosage: Taken orally, 2 boluses each time, 2 to 3 times daily.

Preparation Form: Honeyed bolus.

Package: 6g in each bolus.

Notes: The prescription is quoted from the book *Zheng Zhi Zhun Sheng* compiled by Wang Kentang in the Ming Dynasty.

The effects this drug are antipyresis, anti—bacteria, anti—inflammation and relieving cough as well. It is clinically useful for influenza, bronchitis, etc.

It has a tablet from with the same name, ingredients and actions.

Luohanguo Chongji

Ingredients:

Fructus Momordicae   100%   *Luohanguo*

Actions: Clearing away heat and moistening the lung, removing phlegm and relieving cough.

Indications: Productive cough and asthma caused by lung—heat.

Administration and Dosage: Taken orally after dissolved in boiling water, 1 bag each time, 2 to 3 times daily.

Preparation Form: Granule or powder preparation.

Package: 15g in each bag.

Notes: This drug has the effects of lowering down fever, resisting inflammation, restraining bacteria, removing phlegm, relieving cough, enhancing immunologic function of the body and building up health. It is clinically suitable for cough, sore—throat, aphonia due to common cold, acute or chronic bronchitis.

Chuanbei Pipa Zhengke Chongji

Ingredients:

Folium Eriobotryae   *Pibaye*

Radix Platycodi   *Jiegeng*

Bulbus Fritillariae Cirrhosae   *Chuānbeimu*

Oleum Menthae   *bohenao*

Semen Armeniacae Amarum   *Kuxingren*
etc.

Actions: Relieving cough and removing phlegm.

Indications: Cough with profuse sputum, dyspnea, adverse flow of *Qi,* and dry mouth and tongue.

Administration and Dosage: Taken orally after dissolved in boiling water, 1 bag each time, 3 times daily. For children, the dosage should be reduced.

Preparation Form: Granule or powder preparation.

Package: 10g in per bag.

Notes: This drug is able to stimulate the laryngeal mucous membrane and gastric mucous membrane, reflexly causing excessive secretion of mucous membrane of the respiratory tract to dilute and eliminate phlegm accumulated in the bronchi and tracheas, with phlegm removed and cough relieved. It is clinically good for bronchial asthma, bronchitis and chronic laryngopharyngitis.

Yangyin Qingfei Gao

Ingredients:

Radix Rehmanniae	24.7%	*Dihuang*
Radix Scrophulariae	19.8%	*Xuanshen*
Radix Ophiopogonis	14.8%	*Maimendong*
Bulbus Fritillariae Cirrhosae	9.9%	*Chuanbeimu*
Cortex Moutan	9.9%	*Mudanpi*
Radix Angelicae Sinensis	9.9%	*Danggui*
Herba Menthae	6.2%	*Bohe*
Radix Glycyrrhizae	4.8%	*Gancao*

Actions: Nourishing *Yin* to clear away lung—heart, and relieving sore—throat.

Indications: Cough, thirst, dry throat, aphonia, celosomia, sputum mixed with blood, and swollen pain in the throat due to

Yin deficiency.

Administration and Dosage: Taken orally, 15g each time, twice a day.

Preparation Form: Soft extract.

Package: 30g or 60g in a bottle.

Notes: The prescription is seen in the book *Chong Lou Yu Yue* written by Zheng Meijian in the Qing Dynasty.

The results of pharmacologic experiments showed that this extract possesses remarkably inhibitory actions on Bacillus diphtheriae and greater ability to neutralize diphtheria toxin in vitro. It is clinically efficacious for cough due to common cold, diphtheria, pharyngitis and tonsillitis, and especially for acute tonsillitis.

There is also a pill from with the same ingredients and actions.

Erdong Gao

Ingredients:

Radix Asparagi	50%	*Tianmendong*
Radix Ophiopogonis	50%	*Maimendong*

Actions: Moistening the lung and promoting the production of body fluid to quench thirst.

Indications: Cough, excessive thirst, sore throat, hoarseness, aphonia, and sputum mixed with blood.

Administration and Dosage: Taken orally, 15g each time, twice a day.

Preparation Form: Soft extract.

Package: 60g in each bottle.

Notes: The prescription comes from *Zhang Shi Yi Tong*

written by Zhang Lu in the Qing Dynasty.

This drug has such effects as restraining bacteria, resisting inflammation, increasing secretion of the respiratory tract, and stopping bleeding. Clinically, it can be used in the treatment of whooping cough and pharyngitis, or as an adjuvant in treating pulmonary tuberculosis.

It is contraindicated for cough due to common cold.

Fufang Baibu Zhike Tangjiang

Ingredients:

Radix Stemonae	16.7%	Baibu
Radix Scutellariae	16.7%	Huangqin
Semen Armeniacae Amarum	8.3%	Kuxingren
Pericarpium Citri Reticulatae	16.7%	Chenpi
Radix Platycodi	8.3%	Jiegeng
Cortex Mori Radicis	8.3%	Sangbaipi
Radix Ophiopogonis	4.2%	Maidong
Rhizoma Arisaematis	4.2%	Tiannanxing
Rhizoma Anemarrhenae	4.2%	Zhimu
Radix Glycyrrhizae	4.1%	Gancao
Fructus Aurantii	8.3%	Zhike

Actions: Removing heat from the lung to relieve cough.

Indications: Cough caused by the lung—heat, with yellow and thick sputum.

Administration and Dosage: Taken orally, 10 to 20ml each time, 2 to 3 times daily. For children, the dosage should be reduced.

Preparation Form: Syrup.

Package: 100ml in each bottle.

Notes: This syrup is clinically good for cough due to upper respiratory tract infection, infantile whooping cough, etc.

Runfeibu Gao

Ingredients:

Extractum *Laiyang* Li Inspissatum	*Laiyangli Qiggao*
Radix Codonopsis Pilosulae	*Dangshen*
etc.	

Actions: Invigorating *Qi*, moistening the lung, relieving cough and reducing sputum.

Indications: Chronic cough with dry throat and hoarseness due to lung–dryness.

Administration and Dosage: Taken orally 15g each time, twice daily.

Preparation Form: Soft extract.

Package: 250g in each bottle.

Notes: This drug can remove phlegm, strengthen the stomach, enhance metabolism, aid in digestion and promote absorption of chyle. It is clinically used for chronic bronchitis, bronchial asthma, senile bronchial asthma, etc.

Chuanbei Zhike Tangjiang

Ingredients:

Bulbus Fritillariae Cirrhosae	28.3%	*Chuanbeimu*
Folium Eriobotryae	64.7%	*Pipaye*
Extractum Armeniacae Amarum	1.5%	*Kuxingrenjing*
Mentholum	0.1%	*bohenao*
Radix Platycodi	5.4%	*Jiegeng*

Actions: Moistening the lung, removing phlegm, and relieving cough.

Indications: Cough with short and rapid breath due to common cold.

Administration and Dosage: Taken orally, 10ml each time, 3 times daily. For children, the dosage should be appropriately reduced.

Preparation Form: Syrup.

Package: 100ml in each bottle.

Notes: The drug has the effects of removing phlegm, relieving cough, enhancing secretion of the respiratory tract and promoting elimination of sputum. In clinic, it has been proved to be effective for productive cough due to upper respiratory tract infection and bronchial diseases.

Laiyangli Zhike Tangjiang

Ingredients:

Extractum LaiyangLi Inspissatum	66.3%	*LaiyangliQinggao*
Extractum Glehniae Liquidum	5.1%	*BeisashenLiuqingao*
Extractum Platycodi Liquidum	6.3%	*JiegengLiuqingao*
Extractum Polygalae Liquidum	3.3%	*YuanzhiLiuqingao*
Extractum Lilii Liquidum	2.5%	*BaiheLiuqingao*
Extractum Pruni Armeniacae	3.8%	*Xingrenshui*
Extractum Ephedrae	12.7%	*MahuangTiquye*

Actions: Relieving cough and removing phlegm.

Indications: cough with profuse sputum due to common cold.

Administration and Dosage: Taken orally, 10ml each time, 4 times daily. For children, the dosage should be appropriately reduced.

Preparation Form: Syrup.

Package: 100ml in each bottle.

Notes: The effects of the drug are relieving cough and removing phlegm. It is clinically efficacious for cough with abundant expectoration due to common cold, and acute or chronic bronchitis.

This syrupu has also a granule or powder preparation with the same ingredients and actions, which is to be dissolved in boiling water before administration.

Maxing Zhike Tangjiang

Ingredients:

Herba Ephedrae	15.5%	*Mahuang*
Semen Armeniacae Amarum	15.5%	*Kuxingren*
Gypsum Fibrosum	43.1%	*Shengshigao*
Herba Menthae	15.5%	*bohe*
Radix Glycyrrhizae	10.4%	*Gancao*

Actions: Clearing away heat to promote the dispersing function of the lung, and relieving cough and asthma.

Indications: Cough with profuse sputum or cough with dyspnea.

Administration and Dosage: Taken orally, 10ml each time, 3 times daily. For children the dosage should be appropriately reduced.

Preparation Form: Syrup.

Package: 100ml in each bottle.

Notes: The syrup is known to have the effects of antipyresis, anti−inflammation, and relieving cough and asthma as well.

It is clinically effective for common cold, acute bronchitis, lobar pneumonia, infantile bronchial pneumonia, scarlet fever, urticaria, acute conjunctivitis, bronchial asthma, etc.

Banxia Lu

Ingredients:

Rhizoma Pinelliae	14.2%	*Shengbanxia*
Tinctira Citri Reticulatae	29.6%	*Dingjupi*
Fructus Aurantii	7.4%	*Zhike*
Folium Eriobotryae	8.5%	*Pibaye*
Radix Polygalae	9.1%	*Yuanzhi*
Radix Asteris	8.5%	*Ziyuan*
Herba Ephedrae	5.7%	*Mahuang*
Mentholum	0.5%	*boheyou*
Extractum Pruni Armeniacae	10.8%	*Xingrenshui*
Radix Podophylli	5.7%	*Jiegeng*

Actions: Relieving cough and reducing sputum.

Indications: Productive cough with dyspnea.

Administration and Dosage: Taken orally, 10ml each time, 3 times a day.

Preparation Form: Syrup.

Package: 100ml in each bottle.

Notes: The actions of this drug are restraining bacteria, resisting inflammation, relieving cough and removing phlegm. It is clinically used for various types of cough with profuse sputum, and bronchitis.

This syrup has a granule or powder preparation with the same ingredients and actions, which is to be dissolved in boiling water before administration.

Xingren zhike Tangjiang

Ingredients:

Extractum Pruni Armeniacae	10.6%	*Xingrenshui*
Extractum Polygalae Liquidum	6.1%	*Yuanzhi Liaqingao*
Extractum Podophylli Liquidum	5.3%	*Jiegeng Liuqingao*
Extractum Stemonae Liquidum	5.3%	*Baibu Liuqingao*
Extractum Citri Reticulatae Liquidum		
	3.9%	*Chenpi Liuqingao*
Extractum Glycyrrhizae Liquidum	3.9%	*Gancao Liuqingao*
Sacharum	64.7%	*Shatang*

Actions: Resolving phlegm and relieving cough.

Indications: Abundant expectoration and cough with dyspnea.

Administration and Dosage: Taken orally, 10ml each time, 3 to 4 times daily. For children the dosage should be reduced accordingly.

Preparation Form: Syrup.

Package: 100ml in bottle.

Notes: This drug can relieve cough and remove phlegm. It is clinically suitable for cough due to common cold, laryngitis, pharyngitis, and acute or chronic bronchitis.

Xiaoqinglong Heji

Ingredients:

Herba Ephedrae	12.5%	*Mahuang*
Radix Paeoniae Alba	12.5%	*Baishao*
Ramulus Cinnamomi	12.5%	*Guizhi*
Rhizoma Zingiberis	12.5%	*Ganjiang*

Herba Asari	6.2%	*Xixin*
Fructus Schisandrae	12.5%	*Wuweizi*
Rhizoma Pinelliae	18.8%	*Banxia*
Radix Glycyrrhizae	12.5%	*Gancao*

Actions: Inducing diaphoresis to remove phlegm, and relieving cough and asthma.

Indications: Exogenous wind–cold with such symptoms as fever, anhidrosis, cough with dyspnea and thin sputum.

Administration and Dosage: Taken orally after the bottle is shaked, 15 to 20ml each time, 3 times daily.

Preparation Form: Mixture.

Package: 100ml in each bottle.

Notes: The prescription is cited from the book, *Shang Han Lun* written by Zhang Zhongjing in the Han Dynasty.

This drug produces the effects of lowering fever, tranquilizing pain, removing phlegm, relieving cough and alleviating asthma. It is clinically good for chronic bronchitis, bronchial asthma, senile pulmonary emphysema, combined upper respiratory tract infection and influenza.

Zhigancao Heji

Ingredients:

Radix Glycyrrhizae	9%	*Zhigancao*
Ramulus Cinnamomi	6%	*Guizhi*
Rhizoma Zingiberis Recens	9%	*Shengjiang*
Fructus Jujubae	12.1%	*Dazao*
Semen Sesame Nigyum	9%	*Humaren*
Colla corii Asini	9%	*Ejiao*
Radix Ginseng	6%	*Renshen*

Radix Rehmanniae   30.9%   *Shengdihuang*

Radix Ophiopogonis   9%   *Maidong*

Actions: Supplementing *Qi*, Nourishing *Yin*, enriching the blood and restoring normal pulse.

Indications: Cough due to fever of deficiency type, insufficiency of blood due to deficiency of *Qi*, palpitation, etc.

Administration and Dosage: Taken orally, 15ml each time, 3 times daily.

Preparation Form: Mixture.

Package: 500ml in each bottle.

Notes: The effects of this mixture are antipyresis, anti—inflammation and relief of cough. It can be used to increase immunity of the body, regulate metabolism and the functions of each organ, and promote the hematopoietic ability of the body. It is clinically good for pulmonary tuberculosis, pulmonary emphysema, arrhythmia, and neurasthenia.

Xianzhuli Koufuye

Main Ingredients:

Sucus Bambusae   *Xianzhuli*

Herba Houttuyniae   *Yuxingcao*

Folium Eriobotryae   *Pibaye*

Rhizoma Pinelliae   *Banxia*

Rhizoma Zingiberis Recens   *ShengTiang*

Actions: Removing heat—phlegm.

Indications: Productive cough due to the lung—heat, asthma, oppressed feeling in the chest, appoplexy and stiff tongue.

Administration and Dosage: Taken orally, 15—30ml each time, 2 to 3 times daily.

Preparation Form: Oral Liquid.

Package: 30ml in each bottle.

Notes: The liquid has been proved to exert the effects of lowering fever, relieving cough and removing phlegm. It is clinically efficacious for cough due to common cold, bronchitis, bronchial asthma, etc.

Tankejing

Ingredients:

Semen Armeniacae Amarum	*Xingren*
Radix Platycodi	*Jiegeng*
Radix Glycyrrhizae	*Gancao*
Borneolum	*Longnao*
Radix Polygalae	*Yuanzhi*

Actions: Relieving cough and removing phlegm.

Indications: Short breath, abundant expectoration and cough.

Administration and Dosage: Kept in the mouth or under the tongue, 3—6 times a day, 0.2g each time for adults and appropriate reduction of the dosage for children.

Preparation Form: Powder.

Package: 6g in each box.

Notes: Pharmacological experiments have shown that this drug can relieve cough and asthma by dilating the bronchial smooth muscles to remove their spasm. It may also make phlegm easily expectorated by promoting secretion of the respiratory tract.

Bacteriostatic experiments have suggested that the powder produces more potent inhibition of common bacteria causing diseases in the throat, giving better anti—phlogistic action.

Clinically, it is good for acute or chronic bronchitis, bronchial asthma, pulmonary emphysema, laryngopharyngitis, etc.

It is administrated with caution when pregnant women are treated.

Shedan Chenpi Mo

Ingredients:

Snake Bile	0.02%	*Shedanzhi*
Pericarpium Citri Reticulatae	94.1%	*Chenpi*
Lumbricus	1.9%	*Dilong*
Cinnabaris	1.9%	*Zhusha*
Bombyx Batryticatus	1.9%	*Jiangcan*
Succinum	0.2%	*Hupo*

Actions: Expelling wind, removing phlegm, and relieving convulsion and asthma.

Indications: Mania due to pathogenic wind—heat, mental restlessness, cough and dyspnea.

Administration and Dosage: Taken orally, 0.6g each time, 2 to 3 times daily. For children under 2 years old, the dosage is reduced by half.

Preparation Form: Powder.

Package: 0.6g in each bottle.

Notes: The effects of this drug are relieving fever and cough, and removing phlegm. It is clinically efficacious for cough due to common cold, infantile whooping cough, upper respiratory tract infection of children, etc.

Clinical treatment of 59 cases of whooping cough with the

average course of treatment being 7—10 days, has shown that the total effective rate of this drug is 94.9%.

Shedan Chuanbei Mo

Ingredients:

Snake Bile	14.2%	*Shedanzhi*
Bulbus Fritillariae Cirrhosae	85.8%	*Chuanbeimu*

Actions: Removing heat from the lung to relieve cough and dissolve phlegm.

Indications: Productive cough due to lung—heat.

Administration and Dosage: Taken orally 0.3—0.6g each time, 2—3 times daily. For children, the dosage should be appropriately reduced.

Preparation From: Powder.

Package: 0.6g in each bottle.

Notes: This drug plays the role of relieving cough, removing phlegm and resisting inflammation. It is clinically efficacious for cough due to common cold, infantile whooping cough, etc.

Taohua San

Ingredients:

Gypsum Fibrosum	43.9%	*Shigao*
Bulbus Fritillariae Thunbergii	3.4%	*Beimu*
Rhizoma Pinelliae	43.9%	*Banxia*
Cinnabaris	8.8%	*Zhusha*

Actions: clearing away heat, removing phlegm and relieving cough and asthma.

Indications: Cough and asthma due to lung—heat.

Administration and Dosage: Taken orally, 1 bag each time,

twice daily. For children under 3 years old, the dosage should be reduced proportionally.

Preparation Form: Powder.

Package: 1g in per bag.

Notes: This drug can be used for dilating the bronchial smooth muscules to relieve their spasm and remove phlegm. It is clinically efficacious for pneumonia, acute or chronic bronchitis, etc.

Zihua Dujuan Pian

Ingredient:

Folium et Cacumen Rhododendri mariae 100% *Zihuadujuan*

Actions: Relieving cough and removing phlegm.

Indications: Cough and asthma.

Administration and Dosage: Taken orally, 5 tablets each time, 3 times daily.

Preparation Form: Tablet.

Package: 0.25g in each tablet.

Notes: The tablet of this kind is found to have the effects of removing phlegm and relieving cough, and it is clinically useful for chronic bronchitis.

It is reported that treatment of senile chronic bronchitis of 2921 cases with this remedy for 1—2 courses of treatment has seen its effective rate of 90.2%.

There is also a capsule with the same name, ingrdients and actions.

3.2 Antiasthmatic

Fufang Chuanbeijing Pian

Ingredients:

Bulbus Fritillariae Cirrhosae	35.8%	*Chuanbeimu*
Ephedrine Hydrochloridum	0.5%	*Yansuanmahuangjian*
Pericarpium citri Reticulatae	13.4%	*Chenpi*
Rhizoma Pinelliae	10.8%	*Fabanxia*
Radix Polygalae	7.6%	*Yuanzhi*
Radix Platycodi	13.4%	*Jiegeng*
Fructus Schisandrae	7.6%	*Wuweizi*
Radix Glycyrrhizae	10.8%	*Gancao*

Actions: Stopping cough, resolving phlegm, moistening the lung and relieving asthma.

Indications: Cough with phlegm and asthma, and short and rapid breath due to pathogenic wind—cold.

Administration and Dosage: Taken orally 3—6 tablets each time, 3 times daily. For children, the dosage should be reduced proportionally.

Preparation Form: Sugar—coated tablet.

Package: 0.25g equivalent to 0.5g of the crude drug in each tablet.

Notes: The tablet has the actions of resisting bacteria and inflammation, removing phlegm and dilating the bronchial smooth muscles to relax their spasm. It is clinically good for acute or chronic bronchitis and cough with profuse sputum, but contraindicated for patients with hypertension, heart disease, or coronary sclerosis and pregnant women.

Zhikechuan Reshen Pian

Ingredient:

Radix Physochlainae   100%   *Reshen*

Actions: Relieving cough and asthma, and removing phlegm.

Indications: Dyspnea, oppressed feeling in the chest and productive cough.

Administration and Dosage: Taken orally, 1 to 2 tablets each time, 3 time a day.

Preparation Form: Tablet.

Package: Each tablet contains 0.12mg of hyoscyamine.

Notes: With remarkable action on asthma, this drug can be used to inhibit the glandular secretion of the trachea and bronchial mocosa, reduce phlegm, and relax bronchial spasm. It is clinically efficacious for bronchial asthma and various chronic bronchitis.

It is not to be administrated to patients with glaucoma and pregnant women.

There is also an aerosol with the same name, ingredients and actions.

Chuanshu Pian

Main Ingredients:

Sulphur	*Shenghualiu*
Radix et Rhizoma Rhei	*Dahuang*
Extractum Scutellariae	*Huangqin Tiquwu*

Actions: Relieving asthma and cough and warming the kidney to improve inspiration.

Indications: Dyspnea and oppressed feeling in the chest due

to kidney deficiency.

Administration and Dosage: Taken orally, 2 tablets each time, 3 times daily. For children, the dosage should be appropriatly reduced.

Preparation Form: Sugar-coated tablet.

Package: 0.35g in each tablet.

Notes: This drug has the effects of relieving cough and asthma and is clinically suitable for bronchial asthma, pulmonary emphysema or chronic bronchitis, and for trocheitis with asthma in particular.

Mujiangyou Jiaowan

Ingredient:

Fructus Viticis Negundo   100%   *Mujing*

Actions: Relieving asthma and cough, and removing phlegm.

Indications: Dyspnea, abundant expectoration and cough.

Administration and Dosage: Taken orally, 1 capsule each time, 3 times daily. For serious patients, 2 capsules each time.

Preparation Form: Capsule.

Package: Each capsule contains 1.7mg of Olium Viticis Negundo.

Notes: This drug produces the effects of relieving asthma and cough, and removing phlegm. It is clinically efficacious for bronchiectasis, chronic bronchitis, acute pulmonary abscess, etc.

Yunxiangyou Diwan

Ingredient:

Oleum cymbopogonis   100%   *Yunxiangyou*

Actions: Relieving asthma and cough.

Indications: Cough, abundant expectoration and dyspnea.

Administration and Dosage: Taken Orally after meals, 4 to 6 pills each time, 3 times a day.

Preparation Form: Enteric—coated pill.

Package: Each pill contains 0.2ml of Oleum Cymbopogonis.

Notes: The effects of this pill are relieving asthma and cough, and dilating the bronchial smooth muscles. It is clinically good for chronic bronchitis, bronchial asthma, etc.

There is also a tablet form with the same name, ingredient and actions.

Aiyeyou Qiwuji

Ingredient:

Oleum Artemisiae Argyi   100% *Aiyeyou*

Actions: Relieving asthma and cough, and removing phlegm.

Indications: Cough, abundant expectoration and dyspnea.

Administration and Dosage: Given by nasal or oral inhalation, 2 or 3 times of inhalation each spray, 3 times of spray a day.

Preparation Foirm: Aerosol.

Package: 14ml (equivalent to 3ml of Olium Artemisiae Argyi) in each bottle.

Notes: This drug has the effects of relaxing the bronchial smooth muscles to remove their spasm, relieving cough, resolving phlegm, restraining bacteria and resisting anaphylaxis. It is clinically efficacious for bronchial asthma, bronchitis and thrush.

There is also a capsule with the same name, ingredient and actions.

Baihua Dingchuan Wan

Ingredients:

Bulbus lilii	7.1%	Baihe
Flos Farfarae	3.7%	Kuandonghua
Gypsum Fibrosum	3.7%	Shigao
Radix Trichosanthis	7.1%	Tianhuafei
Radix Scutellariae	7.1%	Huangqin
Cortex Moutan Radicis	7.1%	Mudanpi
Radix Glehniae	3.7%	Beishashen
Radix Asparagi	7.1%	Tianmendong
Radix Ophiopogonis	7.1%	Maimendong
Fructus Schisandrae	3.7%	Wuweizi
Herba Ephedrae	7.1%	Mahuang
Radix Platycodi	7.1%	Jiegeng
Radix Asteris	7.1%	Ziyuan
Semen Armeniacae Amarum	7.1%	Kuxingren
Radix Peucedani	7.1%	Qianhu
Pericarpium Citri Reticulatae	7.1%	Chenpi
Oleum Menthae	0.01%	Bohebing

Actions: Clearing away heat to relieve cough, resolving phlegm to stop asthma.

Indications: Cough, asthma, and dry throat with thirst, all of which are due to wind–heat.

Administration and dosage: Taken orally, 1 bolus each time, twice a day.

Preparation Form: Honeyed bolus.

Package: 9g in each bolus.

Notes: This prescription is cited from the book, *Cheng Fang*

Qie Yong, compiled by *Wu Yilo* in the *Qing* Dynasty.

The bolus is of great use in relieving asthma and cough, and removing phlegm and is beneficial to bronchitis, pneumonia, pulmonary emphysema, etc.

It is contraindicated for patients with cough or asthma due to common cold.

There is also a tablet with the same name, ingredients and actions.

Gejie Dingchuan Wan

Ingredients:

Gecko	0.4%	*Gejie*
Carapax Trionycis	9%	*Biejia*
Rhizoma Coptidis	5.1%	*Huanglian*
Radix Scutellariae	9%	*Huangqin*
Gypsum Fibrosum	9%	*Shigao*
Radix Ophiopogonis	9%	*Maimendong*
Bulbus Lilii	13.5%	*Baihe*
Radix Asteris	13.5%	*Ziyuan*
Semen Trichosanthis	9%	*Gualouzi*
Fructus Perillae	4.5%	*Zisuzi*
Semen Armeniacae Amarum	9%	*Kuxingren*
Radix Glycyrrhizae	9%	*Gancao*

Actions: Nourishing *Yin*, clearing away lung—heat, and relieving cough and asthma.

Indications: Chronic cough, shortness of breath, fever, spontaneous perspiration, night sweat, fullness and oppression in the chest, and inappetence, all due to consumption.

Administration and Dosage: Taken orall, 1 bolus each time,

twice daily.

Preparation Form: Honeyed bolus.

Package: 9g in each bolus.

Notes: The effects of this bolus are as follows: relieving asthma and cough, restraining bacteria, resisting inflammation, and dilating the bronchial smooth muscles. It is useful for pulmonary tuberculosis, senile bronchial asthma, chronic bronchitis, etc.

Zhisou Dingchuan Wan

Ingredients:

Herba Ephedrae	25%	Mahuang
Semen Armeniacae Amarum	25%	Xingren
Gypsum Fibrosum	25%	Shengshigao
Radix Glycyrrhizae	25%	Gancao

Actions: Moistening the lung, resolving phlegm, and relieving cough and asthma.

Indications: Cough with dyspnea due to wind—heat.

Administration and Dosage: Taken orally, 6g each time, twice daily.

Preparation Form: Water—paste pill.

Package: 18g in each bag.

Notes: This prescription is recorded in the book *Shang Han Lun* written by Zhang Zhongjing in the Han Dynasty.

This drug has the effects of relieving asthma and cough, removing phlegm, and resisting inflammation. It is clinically good for acute bronchitis, asthmatic bronchitis, lobar pneumonia, infantile pneumonia, and measles complicated by pneumonia.

Suzi Jiangqi Wan

Ingredients:

Fructus Perillae	10.6%	Suzi
Rhizoma Pinelliae	10.6%	Fabanxia
Cortex Magnoliae Officinalis	10.6%	Houpo
Radix Peucedani	10.6%	Qianhu
Perocarpium Citri Reticulatae	10.6%	Jupi
Lignum Aquilariae Resinatum	7.4%	Chenxiang
Radix Angelicae Sinensis	7.4%	Danggui
Rhizoma Zingiberis Recens	10.6%	ShengJiang
Fructus Jujubae	10.6%	Hongzao
Radix Glycyrrhizae	11.4%	Gancao

Actions: Relieving asthma, and improving inspiration by invigorating kidney—Qi.

Indications: Cough with dyspnea, fullness in the chest, dizziness, poor appetite, constipation and puffiness of the body.

Administration and Dosage: Taken orally on an empty stomach, 3 to 6g each time, twice a day.

Preparation Form: Water—paste pill.

Package: 18g in each bag.

Notes:

This prescription is quoted from the book *Tai Ping Hui Min He Ji Ju Fang* by *Chen Shiwen* in the *Song* Dynasty.

This drug has the effects of relieving asthma and cough, removing phlegm, restraining bacteria, and resisting inflammation. It is clinically efficacious for bronchial asthma, chronic bronchitis, pulmonary emphysema, etc.

Dingchuan Wan

Ingredients:

Semen Ginkgo	31.3%	Baiguo
Semen Armeniacae Amarum	6.3%	Kuxingren
Flos Farfarae	11.3%	Kuandonghua
Cortex Mori	11.3%	Sangbaipi
Fructus Perillae	7.5%	Heisuzi
Herba Ephedrae	11.3%	Mahuang
Rhizoma Pinelliae	11.3%	Banxia
Radix Scutellariae	6.3%	Huangqin
Radix Glycyrrhizae	3.4%	Gancao

Actions: Relieving asthma and sending down abnormally ascending Qi.

Indications: Chronic cough, asthma due to Qi-insufficiency, feeling of oppression in the chest, shortness of breath, and rale in the larynx.

Administration and Dosage: Taken orally, 2 boluses each time, twice daily.

Preparation Form: Honeyed bolus.

Package: 9g in each bolus.

Notes: The effects of this drug are the following: relieving asthma and cough, dilating bronchus, relaxing bronchial spasm, and improving the function of the lung. It is clinically suitable for pulmonary dysfunction due to various diseases, chronic bronchitis and bronchial asthma.

Tanchuan Wan

Ingredients:

Radix Peucedani	*Qianhu*
Semen Armeniacae Amarum	*Xingren*
Herba Asari	*Xixin*
Folium Mori	*Sangye*
Radix Codonopsis Pilosulae	*Dangshen*
Rhizoma Pinelliae	*Banxia*
Flos Osmanthi	*Guihua*
Bulbus Fritillariae Thunbergii	*Beimu*
Radix Asteris	*Ziyuan*
Fructus Perillae	*Zisuzi*
Exocorpium Citri Reticulatae	*Juhong*
Radix Platycodi	*Jiegeng*
Pumice	*Haifushi*
Flos Inulae	*Xuanfuhua*
Radix Glycyrrhizae	*Gancao*
Radix Polygalae	*Yuanzhi*
Poria	*Fuling*
Flos Farfarae	*Kuandonghua*
Fructus Schisandrae	*Wuweizi*
Gypsum Fibrosum	*Shigao*
Radix Paeoniae Alba	*Baishao*
Rhizoma Cynanchi Stauntonii	*Baiqian*
Rhizoma Belamcandae	*Shegan*
Radix Stemonae	*Baibu*
Radix Scutellariae	*Huangqin*
Semen Lepidii seu Descurainiae	*Tinglizi*
Herba Ephedrae	*Mahuang*
Fructus Aristolochiae	*Madouling*
Fructus Ziziphi	*Dazao*

Bulbus Allii Macrostemi	Xiebai
Indigo Naturalis	Qingdai
Concha Meretricis seu Cyclinae	Haige
Rhizoma Zingiberis Recens	Xianqiang
Folium Eriobotryae	Pipaye

Actions: Expelling wind, removing phlegm, and relieving cough and asthma.

Indications: cough due to lung—heat with abundant expectoration, dyspnea, and fullness and distention in the chest and diaphragm.

Administration and Dosage: Taken orally, 6g each time, twice a day. For children the dosage should be reduced proportionally.

Preparation Form: Water—paste pill.

Package: About 1g in every 5 pills.

Notes: This drug acts as an antiasthmatic, an expectorant and an antipyretic. It is clinically efficacious for cough due to upper respiratory tract infection, bronchial atrophy, bronchitis, bronchial asthma, etc.

Xiaokechuan Tangjiang

Ingredient:

Folium Rhododendri Daurici   100%

Actions: Relieving asthma and cough, and removing phlegm.

Indication: Cough due to common cold, and dyspnea.

Administration and Dosage: Taken orally, 7—10ml each time, 3 times daily. For children the dosage should be reduced properly.

Preparation Form: Syrup.

Package: 100ml in each bottle.

Notes: The effects of this syrup are relieving asthma and cough, and removing phlegm. It is clinically useful for simple chronic bronchitis, cough due to common cold, etc.

There are also other dosage forms with the same name, ingredients and actions, such as enteric—coated pill and capsule.

4　Drugs for Acting on Digestive System

4.1　Drugs for strengthening Stomach and Promoting Digestion

Fuzi Lizhong Wan

Ingredients:

Radix Aconiti Flateralis Preparata	15.4%	*Fuzi*
Radix Codonopsis Pilosulae	30.8%	*Dangshen*
Rhizoma Atractylodis Macrocephalae	23.1%	*Baizhu*
Rhizoma Zingiberis	15.4%	*Ganjiang*
Radix Glycyrrhizae	15.4%	*Gancao*

Actions: Warming the middle—*Jiao* to dispel cold, strengthening the spleen to restore *Yang*.

Indications: Diarrhea with undigested food in stools, abdominal pain with vomiting, and cold limbs, all due to worse insufficiency of spleen—*Yang*.

Administration and Dosage: Taken orally, one bolus, or 6g of water—paste pills each time, 2 to 3 times daily.

Preparation Form: Honeyed bolus and water—paste pill.

Package: 9g in each honeyed bolus; 1g in every 20 Water—paste pills.

Notes: This prescription comes from the book *Tai Ping Hui Min He Ji Ju Fang* by Chen Shiwen in the Song Dynasty.

This drug has the effects of strengthening the stomach, resisting inflammation, and enhancing gastrointestinal functions. Clinically, it is good for acute or chronic gastroenteritis, dyspepsia, postoperative gastrointestinal dysfunction, gastric and duodenal ulcer, acute or chronic dysentery, gastrectasia, gastroptosia, ulcerative colitis, intestinal tuberculosis, and neurasthenia which are all due to insufficiency of spleen—*Yang*.

There is also a tablet form with the same name, ingredients and actions.

Muxiang Shunqi Wan

Ingredients:

Rhizoma Cyperi	7.5%	*Xiangfu*
Radix Linderae	7.5%	*Wuyao*
Pericarpium Citri Reticulatae	7.5%	*Chenpi*
Semen Raphani	7.5%	*Laifuzi*
Fructus Aurantii	7.5%	*Zhiqe*
Poria	7.5%	*Fuling*
Radix Aucklandiae	7.5%	*Muxiang*
Fructus Crataegi	7.5%	*Shanzha*
Fructus Hordei Germinatus	7.5%	*Maiya*
Semen Arecae	5.7%	*Binlang*
Pericarpium Citri Reticulatae Viride	5.7%	*Qingpi*
Radix Glycyrrhizae	5.7%	*Gancao*
Massa Fermentata Medicinalis	7.5%	*Liushenqu*

Actions: Checking upward adverse flow of lung—*Qi* or stomach—*Qi* to promote digestion, relieving epigastric distention to regulate the stomach.

Indications: Stagnation of *Qi*, stuffiness in the chest, abdominal distension with pain in the abdomen, anorexia, dyschesia, and constipation.

Administration and Dosage: Taken orally, 3 to 6g each time, 2 to 3 times daily.

Preparation Form: Water-paste pill.

Package: 1g in every 20 pills.

Notes: This prescription is quoted from the book *Shen Shi Zun Sheng Shu* written by Shen Jinao in the Qing Dynasty.

The action of this pill is to strengthen the stomach, protect the liver, and regulate gastrointestinal functions. It is useful in clinical treatment of chronic gastritis, chronic enteritis, chronic hepatitis, early hepatocirrhosis, and dyspepsia which are all due to stagnation of *Qi*.

There is also a tablet from with the same name, ingredients and actions.

Kaixiong Shunqi Wan

Ingredients:

Semen Arecae	24.5%	*Binlang*
Semen Pharbitidis	32.7%	*Qianniuzi*
Pericarpium Citri Reticulatae	8.2%	*Chenpi*
Cortex Magnoliae Officinalis	8.2%	*Houpu*
Radix Aucklandiae	6.1%	*Muxiang*
Rhizoma Sparganii	8.2%	*Sanleng*
Fructus Gleditsiae Abnormalis	4.1%	*Zhuyazao*
Rhizoma Zedoariae	8.2%	*Ezhu*

Actions: Removing stagnation of *Qi* to help digestion, and promoting circulation of *Qi* to relieve pain.

Indications: Fluid and food retention, stagnation of *Qi*, fullness in the chest and hypochondrium, and stomachache.

Administration and Dosage: Taken orally, 3 to 9g each time, once or twice daily.

Preparation Form: Water—paste pill.

Package: 1g in every 20 pills.

Notes: This prescription originates from the book, *Sou Shi Bao Yuan* written by Gong Tingxian in the Ming Dynasty.

This drug can strengthen the stomach to regulate gastrointestinal functions. It is clinically applied to the treatment of chronic gastritis, chronic enteritis, chronic hepatitis, etc.

It is contraindicated for pregnant women and those who are infirm with age.

There is also a tablet form with the same name, ingredients and actions.

Xiangsha Liujun Wan

Ingredients:

Radix Aucklandiae	7.8%	*Muxiang*
Fructus Amoni	8.9%	*Sharen*
Radix Codonopsis Pilosulae	11.1%	*Dangshen*
Poria	22.2%	*Fuling*
Rhizoma Atractylodis Macrocephalae	22.2%	*Baizhu*
Pericarpium Citri Reticulatae	8.9%	*Chenpi*
Rhizoma Pinelliae	11.1%	*Banxia*
Radix Glycyrrhizae	7.8%	*Gancao*

Actions: Invigorating the spleen, improving the flow of *Qi*, eliminating flatulence and regulating the stomach.

Indications: Fullness in the epigastric region, anorexia, loose stools, eructation and vomiting, all of which are due to insufficiency of the spleen and stomach—*Qi*.

Administration and Dosage: Taken orally, 6 to 9g each time, 2 to 3 times daily.

Preparation Form: Water–paste pill.

Package: 1g in every 20 pills.

Notes: This prescription is cited from the book, *Tai Ping Hui Min He Ji Ju Fang* compiled by Chen Shiwen in the Song Dynasty.

The effects of this drug are as follows: Strengthening the stomach, reducing inflammation, stopping vomiting and regulating gastrointestinal functions. It is clinically efficacious for gastric ulcer, duodenal ulcer, gastrectasia, chronic gastritis, chronic disarrhea, gastrointestinal dysfunction, neurasthenia, and common cold of gastrointestinal type, which are all due to deficiency of *Qi*.

There are also other dosage forms with the same name, ingredients and actions, such as tablet and mixture.

Dashanzha Wan

Ingredients:

Fructus Crataegi	77.0%	*Shanzha*
Fructus Hordei Germinatus	11.5%	*Maiya*
Massa Fermentata Medicinalis	11.5%	*Liushenqu*

Actions: Eliminating undigested food, and strengthening and regulating the stomach.

Indications: Indigestion, and fullness in the epigastric region.

Administration and Dosage: Taken orally, 1 to 2 boluses each time, 1 to 3 times daily. For children, the dosage should be decreased by half.

Preparation Form: Honeyed bolus.

Package: 9g in each bolus.

Notes: This drug has the effects of strengthening the stomach to promote digestion. It is clinically used to treat simple dyspepsia, gastrointestinal dysfunction, etc.

It is not to be taken along with sodium bicarbonate, aluminum hydroxide, gastropine or aminophylline.

There is also a granule or powder preparation form with the same name, ingredients and actions, which is to be dissolved in boiling water before administration.

Pingwei Wan

Ingredients:

Rhizoma Atractylodis	29.6%	*Cangzhu*
Radix Glycyrrhizae	11.1%	*Gancao*
Cortex Magnoliae Officinalis	18.5%	*Houpu*
Pericarpium Citri Reticulatae	11.1%	*Chenpi*
Massa Fermentata Medicinalis	29.6%	*Liushenqu*

Actions: Eliminating dampness, invigorating the spleen, promoting circulation of *Qi*, and regulating the stomach.

Indications: Fullness in the epigastric region, nausea, vomiting, and loose stools, all due to incoordination between the spleen and stomach.

Administration and Dosage: Taken orally, 6g each time, twice a day.

Preparation Form: Water—paste pill.

Package: 1g in every 20 pills.

Notes: This prescription comes from the book *Tai Ping Hui Min He Ji Ju Fang* compiled by Chen Shiwen in the Song Dynasty.

The pill of this kind has the effect of strengthening the stomach and gastrointestinal functions. It is clinically effective for hyperhydrochloria, chronic gastritis, gastroatonia, gastroptosis, gastrointestinal neurosis, acute gastritis, bronchial asthma, etc.

It is reported that this drug can be used for treating sore in subrostral lip, inguinal inflammation and cholera.

There is also a tablet form with the same name, ingredients and actions.

Renshen Jianpi Wan

Ingredients:

Radix Ginseng	13.3%	Renshen
Fructus Crataegi	10%	Shanzha
Fructus Hordei Germinatus	13.3%	Maiya
Massa Fermentata Medicinalis	16.8%	Liushenqu
Rhizoma Atractylodis Macrocephalae	13.3%	Baizhu
Pericarpium Citri Reticulatae	13.3%	Chenpi
Fructus Aurantii Immaturus	20%	Zhishi
(fried with bran)	20%	

Actions: Invigorating Qi to strengthen the spleen, and regulating the flow of Qi to promote digestion.

Indications: Dyspepsia, stuffiness in the chest, dyspnea, hypodynamia, borborygmus, abdominal distension, loose stools, all due to the weakness of the spleen and stomach.

Administration and Dosage: Taken orally, 4g of water—paste pill or one bolus of honeyed bolus each time, 2 to 3 times a day.

Preparation Form: Water—paste pill and honeyed bolus.

Package: 1g in every 20 pills, 6g in each bolus.

Notes: This prescription is found in the book, *Yi Fang Ji Jie* compiled by Wang Ang in the Qing Dynasty.

The effect of the drug is strengthening the stomach to regulate gastrointestinal functions. It is clinically efficacious for chronic gastroenteritis, chronic hepatitis, intestinal dysfunction, intestinal tuberculosis, which are all due to spleen deficiency.

Xiangsha Yangwei Wan

Ingredients:

Rhizoma Cyperi	7.6%	*Xiangfu*
Radix Glycyrrhizae	3.2%	*Gancao*
Herba Agastachis	7.6%	*Huoxiang*
Fructus Aurantii Immaturus	7.6%	*Zhishi*
Rhizoma Atractylodis Macrocephalae	10.9%	*Baizhu*
Pericarpium Citri Reticulatae	10.9%	*Chenpi*
Rhizoma Pinelliae	10.9%	*Banxia*
Poria	10.9%	*Fuling*
Radix Aucklandiae	7.6%	*Muxiang*
Fructus Amomi	7.6%	*Sharen*
Fructus Amomi Rotundus	7.6%	*Doukou*
Cortex Magnoliae Officinalis	7.6%	*Houpu*

Actions: Invigorating the spleen, nourishing the stomach, and regulating the flow of *Qi* to resolve dampness and alleviate stagnation in the middle—*Jiao*.

Indications: Fullness in the hypochondriac, stomachache, vomiting, gastric discomfort with acid regurgitation, sallow complexion, and lassitude of limbs, which are all due to the weakness of the spleen and stomach.

Administration and Dosage: Taken orally, 9g in each time, twice a day.

Preparation Form: Water—paste pill.

Package: 3g in every 50 pills.

Notes: This prescription is found in the book *Shou Shi Bao Yuan* compiled by Gong Tingxian in the Ming Dynasty.

This drug has the following effects: strengthening the stomach, reducing inflammation and relieving pain. It is clinically efficacious for chronic gastritis and duodenal ulcer and may act as an adjuvant used to treat chronic hepatitis.

There are also other dosage forms with the same name, ingredients and actions, such as tablet, granule or powder which is to be dissolved in boiling water before administration.

Sijunzi Wan

Ingredients:

Radis Codonopsis Pilosulae	28.6%	*Dangshen*
Poria	28.6%	*Fuling*
Radix Glycyrrhizae	14.2%	*Gancao*
Rhizoma Atractylodis Macrocephalae	28.6%	*Baizhu*

Actions: Invigorating *Qi, streng thening* the spleen, and nourishing the stomach.

Indications: Anorexia and loose stools due to deficiency of *Qi* of the spleen and stomach.

Administration and Dosage: Taken orally, 3 to 6g each time, 3 times a day.

Preparation Form: Vater—paste pill.

Package: 3g in every 50 pills.

Notes: This prescription is cited from the book *Tai Ping Hui Min He Ji Ju Fang* written by Chen Shiwen in the Song Dynasty.

This drug has the effects of strengthening the stomach, promoting digestion, and enhancing immunologic function the body. It is clinically useful for chronic gastroenteritis, gastroatonia, gastroptosia, anaemia and other chronically—wasting diseases, which are all due to deficiency of *Qi* of the spleen and the stomach.

There are also other dosage forms with the same name, ingredients and actions, such as mixture, granule or powder, which is to be dissolved in boiling water before administration.

Liuhe Dingzhong Wan

Ingredients:

Herba Pogostemonis	1.5%	*Guanghuoxiang*
Folium Perillae	1.5%	*Zisuye*
Herba Elsholtziae	1.5%	*Xiangru*
Radix Aucklandiae	3.3%	*Muxiang*
Lignum Santali	3.3%	*Tanxiang*
Cortex Magnoliae Officinalis	4.4%	*Houpu*
Fructus Aurantii	4.4%	*Zhique*
Pericarpium Citri Reticulatae	4.4%	*Chenpi*
Radix Platycodi	4.4%	*Jiegeng*
Radix Glycyrrhizae	4.4%	*Gancao*
Poria	4.4%	*Fuling*
Fructus Chaenomelis	4.4%	*Mugua*
Semen Lablab Album	1.5%	*Baibiandou*
Fructus Crataegi	4.4%	*Shanzha*
Massa Fermentata Medicinalis	17.4%	*Liushenqu*
Fructus Hordei Germinatus	17.4%	*Maiya*
Fructus Glycinae maxae Germinatus	17.4%	*DadouHuangjuan*

Actions: Eliminating summer—heat and dampness, regulating the stomach and promoting digestion.

Indications: Indigestion, fever with chills, headache, oppressed feeling in the chest, nausea, vomiting, diarrhea, abdominal pain, all of which are due to summer—heat and dampness.

Administration and Dosage: Taken orally, 3 to 6g each time, 2 to 3 times a day.

Preparation Form: Water—paste pill or honeyed bolus.

Package: 3g in every 50 pills; 6g in each bolus.

Notes: This prescription originates from the book *Gu Jin Yi Fang Ji Cheng*.

The effects of this drug are strengthening the stomach, preventing or arresting vomiting, and relieving summer—heat. It is clinically indicated for common cold of gastrointestinal type, epidemic diarrhea, acute gastroenteritis in summer, etc.

Compared with this drug, *Huoxiang Zhengqi Shui* is more suitable for the patients with severer vomiting, diarrhea and abdominal pain due to serious summer—heat and dampness.

Qipi Wan

Ingredients:

Radix Ginseng	12%	Renshen
Poria	12%	Fuling
Rhizoma Atractylodis Macrocephalae	12%	*Baizhu*
Radix Glycyrrhizae	6%	*Gancao*
Semen Nelumbinis	12%	*Lianzi*
Pericarpium Citri Reticulatae	6%	*Chenpi*
Fructus Crataegi	6%	*Shanzha*
Rhizoma Dioscoreae	12%	*Shanyao*

Fructus Hordei Germinatus   6%   *Maiya*

Rhizoma Alismatis   6%   *Zexie*

Massa Fermentata Medicinalis   10%   *Liushenqu*

Actions: Strengthening the spleen and stomach, promoting digestion and arresting diarrhea.

Indications: Abdominal pain and distension, vomiting and diarrhea, all due to the weakness of the spleen and stomach.

Administration and Dosage: Taken orally, 1 bolus each time, 2 to 3 times a day. For children, the dosage should be reduced appropriately.

Preparation Form: Honeyed bolus.

Package: 3g in each bolus.

Notes: This prescription is seen in the book *Yi Xue Ru Men* Written by *Li Chan* in the Ming Dynasty.

The bolus of this kind produces the effects of strengthening the stomach, promoting digestion and enhancing gastrointestinal functions. It is clinically efficacious for chronic gastroenteritis, chronic diarrhea, dyspepsia and other chronically—wasting diseases.

There is also a tablet form with the same name, ingredients and actions.

Xiangsha Zhizhu Wan

Ingredients:

Radix Aucklandiae   16.7%   *Muxiang*

Fructus Amomi   16.7%   *Sharen*

Fructus Aurantii Immaturus   16.7%   *Zhishi*

Rhizoma Atractylodis Macrocephalae   50%   *Baizhu*

Actions: Strengthening the stomach, enlivening the spleen,

regulating the flow of *Qi* and soothing the chest oppression.

Indications: Dyspepsia, stagnation of *Qi,* fullness and distension in the epigastric region, vomiting, nausea, and acid regurgitation, all due to insufficiency of the spleen.

Administration and Dosage: Taken orally, 9g each time, once or twice a day.

Preparation Form: Water—paste pill.

Package: 1g in every 20 pills.

Notes: This drug has the effect of strengthening the stomach to regulate gastrointestinal functions. It can be used to treat dyspepsia, gastroptosia and chronic gastritis of children and those infirm with age.

Yueju Wan

Ingredients:

Rhizoma Cyperi	20%	*Xiangfu*
Rhizoma Chuanxiong	20%	*Chuanxiong*
Fructus Gardeniae	20%	*Zhizi*
Rhizoma Atractylodis	20%	*Cangzhu*
Massa Fermentata Medicinalis	20%	*Liushenqu*

Actions:

Regulating the flow of *Qi* to alleviate mental depression and relieving epigastric distension and fullness.

Indications: Stagnation of *Qi,* blood, phlegm, fire, dampness and food, stuffiness in the chest and stomach, eructation, acid regurgitation, and vomiting.

Administration and Dosage: Taken orally, 6 to 9g each time, twice a day.

Preparation Form: Water—paste pill.

Package: 3g in every 50 pills.

Notes: This prescription is cited from the book *Dan Xi Xin Fa* written by Zhu Zhenheng in the Yuan Dynasty.

The effect of the drug is to strengthen the stomach and regulate gastrointestinal functions. It is clinically efficacious for such gastrointestinal diseases as dyspepsia, gastic retention and gastrointestinal neurosis, and such excess syndromes as chronic hepatitis, cholecystitis, dysmenorrhea and mental depression.

Caution is needed when it is used to treat debilitic patients.

Baohe Wan

Ingredients:

Fructus Crataegi	37.3%	*Shanzha*
Massa Fermentata Medicinalis	12.5%	*Liushenqu*
Rhizoma Pinelliae	12.5%	*Banxia*
Poria	12.5%	*Fuling*
Pericarpium Citri Reticulatae	6.3%	*Chenpi*
Fructus Forsythiae	6.3%	*Lianqao*
Semen Raphani	6.3%	*Laifuzi*
Fructus Hordei Germinatus	6.3%	*Maiya*

Actions: Promoting digestion, removing stagnancy and regulating the stomach.

Indications: Indigestion, fullness and distension in the epigastric region, eructation, anorexia, vomiting and diarrhea.

Administration and Dosage: Taken orally, 6 to 9g each time, twice a day. Appropriate reduction of the dosage should be done for children patients.

Preparation Form: Water—paste pill.

Package: 3g in every 50 pill.s

Notes:

This prescription is from the book *Dan Xi Xin Fa* written by Zhu Zhenheng in the Yuan Dynasty.

This drug has the effects of strengthening the stomach and promoting digestion. It is clinically efficacious for dyspepsia, chronic gastritis, acute gastroenteritis, etc.

The pill of this kind is remarkable effective for infantile cough occurring at night with abundant expectoration, which is accompanied by anorexia and abdominal distension.

There is also a tablet form with the same name, ingredients and actions.

Chenxiang Huaqi Wan

Ingredients:

Lignum Aquilariae Resinatum	3.8%	*Chenxiang*
Radix Aucklandiae	7.4%	*Muxiang*
Herba Pogostemonis	14.8%	*Guanghuoxiang*
Rhizoma Cyperi	7.4%	*Xiangfu*
Fructus Amomi	7.4%	*Sharen*
Pericarpium Citri Reticulatae	7.4%	*Chenpi*
Rhizoma Zedoariae	14.8%	*Ezhu*
Massa Fermentata Medicinali	14.8%	*Liushenqu*
Fructus Hordei Germinatus	14.8%	*Maiya*
Radix Glycyrrhizae	7.4%	*Gancao*

Actions: Relieving the depressed liver, removing stagnated food and regulating the stomach.

Indications: Distending pain in the epigastric region, fullness in the chest and diaphragm, inappetence, eructation and acid regurgitation, all due to stagnation of stomach—*Qi* and spleen—*Qi*.

Administration and Dosage: Taken orally, 3 to 6g each time, twice a day.

Preparation Form: Water—paste pill.

Package: 3g in every 50 pills.

Notes: This drug has the actions of regulatinggastrointestinal functions and strengthening the stomech. It is clinically effective for gastrointestinal dysfunction and indigestion both due to *Qi* stagnation.

There is also a tablet form with the same name, ingredients and actions.

Zuojin Wan

Ingredients:

Rhizoma Coptidis	85.7%	*Huanglian*
Fructus Evodiae	14.3%	*Wuzhuyu*

Actions: Purging fire to disperse depressed liver—*Qi* and reg-. ulating the stomach to check the adverse flow of *Qi*.

Indications: Distending pain in the chest, vomiting, acid regurgitation, bitter taste, epigastric upset, and diarrhea due to heat, all of which result from the hyperactive liver—fire attacking the stomach.

Administration and Dosage: Taken orally, 3 to 6g each time, twice a day.

Preparation Form: Water—paste pill.

Package: 3g in every 50 pills.

Notes: This prescription comes from the book *Dan Xi Xin Fa* Written by Zhu Zhenheng in the Yuan Dynasty.

This pill has the actions of antibiosis, anti—inflammation.

antiacid and antiemetic. It may be used in clinic for treating acute and chronic gastritis, hyperhydrochloria, gastric and duodenal ulcer, bacillary dysentery, peritonitis, etc.

Jiuqi Niantong Wan

Ingredients:

Rhizoma Cyperi	13.8%	*Xiangfu*
Radix Aucklandiae	3.5%	*Muxiang*
Rhizoma Alpiniae Officinarum	3.5%	*Gaoliangjiang*
Pericarpium Citri Reticulatae	6.9%	*Chenpi*
Rhizoma Zedoariae	27.4%	*Ezhu*
Radix Curcumae	6.9%	*Yujin*
Rhizoma Corydalis	13.8%	*Yanhusuo*
Semen Arecae	6.9%	*Binlang*
Faeces Trogopterori	13.8%	*Wulingzhi*
Radix Glycyrrhizae	3.5%	*Gancao*

Actions: Regulating the flow of *Qi*, promoting blood circulation cand alleviating pain.

Indications: Distending pain in the chest, hypochondriac and epigastric region, vomiting with acid regurgitation and dysmenorrhea.

Administration and Dosage: Taken orally, 6 to 9g each time, twice daily.

Preparation Form: Water—paste pill.

Package: 1g in every 20 pills.

Notes: This prescription is from the book *Lu Fu Jin Fang* compiled by Gong Tingxian in the Ming Dynasty.

This drug has the effects of regulating gastrointestinal functions, reducing inflammation and relieving pain. It is clinically good for such conditions due to stagnation of cold and *Qi* as chronic gastritis, acute gastroenteritis, chronic hepatitis and dysmenorrhea.

It is constraindicated for pregnant women.

Qingwei Baoan Wan

Ingredients:

Rhizoma Atractylodis Macrocephalae	5.6%	*Baizhu*
Pericarpium Citri Reticulatae	5.6%	*Chenpi*
Mass a Fermentata Medicinalis	5.6%	*Liushenqu*
Fructus Hordei Germinatus	5.6%	*Maiya*
Pericarpium Citri Reticulatae Viride	5.6%	*Qingpi*
Poria	5.6%	*Fuling*
Fructus Aurantii	5.6%	*Zhique*
Radix Glycyrrhizae	5.6%	*Gancao*
Fructus Aurantii Immaturus	5.6%	*Zhishi*
Fructus Amomi	5.6%	*Sharen*
Cortex Magnoliae Officinalis	5.6%	*Houpu*
Semen Arecae	5.6%	*Binlang*
distillers Yeast	11%	*Jiuqu*
Fructus Crataegi	22%	*Shanzha*

Actions: Strengthening the spleen, regulating the stomach, promoting digestion and removing food stagnancy.

Indications: Dyspepsia and fullness in the epigastric region.

Administration and Dosage: Taken orally, 1 bolus each time, twice a day. For Children under one year, 1 / 3 to 1 / 2 bolus is given each time, twice a day.

Preparation Form: Honeyed bolus.

Package: 3g in each bolus.

Notes: This drug has the effect of strengthening the stomach to promote digestion, and is clinically useful for simple dyspepsia, chronic gastroenteritis, etc.

Chenxiang Huazhi Wan

Ingredients:

Lignum Aquilariae Resinatum	8.8%	Chenxiang
Rhizoma Cyperi	70.6%	Xiangfu
Fructus Amomi	8.8%	Sharen
Radix Glycyrrhizae	11.8%	Gancao

Actions: Regulating the flow of Qi, removing food stagnancy, promoting digestion and invigorating the spleen.

Indications: Fullness in the chest, stagnation of Qi and abdominal pain.

Administration and Dosage: Taken orally, 6g each time, twice daily.

Preparation Form: Water-paste pill.

Package: 3g in every 50 pills.

Notes: This prescription originates from the book *Wan Bing Hui Chun* compiled by Gong Tingxian in the Ming Dynasty.

The effect of this drug is regulating gastrointestinal functions to strengthen the stomach. It is indicated clinically for chronic gastritis, chronic hepatitis and gastrointestinal neurosis, which are all due to stagnation of Qi.

Wuji Wan

Ingredients:

Rhizoma Coptidis	46.2%	Huanglian
Radix Paeoniae Alba	46.2%	Baishao

Fructus Evodiae   7.6%   *Wuzhuyu*

Actions: Purging Liver—fire and regulating the stomach and spleen.

Indications: Such ailments caused by incoordination between the liver and spleen as stomachache, acid regurgitation, abdominal pain and diarrhea, and infantile malnutrition as well.

Administration and Dosage: Taken orally, 3 to 6g each time, twice a day.

Preparation Form: Water—paste pill.

Package: 1g in every 20 pills.

Notes: This prescription is seen in the book *Tai Ping Hui Min He Ji Ju Fang* compiled by Chen Shiwen in the Song Dynasty.

This drug has the effects of resisting bacteria, reducing inflammation, strengthening the stomach and arresting diarrhea. It is clinically efficacious for gastritis, acute gastroenteritis, dysentery and infantile lientery, which are all due to incoordination between the liver and spleen.

Dutong Wan

Ingredients:

Fructus Amomi Rotundus (Without shell)	8.5%	*Doukou*
Rhizoma Zingiberis	16.9%	*Ganjiang*
Fructus Amomi	8.5%	*Sharen*
Fructus Piperis Longi	3.4%	*Biba*
Cortex Magnoliae Officinalis	8.5%	*Houpu*
Pericarpium Papaveris	3.4%	*Yingsuke*
Cortex Cinnamomi	8.5%	*Rougui*
Fructus Aurantii Immaturus	16.9%	*Zhishi*

| Radix Aucklandiae | 16.9% | *Muxiang* |
| Radix Linderae | 8.5% | *Wuyao* |

Actions: Warming the middle—*Jiao* to dispel cold, regulating the flow of *Qi* and all eviating pain.

Indications: Cold—pain in the abdomen, fullness in the chest and hypochondriac region, vomiting and acid regurgitation, which are all due to stagnation of *Qi* and cold.

Administration and Dosage: Taken orally, 3g each time, twice a day.

Preparation Form: Water—paste pill.

Package: 1g in every 20 pills.

Notes: This drug is considered as a stomachic, an antiacid or an analgesic. It is clinically suitable for chronic gastritis, atrophic gastritis or enterospasm, which are all due to insufficiency of the spleen—*Yang*.

Xiaobanxia Heji

Ingredients:

| Rhizoma Pinelliae | 62.5% | *Banxia* |
| Rhizoma Zingiberis Recens | 37.5% | *Shengjiang* |

Actions: Preventing or arresting vomiting, lowering the adverse flow of *Qi*.

Indications: Adverse rising of stomach—*Qi*, nausea and vomiting.

Administration and Dosage: Taken orally, 10 to 15ml each time, 3 times a day.

Preparation From: Mixture.

Package: Every bottle contains 100ml.

Notes: This drug has the effects of regulating vegetative

nerve function and strengthening the stomach. It is clinically efficacious for chronic gastroenteritis and vomiting during pregnancy.

4.2 Drugs for Treating Gastric Ulcer

Anwei Pian

Ingredients:

Rhizoma Corydalis	12.6%	Yanhusuo
Alumen	50%	Baifan
Os Sepiae	37.4%	Haipiaoxiao

Actions: Strengthening the spleen and stomach and warming the middle—Jiao to alleviate pain.

Indications: Distension and pain in the epigastric region, erucatation, acid regurgitation, nausea and vomiting or loose stools.

Administration and Dosage: Taken orally, 5 to 7 tablets each time, 3 to 4 times a day.

Preparation Form: Tablet.

Package: 0.6g in each tablet.

Notes: This drug has the effects of relieving hyperacidity, stopping pain and healing ulcer. It is clinically good for gastric or duodenal ulcer, chronic gastritis, hyperhydrochloria, etc.

Liangfu Wan

Ingredients:

Rhizoma Alpiniae Officinarum	50%	Gaoliangjiang
Rhizoma Cyperi	50%	Xiangfu

Actions: Warming the middle—*Jiao* to regulate the stomach, and regulating the flow of *Qi* to alleviate pain.

Indications: Cold stomachache and oppressed feeling in the chest, both of which are caused by stagnation of liver—*Qi* and relieved by warming and pressing.

Administration and Dosage: Taken orally, 3 to 6g each time, twice a day.

Preparation Form: Water—paste pill.

Package: 1g in each 20 pills.

Notes: The prescription is from the book *Liang Fang Ji Ye*.

This drug has the effects of antiinflammation and analgesia. It is clinically useful for chronic gastritis, gastric ulcer, duodenal buld ulcer, chronic hepatitis, gastric neurosis, intercostal neuralgia, dysmenorrhea, etc, which are all due to stagancy of liver—*Qi* and deficiency—cold of the spleen and stomach.

Yuanhu Zhitong Pian

Ingredients:

Rhizoma Corydalis	66.6%	*Yanhusuo*
Radix Angelicae Dahuricae	33.3%	*Baizhi*

Actions: Promoting blood circulation to remove blood stasis, and regulating the flow of *Qi* to alleviate pain.

Indications: Epigastric and hypochondriac distending—pain, headache and dysmenorrhea, which are all due to stagnation of *Qi* and blood.

Administration and Dosage: Taken orally, 4 to 6 tablets each time, 3 times a day.

Preparation Form: Suger—coated tablet.

Package: 0.35g in each tablet.

Notes: This drug has the effects of anti—inflammation and analgesia. Clinically it is suitable for acute and chronic gastritis, enteritis, gastric ulcer, dysmenorrhea, headache, etc., which are all due to stagnancy of *Qi* and blood.

Xiaojianzhong Heji

Ingredients:

Saccharum Granorum	38.3%	*Yitang*
Ramulus Cinnamomi	11.1%	*Guizhi*
Radix Paeoniae Alba	22.2%	*Baishao*
Radix Glycyrrhizae	7.4%	*Gancao*
Rhizoma Zingiberis Recens	11.1%	*Shengjiang*
Fructus Ziziphi Jujubae	11.1%	*Dazao*

Actions: Warming the middle—*Jiao* to nourish deficiency and relieve spasm and pain.

Indications: Distending pain in the epigastric region which is relieved by warming and pressing, gastric discomfort with acid regurgitation, anorexia and palpitation, all due to insufficiency and cold of the spleen—*Yang*.

Administration and Dosage: Taken orally after the bottle is shaken, 20 to 30ml each time, 3 times a day.

Preparation Form: Mixture.

Package: 100ml in each bottle.

Notes: This prescription is found in the book *Shang Han Lun* written by Zhang Zhongjing in the Han Dynasty.

The mixture can strengthen the stomach, inhibit acidity and protect gastrointestinal mucosa. It is clinically beneficial not only to gastric ulcer, duodenal ulcer and enterospasm all of which are due to deficiency—cold of the spleen—*Yang* but also to chronic hepatitis, chronic peritonitis, rhinitis, epistaxis, pulmonary emphysema, prostatomegaly, neurosis, aplastic anemia, etc.

Huangqi Jianzhong Wan

Ingredients:

Radix Astragali	36.4%	Huangqi
Cortex Cinnamomi	18.2%	Rougui
Radix Paeoniae Alba	36.4%	Baishao
Radix Glycyrrhizae	9.0%	Gancao

Invigorating Qi to expell cold, strengthening the stomach to regulate the middle—Jiao.

Indications: Distending pain in the epigastric region which is relieved by warming and pressing, spontaneous perspiration, night sweat and lassitude of limbs, all of which are caused by insufficiency of the spleen—Yang.

Administration and Dosage: Taken orally, 1 bolus each time, 2 to 3 times daily.

Preparation Form: Honeyed bolus

Package: 9g in each bolus.

Notes: This prescription is found in the book Jin Kui Yao Lue Fang Lun by Zhang Zhongjing in the Han Dynasty.

This drug is for resisting inflammation and healing ulcer. It is clinically efficacious for gastric or duodenal ulcer due to insufficieney of the spleen—Yang, cold abscess, chronic hepatitis, chronic peritonitis, neurosism, vegetative nerve functional disturbance, etc.

Hougujun Pian

Ingredient:

Hericium erinaceus   100%   *Hougujun*

Actions: Strengthening the spleen and stomach, regulating *Qi* by alleviation of mental depression and relieving pain.

Indications: Stomachache, fullness in the epigastric region, vomiting, gastric discomfort with acid regurgitation and eructation.

Administration and Dosage: Taken orally, 3 to 4 tablets each time, 3 times a day.

Preparation Form: Sugar—coated tablet.

Package: 0.25g in each tablet.

Notes: This drug has the effects of relieving hyperacidity, alleviating pain and enhancing body immunologic function. It is indicated for gastric or duodenal ulcer, atrophic gastritis and chronic gastritis. It can be used as an accessory drug to treat malignant tumors of the digestive tract such as carcinoma of stomach or esophagus.

It is reported that polysaccharose contained in *Hougujun* Hericium Erinaceus possesses remarkable inhibition of tumor cells, and can enhance cellular immune function, shrink tumor and prolong life.

Weiteling Pian

Main Ingredients:

Rhizoma Corydalis   *Yanhusuo*

Alumen   Baifan

Actions: Warming the middle—*Jiao* to regulate the stomach, relieving flatulence and alleviating pain.

Indications: Fullness in the epigastric region, gastric discomfort with acid regurgitation, nausea, vomiting and inappetence.

Administration and Dosage: Taken orally, 4 to 6 tablets each time, 3 times a day.

Preparation Form: Sugar—coated tablet.

Package: 0.25g in each tablet.

Notes: This drug produces the effects of relieving hyperacidity and relieving pain. It is clinically good for gastric or duodenal ulcer and chronic gastritis.

4.3 Slow—acting Purgative Drugs

Sixiao Wan

Ingredients:

Radix et Rhizoma Rhei	22.2%	*Dahuang*
Fructus Gleditsiae Abnormalis	3.7%	*Zhuyazao*
Semen Pharbitidis	14.8%	*Qianniuzi*
Semen Arecae	14.8%	*Binglang*
Rhizoma Cyperi	14.8%	*Xiangfu*
Semen Pharbitidis	14.8%	*Qianniuzi*
Faeces Trogopterori	14.8%	*Wulingzhi*

Actions: Eliminating excessive fluid to remove phlegm, promoting *Qi* circulation to help digestion, removing stagnancy and relaxing the bowels.

Indications: Stuffiness in the epigastric region, abdominal distension and constipation due to stagnation of *Qi* and accumulation of phlegm and fluid.

Administration and Dosage: Taken orally, 1.5 to 3g each time, twice a day.

Preparation Form: Water—paste pill.

Package: 1g in every 20 pills.

Notes: The pill of this kind has the effects of spasmolysis, analgesia and laxation. It is clinically efficacious for excess syndrome with constipation such as acute gastroenteritis, gastrointestinal spasm, pyloric obstruction and intestinal obstruction.

It is contraindicated for pregnant women.

Binglang Sixiao Wan

Ingredients:

Semen Arecae	13.8%	Binglang
Semen Pharbitidis	27.6%	Qianniuzi
Rhizoma Cyperi	13.8%	Xiangfu
Fructus Gledisiae Abnormalis	3.4%	Zhuyazao
Faeces Trogopterori	13.8%	Wulingzhi
Radix et Rhizoman Rhei	27.6%	Dahuang

Actions: Promoting digestion, removing stagnated food, and inducing diuresis to relieve flatulance.

Indications: Retention of indigested food and fluid with gastric discomfort and acid regurgitation, vomiting, nausea and constipation, all due to stagnation of Qi and accumulation of phlegm.

Administration and Dosage: Taken orally, 9g honeyed bolus each time or 6g water—paste pills each time, 2 to 3 times a day.

Preparation Form: Honeyed bolus and water—paste pill.

Package: 9g in each honeyed bolus and 1g in every 20 water—paste pills.

Notes: This prescription is from the book Gu Jin Yi Fang Ji Cheng compiled by Jiang Tingxi in the Qing Dynasty.

The effect of the drug is to strengthen the stomach and help purgation. It is suitable for excess syndrome such as dyspepsia, constipation, etc.

It should be used with caution for weak persons.

Qingning Wan

Ingredients:

Radix et Rhizoma Rhei	64.5%	Dahuang
Semen Phaseoli Radiati	2.7%	Ludou
Herba Plantaginis	2.7%	Cheqiancao
Rhizoma Atractylodis Macrocephalae	2.7%	Baizhu
Glycine Max	2.7%	Heidou
Rhizoma Pinelliae	2.7%	Banxia
Rhizoma Cyperi	2.7%	Xiangfu
Folium Mori	2.7%	Sangye
Ramulus Persicae	0.4%	Taozhi
Milk	5.4%	Niuru
Cortex Magnoliae Officinalis	2.7%	Houpo
Fructus Hordei Germinatus	2.7%	Maiya
Pericarpium Citri Reticulatae	2.7%	Chenpi
Cacumen Biotae	2.7%	Cebaiye

Actions: Purging gastrointestinal heat to remove stagnancy.

Indications: Indigestion, fullness in the epigastric region and hypochondrium, swelling and pain in the throat, aphthae, boil of the tongue, conjunctival congestion, toothache and constipation.

Administration and Dosage: Taken Orally, 1 bolus each time, once or twice daily.

Preparation Form: Honeyed bolus.

Package: 9g in each bolus.

Notes: This Prescription is quoted from the book *Yin Hai*

Zhi Nan compiled in the Qing Dynasty.

This drug is used as an antiseptic, an antiphlogistic or a purgative. It is clinically efficacious for acute periodontitis, acute conjunctivitis, constipation, etc.

It is contraindicated for pregnant women.

Lanji Wan

Ingredients:

Rhizoma Sparganii	3.8%	*Sanleng*
Semen Arecae	3.8%	*Binglang*
Fructus Aurantii Immaturus	11.4%	*Zhishi*
Pericarpium Citri Reticulatae Viride	7.6%	*Qingpi*
Fructus Crataegi	11.4%	*Shanzha*
Semen Pharbitidis	19%	*Qianniuzi*
Radix et Rhizoma Rhei	19%	*Dahuang*
Pericarpium Citri Reticulatae	11.4%	*Chenpi*
Rhizoma Zedoariae	11.4%	*Ezhu*
Semen Oryaecum Monasco	2.5%	*Hongqu*
Talcum	2.5%	*Huashi*

Actions: Promoting digestion to remove indigested food, relieving flatulence to relax the bowels.

Indications: Retention of food, oppressed—feeling and fullness in the chest, abdominal pain, acid regurgitation, and constipation.

Administration and Dosage: Taken orally by children, 30 pills each time, twice a day; by adults, more pills, each time.

Preparation Form: Water—paste pill.

Package: 1g in each 20 pills.

Notes: This drug has the purgative effect. It is clinically good for chronic gastritis, indigestion, infantile wasting disease, etc.

There is also a tablet form with the same name, ingredients and actions.

Zhishi Daozhi Wan

Ingredients:

Fructus Aurantii Immaturus	13.9%	*Zhishi*
Radix et Rhizoma Rhei	27.8%	*Dahuang*
Rhizoma Coptidis	8.3%	*Huanglian*
Radix Scutellariae	8.3%	*Huangqin*
Massa Fermentata Medicinalis	13.9%	*Liushenqu*
Rhizoma Atractylodis Macrocephalae	13.9%	*Baizhu*
Poria	8.3%	*Fuling*
Rhizoma Alismatis	5.6%	*Zexie*

Actions: Promoting digestion to remove stagnated food, and eliminating dampness and heat.

Indications: Fullness in the chest, dysentery with tenesmus, diarrhea with abdorminal pain, constipation and dark urine, all of which result from dyspepsia and damp—heat.

Administration and Dosage: Taken orally, 6 to 9g each time, twice a day.

Preparation Form: Water—paste pill.

Package: 3g in each 50 pills.

Notes: This prescription was found in the book *Nei Wai Shang Bian Huo Lun* by Li Gao in the Jin Dynasty.

The pill of this kind has the effects of anti—bacteria, anti—inflammation and Laxation. Clinically, it can be used in primary stage of dysentery or for acute gastroenteritis and constipation, both of which are due to damp—heat.

Not fit for weak patients during convalescence from dysentery.

Muxiang Binglang Wan

Ingredients:

Radix Aucklandiae	4.3%	Muxiang
Semen Arecae	4.3%	Binglang
Fructus Aurantii	4.3%	Zhike
Pericarpium Citri Reticulatae	4.3%	Chenpi
Pericarpium Citri Reticulatae Viride	4.3%	Qingpi
Rhizoma Cyperi	13%	Xiangfu
Rhizoma Sparganii	4.3%	Sanleng
Rhizoma Zedoariae	4.3%	Ezhu
Rhizoma Coptidis	4.3%	Huanglian
Cortex Phellodendri	13%	Huangbai
Radix et Rhizoma Rhei	13%	Dahuang
Semen Pharbitidis	17.9%	Qianniuzi
Natrii Sulfas	8.7%	Mangxiao

Actions: Promoting the circulation of Qi to remove stagnancy, purging heat to relax the bowels.

Indications: Retention of food in the stomach and intestine, gastric distention with pain and constipation or dysentery with tenesmus.

Administration and Dosage: Taken orally, 3 to 6g each time, 2 to 3 times a day.

Preparation Form: Water—paste pill.

Package: 3g in every 50 pills.

Notes: This prescription is from the book Yi Fang Ji Jie compiled by Wang Ang in the Qing Dynasty.

This drug has the effects of anti-bacteria, antiinflammation, and purgation. It is clinically indicated for acute enteritis, primary acute bacillary dysentery, indigestion, etc.

It is contraindicated for pregnant woman.

Maren Wan

Ingredients:

Fructus Cannabis	20%	Huomaren
Semen Armeniacae Amarum	20%	Kuxingren
Radix et Rhizoma Rhei	20%	Dahuang
Fructus Aurantii Immaturus	20%	Zhishi
Cortex Magnoliae Officinalis	10%	Houpo
Radix Paeoniae Alba	20%	Baishao

Actions: Relaxing the bowels to relieve constipation.

Indications: Constipation, fullness in the epigastric region and abdominal pain, all due to dryness-heat in the intestine and stomach.

Administration and Dosage: Taken orally, 1 bolus each time, once or twice a day.

Preparation Form: Honeyed bolus.

Package: 9g in each bolus.

Notes: This prescription is from the book *Shang Han Lun* by Zhang Zhongjing in the Han Dynasty.

This bolus has the effects of relieving diarrhea and promoting peristalsis. It is clinically efficacious for habitual constipation, hemorrhoid with constipation, anal fissure, etc.

Not allowed to be taken with enzyme preparations, it is not fit for pregnant women and weak patients with constipation.

There is also a mixture form with the same name, ingredients and actions.

Wuren Runchang Wan

Ingredients:

Fructus Cannabis	7.1%	*Huomaren*
Semen Persicae	7.1%	*Taoren*
Semen Pruni	2.1%	*Yuliren*
Semen Biotae	3.5%	*Baiziren*
Semen Pinus Tabulaeformis	2.1%	*Songziren*
Radix Rehmanniae	28.4%	*Dihuang*
Pericarpium Citri Reticulatae	28.4%	*Chenpi*
Radix et Rhizoma Rhei	7.1%	*Dahuang*
Herba Cistanchis	7.1%	*Roucongrong*
Radix Angelicae Sinensis	7.1%	*Danggui*

Actions: Invigorating *Yin* to nourish blood, relaxing the bowels to relieve constipation.

Indications: Soreness along the spinal column, abdominal distention and constipation, all due to insufficiency of the kidney–*Qi* and impairment of body fluid.

Administration and Dosage: Taken orally, 1 bolus each time, twice daily.

Preparation Form: Honeyed bolus.

Package: 9g in each bolus.

Notes: This dug acts as a laxation, which is clinically efficacious for constipation due to infirm with age or senile, puerperal and postoperative weakness.

4.4 Antidiarrheals

Sishen Wan

Ingredients:

Semen Myristicae	15.4%	*Roudoukou*
Fructus Evodiae	7.7%	*Wuzhuyu*
Fructus Psoraleae	30.7%	*Buguzhi*
Fructus Ziziphi	15.4%	*Dazao*
Fructus Schisandrae	15.4%	*Wuweizi*
Rhizoma Zingiberis Recens	15.4%	*Shengjiang*

Actions: Warming the kidney and spleen, strengthening the intestines to relieve diarrhea.

Indications: Diarrhea before dawn, loose stools, abdominal pain, sore waist and cold limbs, all of which are due to insufficiency of both the spleen and kidney.

Administration and Dosage: Taken orally at bedtime, 9g each time, once or twice a day.

Preparation Form: Water—paste pill.

Package: 3g in every 50 pills.

Notes: This prescription is from the book *Jing Yue Quan Shu* written by Zhang in the Ming Dynasty.

The effects of this pill are resisting inflammation, inducing diuresis and arresting diarrhea. It is clinically suitable for chronic enteritis of deficiency—cold type, intestinal tuberculosis, ulcerative or allergic colitis, etc.

Xianglian Wan

Ingredients:

Rhizoma Coptidis	80%	*Huanglian*

Radix Aucklandiae   20%   *Muxiang*

Actions: Clearing away heat, eliminating dampness, promoting circulation of *Qi* and relieving pain.

Indications: Dysentery of heat type with tenesmus, abdominal pain diarrhea and lassitude of limbs.

Administration and Dosage: Taken orally, 3 to 6g each time, 2 to 3 times a day. Appropriate reduction of the dosage is done for children.

Preparation Form: Water—paste pill.

Package: 1g in every 30 pills.

Notes: This prescription is quoted from the book *Tai Ping Hui Min He Ji Ju Fang* compiled by Chen Shiwen in the Song Dynasty.

The drug has the effects of antisepsis and anti—inflammation. It is clinically efficacious for acute bacillary dysentery and chronic enteritis, especially for fever and diarrhea. In addition, it may be used to treat various diseases due to simple dyspepsia.

It is not fit to be taken with enzyme preparations.

Libiling Pian

Ingredients:

Radix Sophorae Flavescentis   55.6%   *Kushen*
Radix Paeoniae Alba   27.8%   *Baishao*
Radix Aucklandiae   16.6%   *Muxiang*

Actions: Clearing away heat, drying dampness and controlling the intestines to relieve dysentery.

Indications: Abdominal pain and distension, tenesmus, anorexia and loose stools, all due to excessive noxious heat.

Administration and Dosage: Taken orally, 8 tablets each time, 3 times a day. For children, the dosage should be reduced.

Preparation Form: Sugar—coated tablet.

Package: 0.25g in each tablet

Notes: Playing the part in antisepsis and anti—inflammation, this drug is clinically useful for bacillary dysentery, chronic enteritis and gastroenteritis, which do not respond well to antibiotics or respond to them with side effects.

Huangqinsulu Jiaonang

Ingredient:

Radix Scutellariae   100% Huangqin

Actions: Clearing away heat, removing toxic materials and astringing the intestines to stop dysentery.

Indications: Dysentery with bloody stools due to noxious heat, diarrhea with abdominal pain and tenesmus, anorexia and loose stools.

Administration and Dosage: Taken orally, 2 to 4 capsules each time, 2 to 3 times a day.

Preparation Form: Capsule.

Package: 0.2g in each capsule.

Notes: Made from chelate of aluminium of the extract from Huangqin Radix Scutellariae, this drug has the effects of antibiosis, anti—inflammation, and anti—diarrhea. It is clinically good for acute or chronic enteritis, bacillary dysentery, etc.

4.5 Cholagogues

Lidan Pian

Ingredients:

Radix et Rhizoma Rhei	9.5%	*Dahuang*
Radix Scutellariae	4.8%	*Huangqin*
Flos Lonicerae	9.5%	*Jinyinhua*
Radix Aucklandiae	15.9%	*Muxiang*
Herba Lysimachiae	9.5%	*Jinqiancao*
Herba Artemisiae Scopariae	9.5%	*Yinchen*
Radix Bupleuri	9.5%	*Chaihu*
Radix Paeoniae Alba	9.5%	*Baishao*
Natrii Sulfas	3.3%	*Mangxiao*
Rhizoma Anemarrhenae	9.5%	*Zhimu*
Folium Isatidis	9.5%	*Daqingye*

Actions: Dispersing the depressed liver, normalizing the function of the gallbladder, clearing away heat, removing toxic materials, expelling stones and alleviating pain.

Indications: Retention of damp—heat in the interior, stagnantion of liver—Qi,and jaundice.

Administration and Dosage: Taken orally, 4 to 6 tablets each time, 3 times a day.

Preparation Form: Sugar—coated tablet.

Package: 0.23g in each tablet.

Notes: The tablet of this kind can normalize the function of the gallbladder, remove stones, and resist inflammation. It is clinically efficacious for acute or chronic infection of the biliary tract, cholecystitis, calculus of liver and bile duct and cholelithiasis complicated by infection. It is especially suitable for patients with the above disorders who are unable to be operated on.

Experiments have showed that this drug can increase the se-cretion of bile and relax oddi's sphincter, thus leading to the drainage of bile.

Lidan Paishi Pian

Ingredients:

Herba Lysimachiae	22.7%	Jinqiancao
Herba Artemisiae Scopariae	22.7%	Yinchen
Radix Scutellariae	6.8%	Huangqin
Radix Aucklandiae	6.8%	Muxiang
Radix Curcumae	6.8%	Yujin
Radix et Rhizoma Rhei	11.4%	Dahuang
Semen Arecae	11.4%	Binlang
Fructus Aurantii Immaturus	4.5%	Zhishi
Natrii Sulfas	2.4%	Mangxiao
Cortex Magnoliae Officinalis	4.5%	Houpu

Actions: Clearing away heat, removing toxic materials, normalizing the function of the gallbladder and expelling calculi.

Indications: Abdominal pain and distention, and fullness in the chest and hypochondrium, both due to retention of damp—heat in the interior.

Administration and Dosage: Taken orally, 6 to 10 tablets each time, and twice a day for removal of calculus; 4 to 6 tablets each time and twice a day for anti—inflammation.

Preparation Form: Tablet.

Package: 0.25g in each tablet.

Notes: This drug is clinically used for biliary calculi, infection of the biliary tract, and cholecystitis with remarkable curative effects got in treating gallstones.

It is contraindicated for pregnant women.

Xiaoyan Lidan Pian

Ingredients:

Herba Andrographitis	33.3%	*Chuanxinlian*
Ramulus et Folium Picrasmae	33.3%	*Kumu*
Herba Plectranthus Striatus Benth	33.3%	*Xihuangcao*

Actions: Clearing away heat, removing toxic materials, relieving the depressed liver and normalizing the function of the gallbladder.

Indications: Distention and pain in the epigastric region due to dampness and heat in the liver and gallbladder.

Administration and Dosage: Taken orally, 6 tablets each time, 3 times a day.

Preparation Form: Sugar—coated tablet.

Package: 0.3g in each tablet.

Notes: This drug has the effects of reducing inflammation, relieving pain and promoting biliation. It is clinically useful for acute cholecystitis, inflammation of biliary tract, hepatic calculus complicated by infection, etc.

Danshitong Jiaonang

Ingredients:

Herba Artemisiae Capillaris	*Yinchen*
Radix Scutellariae	*Huangqin*
Herba Lysimachiae	*Jinqiancao*
Radix Bupleuri	*Chaihu*
Fructus Aurantii	*Zhique*

Actions: Relieving the depressed liver, normalizing the function of the gallbladder, clearing away heat and removing toxic materials.

Indications: Abdominal distention and pain due to dampness and heat in the liver and gallbladder.

Administration and Dosage: Taken orally, 4 to 6 capsules each time, 3 times a day.

Preparation Form: Capsule.

Package: 0.5g in each capsule.

Notes: The capsule of this kind can relieve inflammation, remove calculi and normalize the function of the gallbladder. It is clinically effective for cholelithiasis, cholecystitis and inflammation of biliary tract.

4.6 Adjuvants Drugs for Treating Liver Diseases

Longdan Xiegan Wan

Ingredients:

Radix Gentianae	14.3%	Longdan
Radix Bupleuri	14.3%	Chaihu
Fructus Gardeniae	7.1%	Zhizi
Radix Scutellariae	7.1%	Huangqin
Semen Plantaginis	7.1%	Cheqianzi
Rhizoma Alismatis	14.3%	Zexie
Radix Angelicae Sinensis	7.1%	Danggui
Caulis Aristolochiae Manshuriensis	7.1%	Mutong
Radix Glycyrrhizae	7.1%	Gancao
Radix Rehmanniae	14.3%	Dihuang

Actions: Clearing away excess—fire from the liver and gallbladder and removing damp—heat from the Liver—gaubladder channel.

Indications: Hypochondriac pain, bitter taste, dizziness, conjunctival congestion, tinnitus and deafness, all of which are due to flaming—up of excess—fire of the liver and gallbladder; deep—colored urine, urodynia and leukorrhea, all due to downward flow of damp—heat in the Liver Channel.

Administration and Dosage: Taken orally, 3 to 6g each time, twice daily.

Preparation Form: Water—paste pill.

Package: 1g in every 20 pills.

Notes: This prescription was recorded in the book *Yi Zhong Jin Jian* written by Wu Qian in the Qing Dynasty.

This drug has such effects as resisting bacteria reducing inflammation and inducing diuresis. In clinic, it can be used for acute conjunctivitis, acute otitis media, acute icterepatitis, acute cholecystitis, acute pyelonephritis, cystitis, orchitis, urethritis, acute pelvic inflammation, vulvitis, orchitis prostatitis, and herpes zosfer.

There is a tablet form with the same name, ingredients and actions.

Shugan Hewei Wan

Ingredients:

Rhizoma Pinelliae	5.5%	*Jiangbanxia*
Radix Glycyrrhizae	5.5%	*Gancao*
Pericarpium Citri Reticulatae Viride	5.5%	*Qingpi*
Pericarpium Citri Reticulatae	5.5%	*Chenpi*
Cortex Magnoliae Officinalis	5.5%	*Houpu*
Radix Paeoniae Alba	5.5%	*Baishao*

Semen Alpiniae Katsumadai	5.5%	Caodoukou
Radix Linderae	5.5%	Wuyao
Massa Fermentata Medicinalis	5.5%	Liushenqu
Radix Curcumae	5.5%	Yujin
Fructus Aurantii	5.5%	Zhike
Radix Angelicae Sinensis	5.5%	Danggui
Semen Arecae	5.5%	Binglang
Fructus Amomi	3.5%	Sharen
Folium Sennae	3.5%	Fanxieye
Radix Bupleuri	3.5%	Chaihu
Fructus Crataegi	18.0%	Shanzha

Actions: Soothing the liver and regulating the stomach.

Indications: Fullness in the chest and hypochondrium, gastric discomfort with acid regurgitation, nausea and vomiting.

Administration and Dosage: Taken orally, 9g each time, twice a day.

Preparation Form: Water–paste pill and sugar–coated pill.

Package: 1g in every 20 pills.

Notes: This drug has the effects of resisting inflammation, normalizing the function of the gallbladder, and protecting damaged liver cells. It is clinically efficacious for chronic hepatitis, cholecystitis, etc.

Shugan Wan

Ingredients:

Fructus Meliae Toosendan	13.2%	Chuanlianzi
Rhizoma Corydalis	8.6%	Yanhusuo
Radix Paeoniae Alba	10.4%	Baishao
Rhizoma Curcumae Longae	8.6%	Pianjiang Huang

Radix Aucklandiae	6.9%	*Muxiang*
Lignum Aquilariae Resinatum	8.6%	*Chenxiang*
Semen Myristicae	5.2%	*Roudoukou*
Fructus Amomi	6.9%	*Sharen*
Cortex Magnoliae Officinalis	5.2%	*Houpu*
Pericarpium Citri Reticulatae	6.9%	*Chenpi*
Fructus Aurantii	8.6%	*Zhique*
Poria	8.6%	*Fuling*
Cinnabaris	2.3%	*Zhusha*

Actions: Relieving the depressed liver, regulating the flow of *Qi* and alleviating pain.

Indications: Fullness in the chest and the hypochondrium, stomachache, gastric discomfort with acid regurgitation, vomiting, and eructation, all of which are due to the stagnation of the liver—*Qi*.

Administration and Dosage: Taken orally, 1 bolus each time, 2 to 3 times a day.

Preparation Form: Honeyed bolus.

Package: 6g in each bolus.

Notes: This product produces the actions of resisting inflammation relieving pain and protecting liver function. It is clinically effective for chronic gastritis, gastric or duodenal buld ulcer, chronic hepatitis, chronic cholangitis, chronic pancreatitis, neurosis due to oppressed liver—*Qi*, portal hypertension and postoperative gastrointestinal dysfunction.

It should be used for pregnant women with caution.

Yunzhi Gantai chongji

Ingredient:

Gakoderma Lucidum   100%   *Yunzhi*

Actions: Relieving the depressed liver, removing stagnancy and regulating the stomach.

Indications: Hypochondriac distending—pain nausea, vomiting and gastric discomfort with acid regurgitation, all due to stagnation of liver—*Qi*.

Administration and Dosage: Taken orally, after being infused in boiling water, 1 bag each time, 2 to 3 times a day.

Preparation Form: Granule or powder.

Package: 5g each bag.

Notes: This drug is the extract from hymenophore of Gakoderma Lucidum, a polyporous fungus, whose active composition is dextran. Pharmacologic experiments have showed that it can enhance immunity of the body, protect liver cells, increase hepatic glycogen, and lower aminotransferase level.

This drug is clinically efficacious for hepatitis B, persisting hepatitis, chronic active hepatitis and chronic tracheitis. Having the marked power to transform AFP of early—stage hepatocarcinoma from positive to negative, it can be used to prevent and treat hepatocarcinoma or inhibit postoperative metastasis of solid tumor of the digestive tract.

Qianggan Wan

Ingredients:

Radix Angeliae Sinensis	*Danggui*
Radix Paeoniae Alba	*Baishao*
Radix Saviae Miltiorrhizae	*Danshen*
Radix Curcumae	*Yujin*
Radix Astragali	*Huangqi*

Radix Codonopsis Pilosulae	Dangshen
Herba Artemisiae Scopariae	Yinchen
Radix Isatidis	Banlangen
Rhizoma Dioscoreae	Shanyao

Actions: Strengthening the spleen, nourishing blood, invigorating Qi, getting rid of stagnancy, inducing diuresis and clearing away heat.

Indications: Such symptoms due to the deficiency of both the spleen and kidney and the stagnation of liver—Qi as fullness and pain in the hypochondrium, nausea and vomiting.

Administration and Dosage: Taken orally, 2 boluses each time, twice a day.

Preparation Form: Honeyed bolus.

Package: 9g in each bolus.

Notes: This drug has the effects of enhancing the immunologic function of the body and protecting liver cells. It is used in clinic for chronic hepatitis, early cirrhosis, fatty liver, toxic hepatitis, etc.

Jigucao Wan

Ingredients:

Herba Abri	Jigucao
Calculus Bovis	Niuhuang
Biles	Danzhi

Actions: Removing heat from the liver to normalize the function of the gallbladder and clearing away heat and toxic materials.

Indications: Fullness and pain in the chest and hypochondrium, acid regurgitation, eructation, nausea and vomiting.

Adminstration and Dosage: Taken orally, 4 capsules each time, 3 times a day.

Preparation Form: Capsule.

Package: 0.5g in each capsule.

Notes: This drug has the effects of anti—inflammation, analgesia and anti—virus. It is clinically efficacious for acute or chronic hepatitis, cholecystitis, etc.

Jiangan pian

Ingredients:

Radix Hemerocallis	13.3%	Xuancaogen
Radix Isatidis	20%	Banlangen
Herba Artemisiae Scopariae	33.4%	Yinchen
Radix Salviae Miltiorrhizae	20%	Danshen
Fructus Ziziphi Jujubae	13.3%	Dazao

Actions: Clearing away heat promoting diuresis.

Indications: Jaundice due to damp—heat, distention and pain in the hypochondrium, feeling of stuffiness in the epigestic region, nausea, vomiting, and gastric discomfort with acid regurgitation.

Administration and Dosage: Taken orally, 8 to 10 tablets each time, once or twice a day. For children, the dosage should be reduced appropriately.

Preparation Form: Tablet.

Package: 0.5g in each tablet.

Notes: With the actions of anti—inflammation, analgesia, and anti—virus. this tablet is good for chronic hepatitis, acute icterohepatitis, etc.

Wurenchun Jiaonang

Ingredient:
Fructus Schisandrae   100%   *Wuweizi*

Actions: Clearing away heat and toxic materials, relaxing the depressed liver and alleviating pain.

Indications: Fullness in the epigastric region, hypochondriac pain, eructation, acid regurgitation and vomiting.

Administration and Dosage: Taken orally, 2 to 4 capsules each time, 2 to 3 times a day.

Preparation Form: Capsule.

Package: Each capsule contains 10mg of B–Schizandrin.

Notes: This drug can lower glutamic–pyruvic transaminase (GPT). It is clinically efficacious for chronic hepatitis, persisting hepatitis, etc.

Yinchen Wuling Wan

Ingredients:

Herba Artemisiae Scapariae	15.9%	*Yinchen*
Poria	7.8%	*Fuling*
Polyporus	7.8%	*Zhuling*
Rhizoma Alismatis	7.8%	*Zexie*
Rhizoma Atractylodis Macrocephalae	7.8%	*Baizhu*
Rhizoma Atractylodis	7.8%	*Cangzhu*
Pericarpium Citri Reticulatae	3.9%	*Chenpi*
Cortex Magnoliae Officinalis	7.8%	*Houpu*
Fructus Hoveniae	7.8%	*Zhijuzi*
Radix Scutellariae	7.8%	*Huangqin*
Fructus Crataegi	7.8%	*Shanzha*

Massa Fermentata Medicinalis	3.9%	*Liushenqu*
Radix Glycyrrhizae	6.1%	*Gancao*

Actions: Clearing away heat, promoting diuresis and invigarating the spleen to relieve flatulence.

Indications: Fullness in the epigastric region, sallow complexion, nausea, inappetence and scanty dark urine, all of which are due to dampness and heat in the liver and the gallbladder.

Administration and Dosage: Taken orally, 6 to 9g each time, 2 to 3 times a day. Appropriate reduction of the dosage is done for children patients.

Preparation Form: Water—paste pill.

Package: 3g in every 50 pills.

Notes: This prescription is from the book *Jin Gui Yao Lue Fang Lun* written by *Zhang Zhongjing* in the *Han* Dynasty.

This drug has the effects of protecting the liver cells from the affection of many kinds of toxic materials, improving liver function and lowering transaminase and icteric index. It is indicated for acute icterohepatitis, toxic hepatitis, nephritis, etc.

Fuganning Pian

Ingredients:

Flos Lonicerae	*Jinyinhua*
Radix Isatidis	*Banlangen*
Cortex Moutan	*Mudanpi*

Actions: Clearing away heat and toxic materials, relieving the depressed liver and regulating the function of the spleen.

Indications: Fullness and pain in the chest and hypochondrium, inappetence, nausea and vomiting, all of which are due to incoordination between the liver and spleen.

Administration and Dosage: Taken orally, 6 tablets each time, 3 times a day.

Preparation Form: Sugar—coated tablet.

Package: 0.3g in each tablet.

Notes: This drug possesses the effect of fighting viruses and lowering transaminases. It is clinically efficacious for hepatitis B, persisting hepatitis, chronic active hepatitis and cirrhosis. Besides, it produces better result in correcting positive surface antigen of chronic hepatitis B.

Yiganling Pian

Ingredient:

Semen Silybum marianum   100%   *Shuifeijizhongzi*

Actions: Relieving the depressed liver and eliminating flatulence to alleviate pain.

Indications: Fullness in the chest and the hypochondrium, nausea and vomiting, all due to dampness and heat in the liver and gallbladder.

Administration and Dosage: Taken orally, 4 to 6 tablets each time, 2 to 3 times a day.

Preparation Form: Tablet.

Package: Each tablet contains 38.5mg Silybin.

Notes: This drug is a made from Silybin which is extracted from the seeds of *Teiji* Silybum Marianum.

With the effects of improving liver function and protecting the liver from being attacked by several toxicants, it is suitable for chronic hepatitis, chronic active hepatitis, early cirrhosis, hyperlipemia, toxic hepatitis, etc.

5 Drugs for Acting on the Blood and Hematopoietic Systems

5.1 Drugs for Nourishing Blood

Ejiao

Ingredients:

Lüpi	donkey—hide	89.3%
Bingtang	crystal sugar	5.9%
Douyou	soya—bean oil	3.0%
Huangjiu	millet wine	1.8%

Actions: Replenishing *Yin*, moisturizing the viscera, tonifying blood and arresting bleeding.

Indications: Deficiency of blood, palpitation, hemoptysis, metrorrhagia and threatened abortion with vaginal bleeding.

Administration and Dosage: Dissolved in boiled water and taken orally, 3—9g each time, once daily.

Preparation Form: Gelatin.

Package: 500g in each box.

Notes: The drug can increase red blood cells and hemoglobin, prevent the disease of granulocyte, raise the absolute value of neutrophil and improve the restorative ability of hemorrhagic anemia. It is clinically indicated for common anemia, leukopenia, dys functional uterine hemorrhage, aplastic anemia and threatened abortion.

Xin Ejiao

Ingredients:

Lüpi	donkey—hide	97.2%
Bingtang	crystal sugar	1.3%
Douyou	soya—bean oil	1.1%
Huangjiu	millet wine	0.4%

Actions: Nourishing *Yin,* enriching blood and arresting bleeding.

Indications: Deficiency of blood, hemoptysis due to pulmonary tuberculosis, antepartum and postpartum deficiency of blood, fatigue, irregular menstruation, etc.

Administration and Dosage: Broken, dissolved through stewing in the decoction or in warm boiled water or millet wine and taken orally, 5—15g each time, once daily.

Preparation Form: Gelatin.

Package: 500g in each box.

Notes: The drug can improve the restorative ability of hemorrhagic anemia, obviously increase red blood cells and hemoglobin and prevent the decrease of granulocyte. It is clinically indicated for common anemia, bloody suptum, leukopenia, menstrual disorder, antepartum and postpartum anemia, etc.

Fufang Ejiao Jiang

Ingredients:

Colla Corii Asini	*Ejiao*
Radix Ginseng	*Renshen*
Rhizoma Rehmanniae Praeparata	*Shudi*

Fructus Crataegi   *Shanzha*

Actions: Benefiting *Qi,* nourishing blood, coordinating the functions of the spleen and stomach.

Indications: Consumptive diseases marked by palpitation, shortness of breath, fatigue, dizziness, insomnia, feeble breath and languor.

Administration and Dosage: Taken orally, 20ml each time, 3 times daily, with 30 days involved in 1 course of treatment. The dosage for children should be reduced properly.

Preparation Form: Extract.

Package: 250ml in each bottle.

Notes: This drug can improve the immuno competence of the body, adjust the central nervous system, regulate visceral functions, promote the digestion and absorption of food, improve hematopoietic function and stop bleeding. It is clinically indicated for leukopenia, iron–deficient and hemorrhagic anemia, etc.

Shandong Ejiao Gao

Ingredients:

Colla Corii Asini	25%	*Ejiao*
Radix Codonopsis Pilosulae	20%	*Dangshen*
Rhizoma Atractylodis Macrocephalae	10%	*Baizhu*
Radix Astragali	20%	*Huangqi*
Fructus Lycii	10%	*Gouqizi*
Radix Paeoniae Alba	5%	*Baishao*
Radix Glycyrrhizae	10%	*Gancao*

Actions: Nourishing blood, arresting bleeding, restoring *Qi* and moisturizing the lung.

Indications: Insufficiency of *Qi* and blood, cough due to consumption, haematemesis due to impairment of the lung, metrorrhagia and excessive fetal movment.

Administration and Dosage: Taken orally, 20 to 25g each time, 3 times a day.

Preparation Form: Extract.

Package: 250g in each bottle.

Notes: This drug can strengthen the resistant ability of the body, promote blood circulation, improve the nutritional status of the body and adjust the function of the nervous system. It is clinically used to treat iron—deficient and malnutritional anemia, leukemia, threatened and habitual abortion, etc.

Huangming Jiao

Ingredients: This drug is a kind of solid gelatin made through decocting, boiling and concentrating cattle hide.

Actions: Nourishing *Yin,* moisturizing dryness, tonifying blood and arresting bleeding.

Indications: Fatigue, constipation, nocturnal emission due to kidney—deficiency, hematemesis, vaginal bleeding during pregnancy, metrorrhagia, etc.

Administration and Dosage: Melted in water for oral use, 10g each time, once or twice daily.

Preparation Form: Gelatin.

Package: 500g in each box.

Notes: This drug can improve general visceral function, adjust organic metabolism, increase the number of red blood cells and the volume of hemoglobin, and arrest bleeding. It is clinically indicated for common anemia, all kinds of haemorrhage, vexation, insomnia and threatened or habitual abortion, etc.

Renshen Guipi Wan

Ingredients:

Radix Ginseng	15.3%	*Renshen*
Radix Angelicae Sinensis	10.7%	*Danggui*
Radix Astragali	10.7%	*Huangqi*
Arillus Longan	10.7%	*Longyanrou*
Radix Aucklandiae	3.1%	*Muxiang*
Radix Polygalae	3.8%	*Yuanzhi*
Semen Ziziphi Spinosae	10.7%	*Suanzaoren*
Poria	10.7%	*Fuling*
Rhizoma Atractylosis Macrocephalae	10.7%	*Baizhu*
Radix Glycyrrhizae	13.7%	*Gancao*

Actions: Invigorating the spleen, tranquilizing the mind, benefiting *Qi* and tonifying blood.

Indications: Deficiency of both the heart and spleen, insufficiency of *Qi* and blood, palpitation, insomnia and menorrhage.

Administration and Dosage: Taken orally, 1 bolus each time, 2—3 times a day.

Preparation Form: Honeyed bolus.

Package: 9g in each bolus.

Notes: This formula is quoted from the book *Ji Sheng Fang* written by Yang Yonghe in the Song Dynasty.

The drug is clinically indicated for neuresthenia, splastic anemia, functional endometrorrhagia, thrombopenic purpura and gastroduodenal ulcer hemorrhage.

There is a tablet form with the same name, ingredients and actions.

Jianxue Chongji

Ingredients:

Radix Astragali   *Huangqi*

Radix Pseudostellariae   *Taizishen*

cotton root   *Mianhua Gen*

Actions: Nourishing blood, invigorating *Qi* and removing blood stasis with new blood generated.

Indications: Fatigue and blood—stagnation both due to deficiency of *Qi*, and numbness of the limbs.

Preparation Form: Powder.

Package: 18g in each bag.

Notes: This drug can improve hamotopoietic function, increase the number of leukocytes, raise the concentration of hematochrome and promote immunologic function. It is clinically indicated for leukopenia caused by radiotherapy or chemotherapy, and occupational and non—reasonable leukopenia through cantaction of organic solvents.

Shengxue Gao

Ingredients:

Radix Rehmanniae Praeparata   *Shudihuang*

Radix Astragali   *Huangqi*

Radix Angelicae Sinensis   *Danggui*

Haematitum   *Daizheshi*

Actions: Benefiting Qi and nourishing blood.

Indications: Blood—deficiency of the heart and liver marked by pale lips and finger—nails, dizziness, palpitation, etc.

Administration and Dosage: Taken orally, twice daily,

10—15g for children of 1—3 years old, 25g for children of 4—7 years old each time.

Preparation Form: Extract.

Package: 250g in each bottle.

Notes: This drug is clinically efficacious for all kinds of anemia.

Jixueteng Pian

Ingredients:

Caulis Spatholobi   100%   *Jixueteng*

Actions: Tonifying blood, activating blood flowing, relaxing muscles and tendons, and dredging the channels.

Indications: Syndrome of wind—dampness marked by soreness of the loins and knees, joint disturbance and vertigo due to blood—deficiency.

Administration and Dosage: Taken orally, 4 tablets each time, 3 times daily.

Preparation Form: Tablet.

Package: 0.25g in each tablet.

Notes: This drug is clinically efficacious for all kinds of anemia, leukopenia, rheumatic arthritis, rheumatoid arthritis and menoxenia.

It is contraindicated for pregnant women.

5.2   Hemostatics

Yunnan Baiyao

Ingredients: omitted

Actions: Activating blood flowing and arresting bleeding.

Indications: Traumatic injury, all kinds of hemorrhage, irregular menstruation, postpartum blood stasis, etc.

Administration and Dosage: Taken orally, 0.2—0.3g each time, twice or three times daily. Or, externally applied to a wound.

Preparation Form: Powder

Package: 8g in each bottle

Notes: This drug is clinically efficacious for hemorrhage due to internal and external injury, spitting blood, nose—bleeding, traumatic injury, etc.

It was reported abroad that two kinds of cellular toxic saponin were dissociated from the drug, which has the activity to inhibit cancer.

It is contraindicated for pregnant women.

Sanqi Pian

Ingredients:

Radix Notoginseng   100% *Sanqi*

Actions: Removing blood stasis, arresting bleeding, relieving pain, and promoting the subsidence of swelling.

Indications: Swelling and pain due to blood stasis caused by traumatic injury, spitting blood, epistaxis, hematochezia and abdominal pain due to postpartum blood stasis.

Administration and Dosage: Taken orally, 3—5 tablets each time, once or twice daily. Or Ground into fine powder after the sweet coat is taken off and applied to the wound.

Preparation Form: Sweet—coated tablet.

Package: 0.3g in each tablet.

Notes: This drug is clinically efficacious for blood stasis, swelling and pain due to wounds, postpartum lower abdominal pain and all kinds of hemorrhage.

It is contraindicated for pregnant women.

There is a powder form with the same name, ingredients and actions.

Heye Wan

Ingredients:

Folium Nelumbinis	27.6%	Heye
Herba Cirsii Japonici	4.1%	Daji
Herba Cephalanoploris	4.1%	Xiaoji
Radix Scutellariae	5.5%	Huangqin
Radix Rehmanniae	8.3%	Dihuang
Petiolus Trachycarpi	8.3%	Zongban
Radix Ranunculus Japonicus	8.3%	Maogen
Fructus Gardeniae	0.7%	Jiaozhizi
Xiangmo China ink stick	5.5%	
Rhizoma Anemarrhenae	5.5%	Zhimu
Radix Scrophulariae	8.3%	Xuanshen
Radix Paeoniae Alba	5.5%	Baishao
Radix Angelicae Sinensis	2.8%	Danggui
Nodus Nelumbinis Rhizomatis	5.5%	Oujie

Actions: Clearing away heat, cooling blood, removing blood stasis and stopping bleeding.

Indications: All kinds of homorrhage due to Yin-deficiency and blood heat marked by hemoptysis, spitting blood, hematuria, metrorrhage, metrostaxis, etc.

Administration and Dosage: Taken orally, one bolus each time, twice daily.

Preparation Form: Honeyed bolus.

Package: 6g in each bolus.

Notes: This drug is clinically efficacious for hemoptysis due to nephritis, functional uterine hemorrhage, etc.

Shihui San

Ingredients:

Herba Cirsii Japonici	10%	Daji
Herba Cephalanoploris	10%	Xiaoji
Cacumen Biotae	10%	Cebaiye
Rhizoma Imperatae	10%	Baimaogen
Radix Rubiae	10%	qiancao
Radix et Rhizoma Rhei	10%	Dahuang
Cortex Trachycarpi	10%	Zonglüpi
Cortex Moutan	10%	Mudanpi
Folium Nelumbinis	10%	Heye
Fructus Gardeniae	10%	Zhizi

Actions: Cooling blood and arresting bleeding.

Indications: Bleeding such as spitting blood and hemoptysis

Administration and Dosgae: Taken orally, 6—9g each time, twice daily.

Preparation Form: Powder.

Package: 18g in each bag.

Notes: The formula is quoted from the book *Shi Yao Shen Shu* written by *Ge Kejiu* in the *Yuan* Dynasty.

This drug is clinically efficacious for all kinds of hemorrhage due to internal injury such as spitting blood, hemoptysis led by pulmonary tuberculosis, functional uterine hemorrhage, etc.

Zanglian Wan

Ingredients:

Rhizoma Coptidis	3.6%	*Huanglian*
Radix Scutellariae	21.4%	*Huangqin*
Radix Paeoniae Rubra	3.7%	*Chishao*
Radix Angelicae Sinensis	7.1%	*Danggui*
Flos Sophorae Immaturus	10.7%	*Huaimi*
Colla Corii Asini	7.1%	*Ejiao*
Fructus Sophorae	14.3%	*Huaijiao*
Radix Sanguisorbae	14.3%	*Diyu*
Herba Schizonepetae	7.1%	*Jingjie*
Radix Rehmanniae	10.7%	*Dihuang*

Actions: Clearing away heat from blood to stop bleeding.

Indications: Hematochezia, anus—dropping pain, and hemorrhage, swelling and pain due to hemorrhoid.

Administration and Dosage: Taken orally, one bolus each time, twice daily.

Preparation Form: Honeyed bolus.

Pakage: 9g in each bolus.

Notes: The formula is quoted from the book *Wai Ke Zheng Zhong* written by *Chen Shigong* in the *Ming* Dynasty.

This drug is clinically efficacious for red—swelling and burning—pain due to hemorrhoid, anal fissure, anal papillitis, constipation and stools with blood.

6　Drugs for Acting on the Urinary System

6.1　Diuretics

Shizo Wan

Ingredients:

Fructus Diospyri Loti	*Heizaorou*
Radix Euphorbiae Kansui	*Gansui*
Radix Knoxiae	*Hongdaji*
Flos Genkwa	*Yuanhua*

Actions: Eliminating retention of fluid.

Indications: Fluid retention characterized by ascites with swelling and distension, hypochondriac pain, dyspnea, rapid breathing, stuffiness in the epigastric region, headache, vertigo and chest—back—drawing pain.

Administration and Dosage: Taken orally on an empty stomach, 2—3g each time, once or twice daily.

Preparation Form: Water—paste pill.

Package: 1g in every 10 pills.

Notes: The formula is quoted from the book *Shang Han Lun* written by *Zhang Zhongjing* in the *Han* Dynasty.

This drug has a potent diuretic effect. It is clinically efficacious for ascites resulting from heptocirrhosis and schistosomiasis, and exudative pleuritis.

It is contraindicated for those with physical weakness and pregnant women, and salt is abstained from in the course of treatment.

Zhouche Wan

Ingredients:

Semen Pharbitidis	34.5%	*Qianniuzi*
Radix et Rhizoma Rhei	17.2%	*Dahuang*
Radix Euphorbiae Kansui	8.6%	*Gansui*
Pericarpium Citri Reticulatae	8.6%	*Chenpi*
Radix Knoxiae	8.6%	*Hongdaji*
Radix Aucklandiae	4.3%	*Muxiang*
Flos Genkwa	8.6%	*Yuanhua*
Calomelas	0.9%	*Qingfen*
Corter Fraxini	8.6%	*Qingpi*

Actions: Promoting circulation of *Qi* and eliminating retention of fluid.

Indications: Edema, fullness in the epigastric region, dyspnea due to fluid retention, constipation and oliguria.

Administration and Dosage: Taken orally, 3g each time, once daily.

Preparation Form: Water—paste pill.

Package: 3g in each bag.

Notes: The formula is quoted from the *Jing Yue Quan Shu* written by *Zhang Jiebin* in the Ming Dynasty.

This drug has a potent diuretic effect. It is clinically efficacious for acute and chronic nephritis, liver cirrhosis, and ascites due to advanced schistosomiasis.

It is cautiously administered to those who are weak,

contraindicated for pregnant women, and not suggested to be used for so long a time for fear that poisoning should occur. In the course of treatment, diet with low or without salt is ordered. Besides, it is not to be taken along with *Gancao* Radix Glycyrrhizae.

Wuling San

Ingredients:

Rhizoma Atractylodis Macrocephalae	18.8%	*Baizhu*
Poria	18.8%	*Fuling*
Rhizoma Alismatis	31.1%	*Zexie*
Polyporus Umbellatus	18.8%	*Zhuling*
Cortex Cinnamomi	12.5%	*Rougui*

Actions: Warming *Yang* to activate the flow of *Qi,* and inducing diuresis to remove dampness.

Indications: Fluid retention marked by edema, dysuria, vomiting, diarrhea, thirst without desire for drink and every kind of watery distension.

Administration and Dosage: Taken orally, 6 to 9g time, twice daily.

Preparation Form: Powder.

Package: 9g in each bag.

Notes: The formula is quoted from the book *Shang Han Lun* written by *Zhang Zhongjing* in the *Han* Dynasty.

This drug has a diuretic function. It is clinically efficacious for edema resulting from acute nephritis, heart disease and malnutrition, and ascites due to liver cirrhosis. It can also be used for urine retention caused by the inhibition of urinary function and the spasm of the bladder sphinctor occurring after abdominal operation, acute gastroenteritis infectious hepatitis and infection of the urinary system.

Sanren Heji

Ingredients:

Semen Armaniacae Amarum	16.7%	*Kuxingren*
Cortex Magnoliae Officinalis	6.7%	*Houpo*
Semen Amomi Cardamomi	6.7%	*Baidoukou*
Medulla Tetrapanacis	6.7%	*Tongcao*
Herba Lophatheri	6.5%	*Danzhuye*
Talcum	20%	*Huashi*
Semen Coicis	20%	*Yiyiren*
Rhizoma Pinelliae	16.7%	*Jiangbanxia*

Actions: Promoting the dispersing function of the lung, regulating the middle—*jiao*, clearing away heat and promoting diuresis.

Indications: Headache, lassitude, choking sensation in the chest, poor appetite, fever appearing after noon, pale tongue and no desire for drink, all of which are due to early damp—warmness in the *Qi* system which has not become dryness but united with summer—heat.

Administration and Dosage: Shaken completely and taken orally, 20 to 30ml each time 3 times daily.

Preparation Form: Mixture.

Package: 500ml in each bottle.

Notes: The formula is quoted from the book *Wen Bin Tiao Bian* written by *Wu Jutong* in the *Qing* Dynasty.

This drug has diuretic, antipyretic and antibacterial effects.

It is clinically efficacious for pyelonephritis, intestinal typhoid, chronic cystitis, bronchopneumonia, fever of unknown reason, postoperative intestinal adhesion and acute gastroenteritis.

Ermiao Wan

Ingredients:

Rhizoma Atractylodis	50%	*Cangzhu*
Cortex Phellodendri	50%	*Huangbei*

Actions: Eliminating dampness and clearing away heat.

Indications: Pyogenic infection and ulceration of the skin in the feet and knees, erysipelas of the shank, abnormal vaginal discharge, scrotal eczema and ecthyma, all due to downward flowing of wetness—heat.

Administration and Dosage: Taken orally, 6—9g each time, twice daily.

Preparation Form: Water—paste pill.

Package: 3g in every 50 pills.

Notes: The formula is quoted from the book *Dan Xi Xin Fa* written by *Zhu Zhengheng* in the *Yuan* Dynasty.

This drug has diuretic, antibacterial, antiviral and anti—inflammatory effects. It is clinically efficacious for surgical infection of feet and knees, erysipelas of low extremities, leuckorrhea, scrotal eczema and ecthyma.

Shenyan Siwei Pian

Ingredients:

Radix Astragali	*Huangqi*
Folium Pyrrosiae	*Shiwei*

Actions: Promting blood circulation to remove blood stasis,

clearing away heat to get rid of toxic materials, tonifying the kidney to supplement *Qi*.

Indications: Pale complexion, low mood, fatigue, headache, vertigo, tinnius, nausea, vomiting, general edema and oliguria or dysuria.

Administration and Dosage: Taken orally after meals, 8 tablets each time, 3 times daily, with a course of treatment involving 3 months. The dosage should be decreased for children properly.

Preparation Form: Tablet.

Package: 0.6g in each tablet.

Notes: This drug is clinically efficacious for chronic glomerulonephritis, renal insufficiency in the stage of decompensation and urinotoxemia.

Hormone, cyclophosphamide and mustargen are kept off in the course of treatment with this drug.

Suoquan Wan

Ingredients:

Fructus Alpiniae Oxyphyllae	33.3%	*Yizhiren*
Rhizoma Dioscoreae	33.3%	*Shanyao*
Radix Linderae	33.3%	*Wuyao*

Actions: Warming and recuperating the kidney—*Yang* and reducing urination by astringents.

Indications: Frequent micturetion and incontinence of urine in children, both due to deficiency—cold.

Administration and Dosage: Taken orally, 6 to 9g each time, twice daily.

Preparation Form: Water—paste pill.

Package: 31g in every 500 pills.

Notes: The formula is quoted from the book *Fu Ren Liang Fang Da Quan* written by *Chen Ziming* in the *Song* Dynasty.

This drug can reduce urine amount, decrease the frequency of urination and adjust the function of the urinary and nervous systems. It is clinically efficacious for polyuria, enuresis, incontinence of urine, and frequent urination, all due to deficiency of the kidney—*Yang*.It also has certain curative effects for diabetes.

6.2 Drugs for Removal of Urinary Calculus

Bazheng Heji

Ingredients:

Semen Plantaginis	12.5%	*Cheqianzi*
Caulis Clematidis Armandii	12.5%	*Mutong*
Radix Glycyrrhizae	12.5%	*Gancao*
Herba Polygoni Avicularis	12.5%	*Bianxu*
Herba Dianthi	12.5%	*Qumai*
Talcum	12.5%	*Huashi*
Fructus Gardeniae	12.5%	*Zhizi*
Radix et Rhizoma Rhei	12.5%	*Dahuang*

Actions: Clearing away heat and inducing diuresis to treat stranguia.

Indications: Syndrome of accumulation of damp—heat in the interior marked by stranguria of heat—type, due to stone or with blood, frequent and dribbling urination with pain, distension in the lower abdomen with eager micturition due to retention of urine, conjuctival congestion and dry throat.

Administration and Dosage: Taken orally, 20 to 25ml each

time, 3 times daily.

Preparation Form: Mixture.

Package: 500ml in each bottle.

Notes: The formula is quoted from the book *Tai Ping Hui Min He Ji Ju Fang written by Chen Shiwen* in the *Song* Dynasty.

This drug has the functions of relieving fever, reducing diuresis and resisting bacteria. It is clinically efficacious for urinary stone, acute and chronic nephritis, pyelonephritis, acute and chronic cystitis, urethritis and postpartum or postoperative urine retention.

It is contraindicated for weak patients and pregnant women.

Fenqing Wulin Wan

Ingredients:

Semen Plantaginis	5.5%	*Cheqianzi*
Radix et Rhizoma Rhei	16.4%	*Dahuang*
Caulis Aristolochiae Manshuriensis	11%	*Guanmutong*
Herba Polygoni	5.5%	*Bianxu*
Radix Scutellariae	11%	*Huangqin*
Talcum	11%	*Huashi*
Polyporus Umbellatus	5.5%	*Zhuling*
Rhizoma Alismatis	5.5%	*Zexie*
Cortex Phellodendri	5.5%	*Huangbai*
Herba Dianthi	5.5%	*Qumai*
Rhizoma Anemarrhenae	5.5%	*Zhimu*
Poria	5.5%	*Fuling*
Radix Glycyrrhizae Praeparata	1.1%	*Zigancao*
Fructus Gardeniae	5.5%	*Jiaozhizi*

Actions: Purging heat to treat stranguria, inducing diuresis and alleviating pain.

Indications: Urgent, frequent, difficult, painful and dripping urination, distention and fullness due to water retention in the lower abdomen and constipation, which are all due to dampness and heat in the urinary bladder.

Administration and Dosage: Taken orally, 6—9g each time, 2 to 3 times daily.

Preapration Form: Water—paste pill.

Package: 3g in every 50 pills.

Notes: The formula is quoted from the book *Tai Ping Hui Min He Ji Ju Fang written by Chen Shiwen* in the *Song* Dynasty.

This drug has antipyretic, diuretic and antibacterial effects. It is clinically efficacious for cystitis, urethritis, acute prostatitis, urinary stones, acute nephritis and pyelonephritis, and filariasis.

It should be cautiously administered to pregnant women.

Shilingtong Pian

Ingredients:

Herba Desmodii Styracifolii   100%   *Guangjinqiancao*

Actions: clearing away damp—heat, inducing diuresis and removing urinary calculus.

Indications: Stranguria due to accumulation of dampness and heat in the lower—*Jiao*.

Administration and Dosage: Taken orally, 5 tablets each time, 3 times daily.

Preparation Form: Tablet.

Package: 0.21g in each tablet with 0.12g of dry drug extract.

Notes: With the effects of inducing diuresis, allaying inflammation, normalizing the function of the gallbladder and removing urinary caculus, this drug is clinically efficacious for urinary stones, urinary infection, gallstones, cholecystitis, icterohepatitis, ascites, nephritic edema and infantile malnutrition.

Sanjin Pian

Ingredients:

Fructus Rosae Laevigatae	*Jinyingzi*
Spora Lygodii	*Haijinsha*
Rhizoma Smilacis Chinae	*Jinganggen*
Radix Tripterygii Wilfordii	*Leigonggen*
Cortex Moutan	*Mudanpi*

Actions: Clearing away heat, removing toxic materials and inducing diuresis to treat stranguria.

Indications: Accumulation of dampness and heat in the lower—*Jiao* marked by such symptoms as frequent, dripping and difficult urination with stabbing pain, oliguria, and contracture of lower abdomen or dragging pain in the lower abdomen.

Administration and Dosage: Taken orally, 5 tablets each time, 3 to 4 times daily.

Preparation Form: Tablet.

Package: 0.5g in each tablet.

Notes: This drug has diuretic, antipyretic, antibacterial and antiinflammatory effects. It is clinically efficacious for acute and chronic pyelonephritis, acute attack of chronic pyelonrphritis, acute cystitis and urinary infection.

Paishi Chongji

Ingredients:

Herba Lysimachiae	*Jingqiancao*

Caulis Lonicerae	Rendongteng
Talcum	Huashi
Radix Glycyrrhizae Praeparata	Zhigancao
Caulis Clematidis Armandii	Mutong
Semen Plantadinis	Cheqianzi
Folium Pyrrosiae	Shiwei
Herba Dianthi	Qumai
Radix Cynanchi Paniculati	Xuchangqing
Fructus Malvae Verticillatae	Donguizi

Actions: Inducing diuresis, and removing urinary caculus.

Indications: Stranguria due to accumulation of dampness and heat in the lower—*Jiao*.

Administration and Dosage: Taken orally, 20g each time, 3 times daily.

Preparation Form: Powder.

Package: 20g in each bag.

Notes: This drug has the effects of removing stone, reducing urinesis, allaying inflammation and arresting pain. It is clinically efficacious for stones such as kidney stones, ureter stones and bladder stones.

7 Drugs for Affecting Metabolic Functions

7.1 Antithyroid Drugs

Haizao Wan

Ingredients:

Sargassum	94.3%	*Haizao*
Yanmei	5.7%	*Yanmei*

Actions: Resolving hard lumps.

Indications: Scrofula and goiter.

Administration and Dosage: Taken orally, 9g each time, twice a day.

Preparation Form: Water—paste pill.

Package: 3g in every 50 pills.

Notes: The prescription is recorded in the book *Zheng Zhi Zhun Sheng* written by Wang Kentang in the Ming Dynasty.

This pill can soften blood vesseles and reduce goiter. It is clinically indicated for thyroid enlargement, thyroma, tuberculous tuberclitis, etc.

Xiakucao Gao

Ingredients:

Spica Prunellae	80.8%	*Xiakucao*
Radix Angelicae Sinensis	1.7%	*Danggui*
Radix Glycyrrhizae	1.0%	*Gancao*

Radix Platycodi	1.0%	Jiegeng
Radix Paeoniae Alba	1.7%	Baishao
Flos Carthami	0.7%	Honghua
Pericarpium Citri Reticulatae	1.0%	Chenpi
Thallus Eckloniae	1.0%	Kunbu
Rhizoma Ligustici Chuanxiong	1.0%	Chuanxiong
Radix Scrophulariae	1.7%	Xuanshen
Rhizoma Cyperi	3.3%	Xiangfu
Bulbus Fritillariae Thunbergii	1.7%	Zhebeimu
Bombyx Batryticatus	1.7%	Jiangyong
Radix Linderae	1.7%	Wuyao

Actions: Clearing away fire, resolving mass, relieving swelling and alleviating pain.

Indications: Scrofula and goitre with swelling and pain, both of which are caused by accumulation of phlegm and heat.

Administration and Dosage: Taken orally, 9—15g each time, twice a day.

Preparation Form: Soft extract.

Package: 60g in each bottle.

Notes: This product can promote thyroid function and resist bacteria, and can be used as diuretic. It is clinically indicated for simple goiter, chronic lymphnoditis, lymphoid tuberculosis, mumps, etc.

7.2   Drugs for Hypoglycemin

Xiaoke Wan

Ingredients:
Radix Astragali   *Huangqi*

Radix Trichosanthis	*Tianhuafen*
Radix Rehmanniae	*Shengdihuang*

Action: Nourishing the kidney—*Yin*, supplementing *Qi* and promoting the production of body fluids.

Indications: Polydipsia, polyphagia, polyuria, emaciation general weakness and acratian, all due to diabetes.

Administration and Dosage: Taken orally, 3 times daily, 5 pills at the lst time, 1 pill added from the 2nd time up to 10 pills each time, with 10 pills kept taken each time and twice daily after the curative effects are achieved.

Preparation Form: Water—paste pills.

Package: 0.25g in each pill.

Notes: This product has the apparent function in reducing the level of blood sugar and treating the symptoms of diabetes. It is clinically indicated for mild, moderate or steady diabetes.

It is to be cautiously used for diabetics with hepatitis.

It is contraindicated for diabetes complicated by serious renal insufficiency, juvenile diabetes, diabetic kerosis diabetes in pregnancy and diabetic coma, and forbidden to be used together with glybenzcyclamide agents.

Yuquan Wan

Ingredients:

Fructus Schisandrae	*Wuweizi*
Radix Rehmanniae	*Shengdihuang*
Radix Ophiopogonis	*Maidong*
Poria	*Fuling*
Radix Hystragali	*Huangqi*
Radix Trichosanthis	*Tianhuafen*

| Radix Puerariae | Gegen |
| Fructus Mume | Wumei |

Actions: Nourishing the kidney—*Yin*, promoting the prodction of body fluid to qench thirst, clearing away heat, removing restlessness, invigorating *Qi* and regulating the funciton of the middle—*Jiao*.

Indications: Polydipsia, polyphagia, emaciation and acratia due to diabetes.

Administration and Dosage: Taken orally, 9g each time, three times a day. One course of treatment involves 30 days.

Preparation Form: Water—paste pill.

Package: 1.5g in every 10 pills.

Notes: This product has the apparent effects of reducing blood and urine sugar. It is clinically used for material metabolic disorder due to the decline of insular function and mild or moderate diabetes.

Xiaokeping Pian

Ingredients:

Radix Ginseng	1.1%	Renshen
Rhizoma Coptidis	1.1%	Huang lian
Radix Trichosanthis	26.9%	Tianhuafen
Radix Asparagi	2.7%	Tiandong
Radix Astragali	26.9%	Huangqi
Radix Salviae Miltiorrhizae	8.0%	Dangshen
Fructus Lycii	6.5%	Gouqizi
Semen Astragli Complanati	8.0%	Shayuanzi
Radix Puerariae	8.0%	Gegen
Rhizoma Anemarrhenae	5.4%	Zhimu

| Galla Chinensis | 2.7% | *Wubeizi* |
| Fructus Schisandrae | 2.7% | *Wuweizi* |

Actions: Supplementing *Qi*, nourishing *Yin*, clearing away heat, purging fire, tonifging the kidney and reducing urination.

Indications: Dysphoria with smothery sensation, polyuria and consumption of *Yin*—fluid due to diabetes.

Administration and Dosage: Taken orally, 6—8 tablets each time,three times a day. One course of treatment involves 30 days.

Preparation Form: Tablet coated with semi—film.

Package: 0.28g in each tablet.

Notes: This tablet can decrease blood sugar and blood liguid and improve the function of the liver and kidney. It is clinically indicated for noninsulin—dependable diabetes.

8 Drugs for Antivirus and Antibacteriats

Angong Niuhuang Wan

Ingredients:

Calculus Bovis	*Niuhuang*
Radix Curcumae	*Yujin*
Rhizoma Coptidis	*Huanglian*
Radix Scutellariae	*Huangqin*
Fructus Gardeniae	*Zhizi*
Concentratum Cornu Bubali	*Shuiniujiao Nongsuofen*
Margarita	*Zhenzhu*
Borneolum Syntheticum	*Bingpian*

Actions: Clearing away heat, removing toxic materials, inducing resuscitation and tranquilizing the mind.

Indications:

Syndrome of heat type due to lingering of pathogenic factors in the pericardium which is marked by high fever, convulsion, coma, delirium and mania or stiff tongue and cold limbs.

Administration and Dosage: Taken orally, 1 bolus each time for those beyond 6 years old, $\frac{1}{4}$ bolus each time for infants below 3 years old, $\frac{1}{2}$ bolus each time for young children between 4 and 6 years old.

Preparation Form: Honeyed bolus

Package: 3g in each bolus

Notes: The prescription is recorded in the book, *Wen Bing Tiao Bian* compiled by Wu Jutong in the Qing Dynasty.

This drug has antibacteria, antiviral antipyretic, antispasmodic and tranquilizing effects. It is clinically efficacious for high fever, coma and convulsion due to encephalitis B, epidemic encephalomyelitis, bacillary dysentery, urinaemia, cerebrovascula accident, viral hepatitis, hepatic coma and infection of nervous system.

It is to be used for pregnant woman with caution.

Jufang Zhibao Dan

Ingredients:

Concentratum Cornu Bubali	*Shuiniujiao Nongsuofen*
Carapax Eretomochelydis	*Daimao*
Succinum	*Hupo*
Benzoinum	*Anxixiang*
Caculus Bovis	*Niuhuang*
Borneolum Snytheticum	*Bingpian*

Actions: Clearing away heat, removing toxic materials, and eliminating phlegm to induce resuscitation.

Indications: Epidemic febrile disease due to stagnation of phlegm and heat in the interior marked by coma, delirium, spasm, clonic convulsion and sudden fright in children.

Administration and Dosage: Taken orally, 1 bolus each time, 1 / 2 bolus each time for children.

Preparation Form: Honeved bolus.

Package: 3g in each bolus.

Notes:

The prescription is recorded in the book *Tai Ping Hui Min He Ji Ju Fang* compiled by Chen Shiwen in the Song Dynasty.

This drug is clinically efficacious for high fever and coma due to acute infectious diseases such as encephalitis B, epidemic encephalomyelitis and typhus, and such diseases as encephalopathy, intracerebal hemorrhage, hematosepsis, heptic coma, and epilepsy.

It is contraindicated for debilitated patients and patients with hypertension.

Zixue Dan

Main Ingredients:

Gypsum Fibrosum	*Shigao*
Calcitum	*Hanshuishi*
Talcum	*Huashi*
Magnetitum	*Cishi*
Radix Scrophulariae	*Xuanshen*
Radix Aucklandiae	*Muxiang*
Lignum Aquilariae Resinatum	*Chenxiang*
Rhizoma Cimicifugae	*Shengma*
Radix Glycyrrhizae	*Gancao*

Actions: Clearing away heat, removing toxic materials, tranquilizing the mind and inducing resuscitation.

Indications: High fever, restlessness, coma, delirium, convulsion, deep—colored urine and constipation due to inward transmission of pathogenic heat.

Administration and Dosage: Taken orally, 1.5—3g each time twice daily; 0.3g each time for an infant of 1 year old with every 0.3 g added whenever it becomes 1 year older until it is 5.

Preparation Form: Powder.

Package: 1.5g in each bottle.

Notes: The prescription is recorded in the book *Tai Ping Hui Min He Ji Ju Fang* compiled by Chen Shiwen in the Song Dynasty.

This drug is clinically efficacious for acute eruptive illnesses such as typhus and measles, and high fever and coma due to encephalitis B and epidemic encephalomyelitis.

It is contraindicated for pregnant woman.

Niuhuang Jiedu Pian

Ingredients:

Calculus Bovis	0.6%	*Niuhuang*
Realgar	6.4%	*Xionghuang*
Gypsum Fibrosum	25.7%	*Shigao*
Radix et Rhizoma Rhei	25.7%	*Dahuang*
Radix Scutellariae	19.2%	*Huangqin*
Radix Platycodi	12.8%	*Jiegeng*
Borneolum Syntheticum	3.2%	*Bingpian*
Radix Glycyrrhizae	6.4%	*Gancao*

Actions: Clearing away heat, removing toxic materials, expelling wind and relieving pain.

Indications: Syndrome due to fire and heat in the interior marked by swollen and painful throat and gingiva, aphthous stomatitis, conjunctival congestion and tinnitus.

Administration and Dosage: Taken orally, 1.2g each time, once or twice a day.

Preparation Form: Tablet.

Package: 0.4—0.6g in each tablet.

Notes: The prescription is recorded in the book *Bian Zheng Zhun Sheng Hao You Ji* compiled in the Ming Dynasty.

This drug has the effects of antisepsis, antiinflammation and analgesia. It is clinically efficacious for acute pharynglaryngitis. acute tonsillitis. periodontitis, mumps, etc.

Contraindicated for pregnant women, it should not be taken along with enzyme products.

Qingwen Jiedu Wan

Ingredients:

Folium Isatidis	8.3%	*Daqingye*
Fructus Forsythiae	6.3%	*Lianqiao*
Radix Scrophulariae	8.3%	*Xuanshen*
Radix Trichosanthis	8.3%	*Tianhuafen*
Radix Platycodi	6.3%	*Jiegeng*
Fructus Arctii	8.3%	*Niubangzi*
Rhizoma seu Radix Notopterygii	6.3%	*Qianghuo*
Radix Ledebouriellae	4.2%	*Fangfeng*
Radix Puerariae	8.3%	*Gegen*
Radix Bupleuri	4.2%	*Chaihu*
Radix Scutellariae	8.3%	*Huangqin*
Radix Angelicae Dahuricae	4.2%	*Baizhi*
Rhizoma Chuanxiong	4.2%	*Chuanxiong*
Radix Paeoniae Rubra	4.2%	*Chishao*
Herba Lophatheri	8.3%	*Danzhuye*
Radix Glycyrrhizae	2%	*Gancao*

Actions: Driving away pathogens and removing toxic materials.

Indications: Epidemic febrile diseases caused by

exopathogens marked by chills, high fever, headache, anhidrosis, thirst, dry throat, mumps and infection with swollen head.

Administration and Dosage: Taken orally, 2 boluses each time, twice a day.

Preparation Form: Honeyed bolus.

Package: 9g in each bolus.

Notes: The prescription is recorded in the book *Zhen Fang Hui Lu*.

This drug is clinically efficacious for upper respiratory tract infection, acute bronchitis, pneumonia, etc.

It is to be cautiously used for pregnant woman.

Wanshi Niuhuang Qiangxin Wan

Ingredients:

Calculus Bovis	1.7%	*Niuhuang*
Cinnabaris	10.2%	*Zhusha*
Rhizoma Coptidis	33.9%	*Huanglian*
Radix Scutellariae	20.3%	*Huangqin*
Fructus Gardeniae	20.3%	Zhizi
Radix Curcumae	13.6%	Yujin

Actions: Clearing away heat, removing toxic materials, tranquilizing the mind and allaying excitement.

Indications: Syndrome due to accumulation of heat in the interior marked by dysphoria, coma, delirium, and high fever and convulsion in infants.

Administration and Dosage: Taxen orally, 1 bolus each time, twice or 3 times a day.

Preparation Form: Honeyed bolus.

Package: 1.5g in each bolus.

Notes: The prescription is recorded in the book *Dou Zhen Shi Yi Xin Fa* compiled by Wang Chuan in the Ming Dynasty.

This drug is clinically efficacious for primary hypertension, uremic coma, hepatic coma, etc.

Yinqiao Jiedu Pian

Ingredients:

Flos Lonicerae	17.9%	Jinyinhua
Fructus Forsythiae	17.9%	Lianqiao
Herba Menthae	10.7%	Bohe
Herba Schizonepetae	7.2%	Jingjie
Semen Sojae Praeparatum	8.9%	Dandouchi
Fructus Arctii	10.7%	Niubangzi
Radix Platycodi	10.7	Jiegeng
Herba Lophatheri	7.2%	Danzhuye

Radix Glycyrrhizae]8.9% Gancao

Actions: Clearing away heat and removing toxic materials.

Indications: common cold due to wind heat marked by fever, headache, cough, dry month, and swollen and painful throat.

Administration and Dosage: Taken Orally, 4 tablets each time, twice or 3 times a day.

Preparation Form: Tablet.

Package: 1g in each tablet. drug.

Notes: The prescription is recorded in the book *Wen Bing Tiao Bian* compiled by Wu Jutong in the Qing Dynasty.

This drug has the effects of antisepsis, andtivirus and treating diuresis. It is clinically efficacious for common cold, influenza, upper respiratory tract infection, mumps, acute bronchitis, pneumonia, etc.

Xiling Jiedu Pian

Ingredients:

Herba Menthae	*Bohe*
Herba Schizonepetae	*Jingjie*
Fructus Forsythiae	*Lianqiao*
Flos Lonicerae	*Jinyinhua*
Fructus Arctii	*Niubangzi*
Herba Lophatheri	*Danzbuye*
Semen Sojae Praeparatum	*Dandouchi*
Radix Platycodi	*Jiegeng*
Radix Glycyrrhizae	*Gancao*
Corun Antelopis	*Lingyangjiao*
Borneolum Syntheticcum	*Bingpian*

Actions: Clearing away heat to relieve exterior syndrome.

Indications: Fever, headache, cough, swollen and painful throat due to common cold.

Administration and Dosage: Taken orally, 4 tablets each time, 3 times a day.

Preparation Form: Tablet.

Package: 0.25g in each tablet.

Notes: This drug is clinically efficacious for common cold of wind—heat type, upper respiratory tract infection, acute bronchitis, pneumonia, etc.

Xiling Ganmao Pain

Main Ingredients:

Cornu Antelopis	*Lingyangjiao*
Caulis Lonicerae	*Rendongteng*

Flos Chrysanthemi Indici   *Yejuhua*

Rhizoma Menispermi   *Beidougen*

Actions: Clearing away heat and removing toxic materials.

Indications: Headache and cough, swollen and painful throat due to common cold of wind type.

Administration and Dosage: Taken orally, 3–4 tablets each time, 3 ti mes a day.

Preparation Form: Tablet.

Package: 0.3g in each tablet.

Notes: This drug is clinically efficacious for upper respiratory tract infection, acute bronchitis, pneumonia, etc.

Lingqiao Jiedu Pian

Ingredients:

Flos Lonicerae	17.1%	*Jinyinhua*
Fructus Forsythiae	17.1%	Lianqiao
Radix Platycodi	11.4%	*Jiegeng*
Fructus Arctii	11.4%	*Niubangzi*
Herba Menthae	11.4%	*Bohe*
Herba Lophatheri	8.5%	*Danzhuye*
Herba Schizonepetae	8.5%	*Jingjie*
Semen Sojae Preparatum	7.1%	*Dandouchi*
Cornu Antelopis	0.4%	*Lingyangjiao*
Radix Glycyrrhizae	7.1%	*Gancao*

Actions: Dispelling wind, relieving exterior syndrome, clearing away heat and removing toxic materials.

Indications: Symptoms at the onset of common cold such as fever, chills, sore and weak limbs, headache, cough, and swollen and painful throat.

Administration and Dosage: Taken orally, 4—6 tablets each time, twice a day.

Preparation Form: Tablet.

Package: 0.3g in each tablet.

Notes: This drug is clinically efficacious for common cold of wind—heat type, upper respiratory tract infection, pneumonia, etc.

Lianqiao Baidu Wan

Ingredients:

Fructus Forsythiae	7.3%	Lianqiao
Flos Lonicerae	7.3%	Jinyinhua
Radix et Rhizoma Rhei	7.3%	Dahuang
Fructus Gardeniae	5.5%	Zhizi
Radix Scutellariae	5.5%	Huangqin
Caulis Aristolochiae	5.5%	Mutong
Herba Taraxaci	5.5%	Pugongying
Herba Violae	5.5%	Diding
Radix Trichosanthis	3.3%	Tianhuafen
Radix Scrophulariae	5.5%	Xuanshen
Fritillariae Thunbergii	5.5%	Zhebeimu
Radix Ledebouriellae	5.5%	Fangfeng
Radix Angelicae Dahuricae	5.5%	Baizhi
Radix Paeoniae Rubra	5.5%	Chishao
Radix Platycodi	5.5%	Jiegeng
Periostracum Cicadae	3.3%	Chantui
Cortex Dictamni	5.5%	Baixianpi
Radix Glycyrrhizae	5.5%	Gancao

Actions: Clearing away heat, removing toxic materials, relieving swelling and alleviating pain.

Indications: Swelling and pain due to early skin and external diseases, ulcerated sore or bois with burning sensation and pus, and pain and itch due to erysipelas, furuncle, scabies and tinea.

Administration and Dosage: Taken orally, 9g each time, twice daily.

Preparation Form: Water—paste pill.

Package: 3g in every 50 pills.

Notes: The prescription is recorded in the book *Zheng Zhi Zhun Sheng* compiled by Wang Kentang in the Ming Dynasty.

This drug is clinically efficacious for various suppurative dermatitis, dermatophyte, beriberi, etc.

Huanglian Shangqing Wan

Ingredients:

Radix et Rhizoma Rhei	10.8%	Dahuang
Radix Scutellariae	10.8%	Huangqin
Radix Paeoniae Rubra	10.8%	Chishao
Fructus Gardeniae	6.7%	Zhizi
Fructus Forsythiae	6.7%	Lianqiao
Radix Angelicae Sinensis	6.7%	Danggui
Rhizoma Chuanxiong	6.7	Chuanxiong
Herba Menthae	6.7%	Bohe
Herba Schizonepetae	6.7%	Jingjie
Flos Chrysanthemi	5.4%	Juhua
Radix Trichosanthis	5.4%	Tianhuafen
Radix Platycodi	2.8%	Jiegeng
Radix Scrophulariae	2.8%	Xuanshen
Rhizoma Coptidis	5.4%	Huanglian

Cortex Phellodendri   2.8%   *Huangbai*

Radix Glycyrrhizae   2.8%   *Gancao*

Actions: Removing fire, expeling wind, and relaxing the bowels to purge heat.

Indications: Syndrome due to heat of excess type in the stomach and intestines marked by dizziness, tinnitus, aphthae, swollen and painful gum and throat, epidemic hemorrhagic conjunctivitis, constipation and deep—colored urine.

Administration and Dosage: Taken orally, 9g each time, once a day.

Preparation Form: Water—paste pill.

Package: 3g in every 50 pills.

Notes: The prescription is recorded in the book *Wan Bing Hui Chun* compiled by Gong Tingxian in the Ming Dynasty.

This drug has the effects of resisting inflammation, relieving pain and lowering down fever. It is clinically efficacious for acute pharyngolaryngitis, mumps, periodontitis and various infective eye troubles.

It is contraindicated for pregnant women.

Niuhuang Shangqing Wan

Ingredients:

Calculus Bovis	0.3%	*Niuhuang*
Herba Menthae	4.8%	*Bohe*
Flos Chrysanthemi	6.4%	*Juhua*
Herba Schizonepetae	2.6%	*Jingjie*
Radix Angelicae Dahuricae	2.6%	*Baizhi*
Rhizoma Chuanxiong	2.6%	*Chuanxiong*
Fructus Gardeniae	8%	*Zhizi*

Rhizoma Coptidis	2.6%	*Huanglian*
Cortex Phellodendri	1.6%	*Huangbai*
Radix Scutellariae	8%	*Huangqin*
Radix et Rhizoma Rhei	12.9%	*Dahuang*
Fructus Forsythiae	8%	*Lianqiao*
Radix Paeoniae Rubra	2.6%	*Chishao*
Radix Angelicae Sinensis	8%	*Danggui*
Radix Rehmanniae	10.3%	*Dihuang*
Radix Platycodi	2.6%	*Jiegeng*
Gypsum Fibrosum	12.9%	*Shigao*
Borneolum Syntheticum	1.6%	*Bingpian*
Radix Glycyrrhizae	1.6%	*Gancao*

Actions: Clearing away heat, purging fire, dispelling wind and relieving pain.

Indications: Headache, vertigo, conjunctival congestion, tinnitus, swollen and painful throat, aphthae, swollen and painful gum, and dry stools.

Administration and Dosage: Taken orally, 1 bolus each time, twice a day.

Preparation Form: Honeyed bolus

Package: 6g in each bolus

Notes: The prescription is recorded in the book *Yi Xue Ru Men* compiled by Li Chan in the Ming Dynasty.

This drug has the effects of resisting inflammation, lowering down fever and relieving pain. It is clinically efficacious for common cold of wind—heat type, upper respiratory tract infection, periodontitis, etc.

Chuanxiong Chatiao San

Ingredients:

Rhizoma Chuanxiong	16.3%	*Chuanxiong*
Radix Angelicae Dahuricae	8.2%	*Baizhi*
Rhizoma seu Radix Notopterygii	8.2%	*Qianghuo*
Herba Asari	4.1%	*Xixin*
Radix Ledebouriellae	6.1%	*Fangfeng*
Herba Menthae	32.7%	*Bohe*
Herba Schizonepetae	16.3%	*Jingjie*
Radix Glycyrrhizae	8.1%	*Gancao*

Actions: Despelling wind and relieving pain.

Indications: Headache, chills, fever, and stuffy nose due to attack of exopathic wind.

Administration and Dosage: Taken orally, 3—6g each time, twice daily.

Preparation Form: Powder.

Package: 30g in each bag.

Notes: The prescription is recorded in the book *Tai Ping Hui Min He Ji Ju Fang* compiled by Chen Shiwen in the Song Dynasty.

This drug has the effects of allaying inflammation and relieving pain. It is clinically efficacious for common cold of wind—cold type, rhinitis, nasosinustitis and nervous headache.

Sangju Ganmao Pian

Ingredients

Folium Mori	21.2%	*Sangye*
Flos Chrysanthemi	8.4%	*Juhua*

Oleum Menthae	0.1%	Boheyou
Semen Armeniacae Amarum	16.9%	Kuxingren
Radix Platycodi	16.9%	Jiegeng
Fructus Forsythiae	12.8%	Lianqiao
Rhizoma Phragmitis	16.9%	Lugen
Radix Glycyrrhizae	6.8%	Gancao

Actions: Dispelling wind, removing heat and ventilating the lung to relieve cough.

Indications: Early common cold due to wind and heat marked by headache, cough, dry mouth and painful throat.

Administration and Dosage: Taken orally, 4–8 tablets each time, twice or 3 times a day.

Preparation Form: Tablet.

Package: 0.6g in each tablet.

Notes: The prescription is recorded in the book *Wen Bing Tiao Bian* compiled by Wu Jutong in the Qing Dynasty.

This drug is clinically efficaious for common cold, upper respiratory tract infection, bronchitis, pneumonia and acute tonsillitis.

Fufang Daqingye Zhusheye

Ingredients:

Folium Isatidis	44.5%	Daqingye
Flos Lonicerae	22.2%	Jinyinhua
Rhizoma seu Radix Notopterygii	11.1%	Qianghuo
Rhizoma Bistortae	11.1%	Quanshen
Radix et Rhizoma Rhei	11.1%	Dahuang

Actions: Eliminating pathogens and removing toxic materials.

Indications: Fever, cough, dyspnea and swollen and painful throat due to epidemic febrile disease.

Administration and Dosage: Given through intramuscular injection, 2—4ml each time, once or twice a day.

Preparation Form: Injection.

Package: 2ml in each ampule.

Notes: This drug is clinically efficacious for influenza, epidemic encephalomyelitis, mumps, upper respiratory tract infection and virus—pneumonia.

Ganmao Jiere Chongji

Ingredients:

Herba Ephedrae	8.1%	Mahuang
Flos Chrysanthemi	8.1%	Juhua
Rhizoma Atractylodis Macrocephalae	8.1%	Baizhu
Rhizoma seu Radix Notopterygii	8.1%	Qianghuo
Radix Ledebouriellae	8.1%	Fangfeng
Rhizoma Zingiberis Recens	5.4%	Shengjiang
Gypsum Fibrosum	27.1%	Shigao
Radix Puerariae	16.2	Gegen
Ramulus Uncariae cum Uncis	10.8%	Gouteng

Actions: Dispelling wind and clearing away heat.

Indications: Aversion to cold, fever, aching of limbs, dizziness and headache due to common cold.

Administration and Dosage: Taken orally, 1—2 bag each time, 3 times daily.

Preparation Form: Granule or power dissolvable in water.

Package: 15g in each bag.

Notes: This drug is clinically efficacious for upper

respiratory tract infection, influenza, bronchitis, innominatal—fever, etc.

Niuhuang Xiaoyan Wan

Ingredients:

Calculus Bovis	9.7%	*Niuhuang*
Radix et Rhizoma Rhei	19.2%	*Dahuang*
Radix Trichosanthis	19.2%	*Tianhuafen*
Indigo Naturalis	7.7%	*Qingdai*
Venenum Bufonis	5.8%	*Chansu*
Realgar	19.2%	*Xionghuang*
Concha Margaritifera Usta	19.2%	*Zhenzhumu*

Actions: Clearing away heat, removing toxic materials, reducing swelling and alleviating pain.

Indications: Swollen and painful throat, furuncle, carbuncle, and skin and external diseases.

Administration and Dosage: Taken orally, 10 pills each time, 3 times a day, or ground into powder, mixed well with water and applied to the affected part.

Preparation Form: Water—paste pill

Package: 0.3g in every 60 pills.

Notes: This drug is clinically efficacious for upper respiratory tract infection, laryngopharyngitis, multiple abscess, etc.

Ganmao Qingre Chongji

Ingredients:

Herba Schizonepetae	16.9%	*Jingjie*
Herba Menthae	5.1%	*Bohe*

Radix Ledebouriellae	8.5%	*Fangfeng*
Radix Bupleuri	8.5%	*Chaihu*
Folium Perillae	5.1%	*Zisuye*
Radix Puerariae	8.5%	*Gegen*
Radix Platycodi	5.1%	*Jiegeng*
Semen Armeniacae Amarum	6.8%	*Kuxingren*
Radix Angelicae Dahuricae	5.1%	*Baizhi*
Herba Violae	16.9%	*Kudiding*
Rhizoma Phragmitis	13.5%	*Lugen*

Actions: Expelling wind, dispersing cold, relieving exterior syndrome and clearing away heat.

Indications: Headache, fever, aversion to cold, general ache, stuffy nose with running clear discharge, cough and dry throat due to common cold of wind cold type.

Administration and Dosage: Taken orally, 12g each time, twice a day.

Preparation Form: Granule or powder dissolvable in water.

Package: 12g in each bag.

Notes: This drug is clinically efficacious for common cold of wind—cold type and upper respiratory tract infection.

Fangfeng Tongsheng Wan

Ingredients:

Radix Ledebouriellae	3.8%	*Fangfeng*
Herba Schizonepetae	1.9%	*Jingjie*
Herba Menthae	3.8%	*Bohe*
Herba Ephedrae	3.8%	*Mahuang*
Radix et Rhizoma Rhei	3.8%	*Dahuang*
Natrii Sulfas	3.8%	*Mangxiao*

Fructus Gardeniae	1.9%	Zhizi
Talcum	22.6%	Huashi
Radix Platycodi	7.5%	Jiegeng
Gypsum Fibrosum	7.5%	Shigao
Rhizoma Chuanxiong	3.8%	Chuanxiong
Radix Angelicae Sinensis	3.8%	Danggui
Radix Paeoniae Alba	3.8%	Baishao
Radix Scutellariae	7.5%	Huangqin
Fructus Forsythiae	3.8%	Lianqiao
Radix Glycyrrhizae	15%	Gancao
Rhizoma Atractylodis Macrocephalae	1.9%	Baizhu

Actions: Relieving exterior syndrome, clearing away interior heat and removing toxic materials.

Indications: Aversion to cold, high fever, headache, dry throat, oliguria with reddish urine and dry stools due to exogenous cold of excess type in the exterior and endogenous heat of excess type in the interior, early scrofula, rubella, and sore due to dampness.

Administration and Dosage: Taken orally, 6g each time, twice daily.

Preparation Form: Water–paste pill.

Package: 3g in every 50 pills.

Notes: The prescription is recorded in the book *Xuan Ming Lun Fang* compiled by Liu Wansu in the Jin Dynasty.

This drug is clinically efficacious for common cold with fever, pyogenic infection of skin, urticaria, adiposis, hypertension, etc.

Jiuwei Qianghuo Wan

Ingredients:

Rhizoma sue Radix Notopterygii	15%	Qianghuo
Radix Ledebouriellae	15%	Fangfeng
Rhizoma Atractylodis	15%	Cangzhu
Herba Asari	5%	Xixin
Rhizoma Chuanxiong	10%	Chuanxiong
Radix Angelicae Dahuricae	10%	Baizhi
Radix Scutellariae	10%	Huangqin
Radix Rehmanniae	10%	Dihuang
Radix Glycyrrhizae	10%	Gancao

Actions: Inducting diaphoresis to eliminate dampness.

Indications: Aversion to cold, fever, anhidrosis, headache, dry mouth, and aching limbs.

Administration and Dosage: Taken orally, 6—9g each time, twice or 3 times a day.

Preparation Form: Water—paste pill

Package: 31g in every 500 pills.

Notes: The prescription is recorded in the book *Ci Shi Nan Zhi* compiled by Wang Haogu in the Yuan Dynasty.

This drug is clinically efficacious for common cold of wind—cold type, influenza, upper respiratory tract infectin, rheumatic arthritis, etc.

Yinhuang Pian

Ingredients:

Extractum Lonicerae Inspissatum	56%	Jingyinhuagao
Baicalein	44%	Huangqinsu

Actions: Clearing away heat and removing toxic materials.

Indications: Skin and external diseases, dysentery, erysipelas and swollen and painful throat.

Administration and Dosage: Taken orally, 4—6 tablets each time, 4 times a day.

Preparation Form: Tablet.

Package: Each tablet contains not less than 18mg of chlorogenic acid and 36mg baiclin.

Notes: This drug has the effects of antibacteria antiinflammation, antivirus, and diuresis. It is clinically efficacious for upper respiratory tract infection, acute enteritis, bacillary dysentery, pneumonia, etc.

Ganmao Chongji

Ingredients:

Caulis Lonicerae	31.6%	Rendongteng
Radix Isatidis	22.6%	Banlangen
Radix Peucedani	10.1%	Qianhu
Radix Platycodi	10.1%	Jiegeng
Radix Puerariae	10.1%	Gegen
Radix Glycyrrhizae	10.1%	Gancao
Fructus Arctii	5.1%	Niubangzi
Menthol	0.3%	Bohenao

Actions: Clearing away heat, removing toxic materials and ventilating the lung to resolve phlegm.

Indications: Headache, cough and swollen and painful throat due to common cold of wind—heat type.

Administration and Dosage: Taken orally, 1—2 bags each time, 3 times daily. For children, the dosage should be reduced properly.

Preparation Form: Granule or powder dissolvable in water.

Package: 15g in eath bag.

Notes: This drug is clinically efficacious for upper respiratory tract infection, acut mumps, epidemic cerebrospinal meningtis, etc.

Fenghan Ganmao Chongji

Ingredients:

Ramulus Cinnamomi	*Guizhi*
Radix Angelicae Dahuricae	*Baizhi*
Herba Schizonepetae	*Jingjie*
Rhizoma seu Radix Notopterygii	*Qianghuo*
Radix Paeoniae Alba	*Baishao*
Radix Puerariae	*Gegen*
Semen Armeniacae Amarum	*Xingren*

Actions: Inducing diaphoresis to dispel cold, clearing away heat to relieve cough.

Indications: Aversion to cold, fever, headache, stiffness of nape, general aching and cough due to common cold of wind—cold type.

Administration and Dosage: Taken orally, 1 bag each time, 3 times a day.

Preparation Form: Granule or powder dissolvable in water.

Package: 12g in each bag.

Notes: This drug is clinically efficacious for common cold of wind—cold type, upper respiratory tract infection, bronchitis and pneumonia.

Fanggan Pian

Main Ingredients:

Radix Astragali   *Huangqi*

Rhizoma Astractylodis Macrocephalae   *Baizhu*

Actions: Replenishing *Qi* to invigorate the spleen, normalizing the functioning of the body to strengthen superficial resistance, and suppressing sweating.

Indications: Dizziness, lassitude, swollen and painful throat, spontaneous perspiration and dyspnea due to general deficiency of *Qi* and attack of wind.

Administration and Dosage: Taken orally, 5—7 tablets each time, twice daily.

Preparation Form: Tablet.

Package: 0.32g in each tablet.

Notes: This drug is clinically efficacious for common cold due to general deficiency, upper respiratory tract infection, bronchial asthma,etc.

Banlangen Gantangjiang

Ingredient:

Radix Isatidis   100%   *Banlangen*

Actions: Clearing away heat from blood, removing toxic materials and promoting subsidence of swelling.

Indications: Flushed face with edema, swollen and painful throat, thirst, dysphoria and measles.

Administration and Dosage: Taken orally, 5g each time, 6 times a day.

Preparation Form: Cranule.

Package: 10g in each bag.

Notes: This drug has the effects of broad-spectrum antisepsis and antivirus. It is clinically efficacious for epidmic mumps, epidemic encephalomyelitis, infective hepatitis, upper respiratory tract infection, etc.

Fufang Chaihu Zhusheye

Ingredients:

Radix Bupleuri	91%	Chaihu
Herba Asari	9%	Xixin

Actions: Clearing away damp-heat, inducing diaphoresis and alleviating pain.

Indications: Headache, cough and general aching due to affection of wind.

Administration and Dosage: Given through intramuscular injection, 2-4ml each time, once or twice daily.

Preparation Form: Injection.

Package: 2ml in each ample.

Notes: This drug is clinically efficacious for common cold, upper respiratory tract infection, bronchopneumonia, herpes simplex, viral keratitis, etc.

Xiougju Shangqing Wan

Ingredients:

Radix et Rhizoma Rhei	8.6%	Dahuang
Fructus Gardeniae	8.6%	Zhizi
Rhizoma Chuanxiong	8.6%	Chuanxiong
Radix Ledebouriellae	8.6%	Fangfeng
Radix Platycodi	8.6%	Jiegeng

Flos Chrysanthemi	8.6%	*Juhua*
Radix Scutellariae	8.6%	*Huangqin*
Herba Schizonepetae	4.3%	*Jingjie*
Herba Menthae	4.3%	*Bohe*
Talcum	5.6%	*Huashi*
Radix Glycyrrhizae	12.8%	*Gancao*
Cortex Phellodendri	12.8%	*Huangbai*

Actions: Expelling wind and clearing away heat.

Indications: Headache, dizziness, epidemic hemorrhagic conjunctivitis, stuffy nose and tinnitus due to wind heat in the upper—*Jiao*.

Administration and Dosage: Taken orally, 6g each time, twice a day.

Preparation Form: Water—paste pill.

Package: 1g in every 20 pills.

Notes: The prescription is recorded in the book *Tai Ping Hui Min He Ji Ju Fang* compiled by Chen Shiwen in the Song Dynasty.

This drug is clinically efficacious for upper respiratory tract infection, nervous headache, nasosinusitis, rhinitis, ophthalmia, and hypertension.

Qingxuan Wan

Ingredients:

Rhizoma Chuanxiong	28.6%	*Chuanxiong*
Radix Angelicae Dahuricae	28.6%	*Baizhi*
Herba Menthae	14.3%	*Bohe*
Herba Schizonepetae	14.3%	*Jingjie*
Gypsum Fibrosum	14.2%	*Shigao*

Acitons: Expelling wind and clearing away heat.

Indications: Dizziness, migraine, headache, stuffy nose and toothache due to wind—heat.

Administration and Dosage: Taken orally, 1—2 boluses each time, twice daily.

Preparation Form: Honeyed bolus.

Package: 6g in each bolus.

Notes: The prescription is recorded in the book *Wei Sheng Bao Jian* compiled by Luo Tianyi in the Yuan Dynasty.

This drug is clinically efficacious for headache due to common cold, nasosinusitis, rhinitis, prosopalgia, hypertension, etc.

Kangjun Xiaoyan Pian

Ingredients:

Flos Lonicerae	17.8%	*Jinyinhua*
Folium Isatidis	17.8%	*Daqingye*
Radix Stemonae	17.8%	*Baibu*
Herba Lysimachiae	17.8%	*Jinqiancao*
Rhizoma Anemarrhenae	14.6%	*Zhimu*
Radix Scutellariae	8.9%	*Huangqin*
Radix et Rhizoma Rhei	5.3%	*Dahuang*

Actions: Clearing away heat and removing toxic materials.

Indications: Swollen and painful throat due to affection of exopathogenic wind—heat, skin and external diseases, and symptoms due to damp—heat in the lower—Jiao.

Administration and Dosage: Taken orally 4—8 tablets each time, 3 times daily.

Preparation Form: Tablet.

Package: 0.25g in each tablet.

Notes: This drug is clinically efficacious for upper respiratory tract infection, periodontitis, pyogenic infection of skin, inflammation due to trauma, etc.

Qianliguang Pian

Ingredient:

Herba Senecionis Scandentis   100%   *Qianliguang*

Actions: Clearing away heat and removing toxic materials.

Indications: Swelling and pain of throat due to endogenous dampness and exogenous pathogens, and diarrhea due to damp—heat.

Administration and Dosage: Taken orally, 3—5 tablets each time, 3 times daily.

Preparation Form: Tablet.

Package: 2g in each tablet.

Notes: This drug is clinically efficacious for upper respiratory tract infection, lobar pneumonia, acute enteritis, acute appendicitis, acute bacillary dysentery and trichomonal vaginitis.

Sijiqing Pian

Ingredient:

Folium Ilicis Chinensis   100%   *Sijiqing*

Actions: Clearing away heat and removing toxic materials.

Indications: Cough due to lung—heat, swelling and pain of throat, dribbling and difficult and pain ful micturition, scald, furuncle and carbuncle.

Administration and Dosage: Taken orally, 5 tablets each time, 3 times a day.

Preparation Form: Tablet.

Package: 4g in each tablet.

Notes: This drug has the effects of broad—spectrum antisepsis. It is clinically efficacious for acute or chronic tonsillitis, acute or chronic bacillary dysentery, enteritis, urinary tract infection, traumatic infection, etc.

Jinyinhua Lu

Ingredient:

Flos Lonicerae   100%   JInyinhua

Actions: Clearing away heat and removing toxic materials.

Indication: Disphoria and thirst due to summer—heat, eruptive disease, large carbuncle, and fetal toxins in infants.

Administration and Dosage: Taken orally, 30—50ml each time, twice or 3 times daily.

Preparation Form: Distillate.

Package: 500ml in each bottle.

Notes: This drug is clinically efficacious for summer hidradenitis, infection due to skin papule, heatstroke, dry mouth and, skin infection of the newborn.

Yili   Zhu

Main Ingredients:

Calculus Bovis	Niuhuang
Resina Olibani	Ruxiang
Myrrha	Moyao
Margarita	Zhenzhu
Venenum Bufonis	Chansu
Borneolum Syntheticum	Bingpian

Actions: Promoting blood circulation, reducing swelling and

removing toxic materials.

Indications: Swelling and pain due to early carbuncle, furuncle, skin and external diseases, acute mastitis and breast carcinoma, all of which have not broken or have suppurated.

Administration and Dosage: Taken orally, 1.5g each time, once a day.

Preparation Form: Water—paste pill.

Package: 3g in every 50 pills.

Notes: The prescription is recorded in the book *Liang Fang Ji Ye* compiled by Xie Yunqing in the Qing Dynasty.

This drug is clinically efficacious for mastadenitis, multiple abscess and pyogenic infection of skin.

Gegen Qinlian Pian

Ingredients:

Radix Puerariae	50%	*Gegen*
Radix Scutellariae	18.8%	*Huangqin*
Rhizoma Coptidis	18.7%	*Huanglian*
Radix Glycyrrhizae	12.5%	*Gancao*

Acitons: Relieving exterior syndrome and clearing away interior heat.

Indications: Fever, dyspnea, sweating, restlessness, thirst, abdominal pain and diarrhea.

Preparation Form: Tablet.

Administration and Dosage: Taken orally, 3—4 tablets each time, 3 times daily.

Package: 0.3g in each tablet.

Notes: The prescription is recorded in the book *Shang Han Lun* compiled by Zhang Ji in the Han Dynasty.

This drug is clinically efficacious for acute gastroenteritis, bacillary dysentery, etc.

9 Antirheumatics

Fengliaoxing Yaojiu

Ingredients:

Caulis Erycibae	*Dinggongteng*
Radix Angelicae Dahuricae	*Baizhi*
Cortex Acanthopanacis Radicis	*Wujiapi*
Herba Ephedrae	*Mahuang*
Fructus Artemisiae Chinghao	*Qinghaozi*
Radix Angelicae Sinensis	*Dangguiwei*
Ramulus Cinnamomi	*Guizhi*
Fructus Foeniculi	*Xiaohuixiang*
Rhizoma Ligustici Chuanxiong	*Chuanxiong*
Radix Clematidis	*Weilingxian*
Radix Stephaniae Tetrandrae	*Fangji*
Fructus Gardeniae	*Zhizi*
Rhizoma seu Radix Notopterygii	*Qianghuo*
Radix Angelicae Pubescentis	*Duhuo*

Actions: Dispelling wind to remove obstruction in the channels, dispersing cold to relieve pain.

Indications: Arthralgia due to wind—cold—dampness, numbness of Limbs, soreness of tendons and bones and debility of the tower back and knees.

Administration and Dosage: Taken orally, 15ml each time, 3 times a day.

Preparation Form: Medicated alcohol

Package: 500ml in each bottle.

Notes: This medicated alcohol has the effects of struggling against inflammation and rheumatism, improving microcirculation, eliminatin swelling and relieving pain. It is clinically used to treat rheumatic and rheumatoid arthritis (arthralgia due to wind—cold—dampness), swelling and pain due to injury.

Wujiapi Yaojiu

Ingredients:

Rhizoma Polygonati Odorati	23.2%	Yuzhu
Radix Codonopsis Pilosulae	8.7%	Dangshen
Rhizoma Curcumae Longae	8.7%	Jianghuang
Cortex Acanthopanacis Radicis	5.8%	Wujiapi
Pericarpium Citri Reticulatae	5.8%	Chenpi
Flos Chrysanthemi	2.9%	Jühua
Flos Carthami	2.9%	Honghua
Radix Achyranthis Bidentatae	2.9%	Niuxi
Rhizoma Atractylodis Macroscephalae	2.2%	Baizhu (Fuchao)
Radix Angelicae Dahuricae	2.2%	Baizhi
Radix Angelicae Sinensis	1.4%	Danggui
Caulis Sinomenii	1.4%	Qingfengteng
Rhizoma Chuanxiong	1.4%	Chuanxiong
Radix Clematidis	1.4%	Weilingxian
Lignum Santali	1.4%	Tanxiang
Caulis Piperis Kadsurae	1.4%	Haifengteng
Semen Myristicae	1.1%	Roudoukou
Radix Angelicae Pubescentis	0.7%	Duhuo

Radix Aconiti Kusnezoffii	0.7%	*Caowu*
Fructus Amomi Rotundus	0.7%	*Doukou*
Flos Caryophylli	0.7%	*Dingxiang*
Fructus Amomi	0.7%	*Sharen*
Radix Aucklandiae	0.7%	*Muxiang*
Cortex Cinnamomi	0.7%	*Rougui*
Fructus Gardeniae	16.4%	*Zhizi*
Fructus Chaenomelis	1.4%	*Mugua*
Radix Aconiti	0.7%	*Chuanwu*

Acitons: Relaxing tendons, promoting blood circulation, and expelling dampness and wind.

Indications: Flaccidity due to wind–dampness, muscular contracture of hands and feet, numbness of limbs, pain in the loins and knees, and wetness and cold of scrotum.

Administration and Dosage: Taken orally, 10 to 15ml each time, twice daily.

Preparation Form: Medicated alcohol

Package: 500ml in each bottle.

Notes: This medicated alcohol has the effects of resisting inflammation, relieving pain, struggling against rheumatism and improving microcirculation. Clinically, it is administered to treat rheumatic and rheumatoid arthritis and senile numbness of limbs.

This sort of alcohol has stronger nourishing effects than *Fengliaoxing Yaojiu*. When it is used to treat patients who are old or weak, better curative effects will be achieved.

Guogong Jiu

Ingredients:

Rhizoma Polygonati Odorati *Yüzu*

Pericarpium Citri Reticulatae	*ChenPi*
Semen Oryzae cum Monasco	*Hongqu*
Cortex Cinnamomi	*Rougui*
Flos Cryophylli	*Dingxiang*
Fructus Amomi	*Sharen*
Semen Myristicae	*Roudoukou*
Radix Aucklandiae	*Muxiang*
Lignum Santali Albi	*Tanxiang*
Radix Rehamanniae	*Dihuang*
Herba Erodii seu Gerantii	*Laoguancao*
Radix Angelicae Sinensis	*Danggui*
Radix Achyranthis Bidentatae	*Niuxi*
Fructus Aurantii	*Zhique*
Radix Ophiopogonis	*Maimendong*
Radix Atractylodis Macrocephalae	*Baizhu*
Rhizoma Atractylodis	*Cangzhu*
Semen Arecae	*Binlang*
Rhizoma Chuanxiong	*Chuanxiong*
Fructus Chaenomelis	*Mugua*
Radix Angelicae Dahuricae	*Baizhi*
Cortex Moutan Radicis	*Danpi*
Rhizoma seu Radix Notopterygii	*Qianghuo*
Cortex Magnoliae Officinalis	*Houpu*
Herba Agastachis	*Huoxiang*
Flos Carthami	*Honghua*
Radix Angelicae Pubescentis	*Duhuo*
Fructus Lycii	*Gouqizi*
Radix Paeoniae Alba	*Baishao*
Fructus Psoraleae	*Buguzhi*

Fructus Citri Sarcodae	*Fusou*
Fructus Crataegi	*Shanzha*
Fructus Gardeniae	*Zhizi*
Cortex Periplocae Radicis	*Xiangjiapi*
Radix Ledebouriellae	*FangFeng*
Radix Arnebiae Seu Lithospermi	*Zicao*
Mel	*Fengmi*

Actions: Expelling wind and removing dampness, nourishing blood and activating the collaterals.

Indications: Arthralgia due to wind—cold—dampness marked by numbness of limbs and pain of joints.

Administration and Dosage: Taken orally, 10ml to 15ml each time, twice daily.

Preparation Form: Medicated alcohol.

Package: 250ml in each bottle.

Notes: This alcohol has the effects of resisting bacteria and inflammation, promoting microcirculation and nourishing the body. It is clinically used to treat rheumatic arthritis, rheumatoid arthritis and senile numbness of limbs. Taking it with Asprine or Sodium salicylate is not allowed.

Fengshi Yaojiu

Ingredients:

Radix Aconiti Kusnezoffii	0.9%	*Caowu*
Flos Carthami	0.9%	*Honghua*
Semen Oryzae cum Monasco	1.3%	*Hongqu*
Herba Erodii seu Geranii	0.9%	*Laoguancao*
Cortex Lycii	0.4%	*Digupi*
Semen Coicis	0.9%	*Yiyiren*

Rhizoma Atractylodis Macrocephatae	0.4%	*Baizhu*
Herba Ephedrae	0.9%	*Mahuang*
Rhizoma Zingiberis	0.4%	*Shengjiang*
Ramulus Cinnamomi	0.4%	*Guihzi*
Radix Stephaniae Tetrandrea	0.4%	*Fangji*
Radix Astragali	0.4%	*Huangqi*
Semen Strychni	0.4%	*Maqianzi*
Radix Paeoniae Rubra	0.4%	*Chishao*
Cortex Cinnamomi	0.4%	*Rougui*
SemenAlpiniae Katsumadai	0.4%	*Caokou*
Cortex Periplocae Radicis	0.4%	*Xiangjiapi*
Radix Clematidis	0.4%	*Weilingxian*
Fructus Chaenomelis	0.4%	*Mugua*
Radix Salviae Miltiorrhizae	0.4%	*Danshen*
Rhizoma Dioscoreae	0.4%	*Shanshao*
Rhizoma Atractylodis	0.4%	*Cangzhu*
Exocarpium Citri Reticulatae	0.2%	*Juhong*
Rhizoma Aipinae Officinarum	0.4%	*Gaoliangjiang*
Alcohol	87.1%	*Baijiu*

Actions: Expelling wind and removing dampness, clearing and activating the channels and collaterals.

Indications: Pain in the loins and legs, muscular contraction of hands and feet, hemiparalysis, and arthralgia due to wind—dampness.

Administration and Dosage: Taken orally, 15ml to 25ml each time, twice daity

Preparation Form: Medicated alcohol.

Notes: With the effects of resisting rheumatism and inflammation, relieving pain and improving microcirculation, this medicated alcohol is suitable for the treatment of rheumatic arthritis and palsy.

Package: 250ml in each bothe.

Taking it with Asprine and Sodium salicylate, is not allowed.

Shujn Huoluo Jiu

Ingredients:

Fructus Chaenomelis	4.1%	Mugua
Ramulus Loranthi	6.8%	Sangjisheng
Rhizoma Polygonati Odorati	21.6%	Yuzhu
Radix Dipsaci	2.7%	Xuduan
Radix Cyathulae	8.2%	Chuanniuxi
Radix Angelicae Sinensis	4.1%	Danggui
Rhizoma Chuanxiong	5.4%	Chuanxiong
Flos Carthami	4.1%	Honghua
Radix Angelicae Pubescentis	2.7%	Duhuo
Rhizoma seu Radix Notopterygii	2.7%	Qianghuo
Radix Ledebouriellae	5.4%	Fangfeng
Rhizoma Atractylodis Macrocephalae	8.2%	Baizhu
Exrementum Bombycis	5.4%	Cansha
Semen Oryzae cum Monasco	16.2%	Hongqu
Radix Glycyrrhizae	2.7%	Gancao

Actions: Expelling wind, removing dampness, relaxing muscles and tendons, and activating the collaterats.

Indications: Arthralgia due to wind—cold—dampness, pain of tendons and bones and numbness of limbs.

Administration andDosage:

Taken orally, 20ml to 30ml each time, twice a day.

Preparation Form: Medicated alcohol.

Package: 250ml in each bottle.

Notes: This medicated alcohol can resist rheumatism and inflammation, relieve pain and improve microcirculation.

Goupi Gao

Ingredients:

Fructus Aurantii	Zhique
Pericarpium Citri Reticulatae Viride	Qingpi
Semen Hydnocarp	Dafengzi
Halloysitum Rubrum	Chishizhi
Radix Paeoniae Rubra	Chishao
Rhizoma Gastrodiae	Tianma
Radix Glycyrrhizae	Gancao
Radix Linderae	Wuyao
Radix Achyranthis Bidentatae	Niuxi
Rhizoma seu Radix Notopterygii	Qianghuo
Cortex Phellodendri	Huangbai
Fructus Psoraleae	Buguzhi
Radix Clematidis	Weilingxian
Radix Aconiti	Shengchuanwu
Radix Dipsaci	Xuduan
Radix Ampelopsis	Bailian
Semen Persicae	Taoren
Radix Aconiti Praeparata	Shengfuzi
Rhizoma Chuanxiong	Chuanxiong
Radix Aconiti Kusnezoffii	Shengcaowu
Cortex Eucommiae	Duzhong
Radix Polygalae	Yuanzhi
Rhizoma Cyperi	Xiangfu

Rhizoma Atractylodis Macrocephalae	*Baizhu*
Fructus Meliae Toosendan	*Chuanlianzi*
Bombyx Batryticatus	*Jiangcan*
Fructus Foeniculi	*Xiaohuixiang*
Fructus Cnidii	*Shechuangzi*
Radix Angelicae Sinensis	*Danggui*
Herba Asari	*Xixin*
Semen Cuscutae	*Tusizi*
Pericarpium Citri Reticulatae	*Chenpi*
Caulis Sinomenii	*Qingfengteng*
Radix Aucklandiae	*Muxiang*
Cortex Cinnamomi	*Rougui*
Calomeas	*Qingfen*
Catechu	*Ercha*
Flos Caryophylli	*Dingxiang*
Resina Olibani	*Ruxiang*
Myrrha	*Moyao*
Resina Draconis	*Xuejie*
Camphora	*Zhangnao*

Actions: Expelling wind, clearing away cold, relaxing muscles and tendons, promoting blood circulation and alleviating pain.

Indications: Arthralgia due to wind—cold—dampness, pain in the shoulders, arms, loins and legs, numbness of limbs, and sprain due to injury.

Administration and Dosage: Softened through heating and applied to the affected area.

Preparation Form: Black plaster.

Package: 15g or 30g included in each piece of this plaster.

Notes: The effects of this plaster are bacteriostasis, anti—inflammation, anagesia and microcirculation—improvement. It is clinically used for rheumatalgia, neuralgia, pain and swelling due to sprain.

Jinbuhuan Gaoyao

Ingredients:

Radix Angelicae Sinensis	*Danggui*
Radix Angelicae Pubescentis	*Duhuo*
Rhizoma Atractylodis	*Cangzhu*
Cortex Eucommiae	*Duzhong*
Radix Aconiti	*Chuanwu*
Rhizoma Alpiniae Officinari	*Gaoliangjiang*
Radix Gentianae Macrophyllae	*Qinjiao*
Radix Angelicae Dahuricae	*Baizhi*
Rhizoma seu Radix Notopterygii	*Qianghuo*
Rhizoma Zingiberis	*Ganjiang*
Herba Schizonepetae	*Jingjie*
Radix Ledebouriellae	*Fangfeng*
Rhizoma Chuanxiong	*Chuanxiong*
Radix Scrophulariae	*Xuanshen*
Radix Glycyrrhizae	*Gancao*
Myrrha	*Moyao*
Resina Olibani	*Ruxiang*
Os Oraconis	*Longgu*
Os Sepiellae seu Sepiae	*Haipiaoxiao*
Radix Aconiti Kusnezoffii	*Caowu*
Radix Rehmanniae	*Dihuang*
Herba Ephedrae	*Mahuang*

Cortex Cinnamomi	Rougui
Resina Draconis	Xuejie

Actions: Expelling wind and promoting blood circulation, eliminating swelling and alleviating pain.

Indications: Arthralgia due to wind—cold—dampness, numbness of limbs, pain in the loins and legs, traumatic injury and pain of muscles and joints.

Administration and Dosage: Soflened through heating and applied to the affected area.

Preparation Form: Black plaster.

Package: 10g of this plaster included in each piece of it.

Notes: With the effects of resisting rheumatism, relieving swelling, stopping pain and promoting microcirculation, this plaster is clinically used for the treatment of rheumatic arthritis, neuralgia and sprain—pain.

Fengshi Zhitong Gao

Ingredients:

Resina Olibani	Ruxiang
Myrrha	Moyao
Camphora	Zhangnao
Menthol	Bohenao
Radix Aconiti	Chuanwu
Herba Schizonepetae	Jingjie
Rhizoam Zingiberis	Ganjinag
Borneolum Syntheticum	Bingpian
Herba Menthae	Behe
Flos Caryophylli	Dingxina
Flos Carthami	Honghua

Radix Aconiti Kusnezoffii	*Caowu*
Radix Ledebouriellae	*Fangfeng*
Flos Lonicerae	*Jinyinhua*
Radix Angelicae Singensis	*Danggui*

Actions: Expelling wind, removing dampness, eliminating blood stasis and alleviating pain.

Indications: Pain of the loins, shoulders, extremities and muscles due to wind—cold—dampness.

Administration and Dsoage: Applied to the affected area which has been washed clean and wiped.

Preparation Form: Rubber plaster.

Package: Each piece of it is 5 × 7cm.

Notes: This drug has the effects of anti—rheumatism, anti—inflammation, analgesia and microcirculation—improvement.It is clinically efficacious for pain of loins, shoulders, extremities, joints and muscles, which is caused by rheumatic orrheumatoid arthritis and muscle—fiber inflammation. It should be cautious to apply this drug to those who are hypersensitive to adhesive plaster.

Shangshi Qutong Gao

Ingredients:

Rhizoma Zingiberis	19.3%	*Ganjiang*
Rhizoma Atractylodis	14.3%	*Cangzhu*
Rhizoma Chuanxiong	7.1%	*Chuanxiong*
Herba Ephedrae	7.1%	*Mahuang*
Fructus Illicii Veri	4.6%	*Bajiaohuixiang*
Camphora	2%	*Zhangnao*
Borneolum Syntheticum	2%	*Bingpian*

Radix Angelicae Dahuricae	9.1%	*Baizhi*
Radix Angelicae Sinesis	14.3%	*Danggui*
Radix Aconiti Kusnezoffii	7.1%	*Caowu*
Rhizoma Kaempferiae	5.8%	*Shannai*
Oil of Llicis Pedunculosae	3%	*Dongqingyou*
Menthol	4.1%	*Bohenao*

Actions: Expelling wind, removing dampness and alleviating pain.

Indications: Rheumatalgia, numbness of limbs, headache, and swelling and pain due to sprain.

Administration and Dosage: Applied to the affected area which has been washed clean and wiped.

Preparation Form: Rubber plaster

Package: Each piece of this plaster is 5 × 6.5cm.

Notes: This plaster has the effects of anti—rheumatism, anti—inflammation, analgesia and microcirculation—improvement. It is clinically efficacious for rheumatic arthritis, muscle—fiber inflammation, muscular injury due to pulling—force and neuritis. It is forbidden to use this plaster for those who are hypersensitive to adhesive plaster or suffering from skin—exudate, traumatic bleeding and suppuration.

Yanghe Jienjing Gao

Ingredients:

Fructus Arctii	*Niubangzi*
Caulis Lmpatients	*Fengxiantougucao*
Ramulus Cinnamomi	*Guizhi*
Radix Angelicae Sinensis	*Danggui*
Radix Aconiti	*Shengfuzi*

Radix Aconiti	*Shengchuanwu*
Radix et Rhizoma Rhei	*Dahuang*
Radix Aconiti Kusnezoffii	*Shengcaowu*
Lumbricus	*Dilong*
Bombyx Batryticatus	*Jiangcan*
Radix Angelicae Dahuricae	*Baizhi*
Rhizoma Bletillae	*Baiji*
Radix Dipsaci	*Xuduan*
Herba Schizonepetae	*Jingjie*
Radix Aucklandiae	*Muxiang*
Pericarpium Citri Reticulatae	*Chenpi*
Cortex Cinnamomi	*Rougui*
Myrrha	*Moyao*
Radix Paeoniae Rubra	*Chishao*
Radix Ampelopsis	*Bailian*
Rhizoma Chuanxiong	*Chuanxiong*
Radix Ledebouriellae	*Fangfeng*
Faeces Trogopterorum	*Wulingzhi*
Resina Boswelliae Carterii	*Xiangmuyuan*
Fructus Citri	*Xiangyuan*
Styrax	*Suhexiang*

Actions: Warming *Yang* and expelling dampness, reducing swelling and removing masses.

Indications: Deep—rooted carbuncle of *Yin* type, unburst scrofula, and numbness and pain due to cold—dampness.

Administration and Dosage: Used externally, softened through heating and applied to the affected area.

Preparation Form Black plaster

Package: 1.5g, 3g or 6g included in each piece of it.

Notes: The effects of this plaster are anti—bacteria, anti—inflammation, anti—tuberculosis and anti—rheumatism. It is clinically efficacious for bone tuberculosis, tuberculosis of peritoneum, scrofula, thromboangiitis, chronic rheumatic arthritis and muscle—fiber inflammation.

It can't beu sed for pyogenic infection and ulceration of skin with swelling and pain.

Shangshi Baozhen Gao

Ingredients:

Extract of Herba Cymbopogonis	*Yunxiangjingao*
Camphora	*Zhangnao*
Fluid extract of Co. Xixin	*Fufongxixinjingao*
Menthol	*Bohenao*
Oil of Licis Pedunculosae	*Dongqingyou*

Actions: Expelling wind and dampness, removing stagnation of *Qi* by warming the channels.

Indications: Traumatic injury, rheumatic neuralgia, omalgia, dorsalgia and lumbago.

Administration and Dosage: Applied to the affected area with dress change done every 4 to 5 days.

Preparation Form: Plaster.

Package: 2 pieces of it in each bag.

Notes: This plaster has the effects of anti—inflammation, anti—rheumatism and microcirculatory improvement. It is clinically efficacious for rheumatic arthritis, pain of loins and kness, muscular tension, rheumatic neuralgia and traumatic pain.

It is contraindicated for pregnant women.

Shangshi Zhitong Gao

Ingredients:

Borneolum Syntheticum	*Bingpian*
Fluid extract of *Shang Shi Zhi Tong*	*Shang Shi Zhi Tong liu jin gao*
Extract of Herba Cymbopogonis	*Yunxiangjingao*
Camphora	*Zhangnao*

Actions: Expelling wind—dampness, promoting blood circulation and stopping pain.

Indications: Arthrlagia due to wind—cold—dampness, muscular tension, numbness of limbs and muscular injury due to pulling—force.

Administration and Dosage: Stuck to the affected area.

Preparation Form: Plaster.

Package: 5 pieces of it in each bag.

Notes: This drug has the effects of resisting bacteria, reducing inflammation, eliminating swelling, relieving pain, and improving local microcirculation. It is clinically efficacious for rheumatic arthitis, muscle—fiber inflammation, and sprain and sorness of muscles.

Replace the applied plaster with a new one every 8 to 10 hours later because of its short—run effect. It is not suitable for those who are sensitvie to plaster or have local wound.

Zhenjiang Gaoyao

Ingredients:

Radix Aconiti	*Chuanwu*
Radix Aconiti Kusnezoffii	*Caowu*

Zaocys   *Wushaoshe*

Rhizoma seu Radix Notopterygii   *Qianghuo*

Actions: Expelling wind and stopping pain, relaxing tendons and promoting blood circulation.

Indications: Pain of muscles and joints, traumatic injury, numbness of limbs and arthralgia.

Administration and Dosage: Heated up to softness and applied to the affected part.

Preparation Form: Black plaster.

Package: 25g contained in each piece.

Notes: This plaster has the effects of anti—inflammation, analgesia, anti—rheumatism and microcirculatory improvement. It is clinincally used for rheumatic arthritis, rheumatoid arthritis, neuritis, muscle—fiber inflammation and numbness of limbs in the aged.

Xiaoluotong Pian

Ingredients:

Ramulus Genkwae   99%   *Yuanhuatiao*

Semen Phaseoli Aurei   1%   *Lüdou*

Actions: Expelling wind, removing dampness, reducing swelling and alleviating pain.

Indications: Arthralgia due to wind—cold—dampness.

Administration and Dosage: Taken orally. 3 to 4 tablets each time, three times a day.

· Preparation Form: Sugar—coated tablet.

Package: 0.25g in each tablet.

Notes: This drug has the effects of antisepsis, anti—inflammation, analgesia, detumescence, and promotion of microcirculation in the joints. It is clinically used for rheumatic arthritis, expecially for relieving the swelling and alleviating the pain in its acute stage.

Duhuo Jisheng Wan

Ingredients:

Radix Angelicae Pubescentis	7.4%	Duhuo
Radix Gentianae Macrophyllae	7.3%	Qinjiao
Herba Asari	7.3%	Xixin
Radix Ledebouriellae	7.3%	Fangfeng
Cortex Eucommiae	7.3%	Duzhong
Radix Achyranthis Bidentatae	7.3%	Ninxi
Radix Angelicae Sinensis	7.3%	Dangui
Radix Paeoniae Alba	4.9%	Baishao
Radix Codonopsis	4.9%	Dangshen
Radix Glycyrrhizae	4.9%	Gancao
Herba Taxilli	7.3%	Sangjisheng
Radix Rehmanniae Preparata	7.3%	Shudihuang
Rhizoma Chuanxiong	7.3%	Chuanxiong
Poria	4.9%	Fuling
Cortex Cinnamomi	7.3%	Rougui

Action: Nourishing blood, relaxing tendons, expelling wind and eliminating dampness.

Indications: Asthenia of the liver and kidney, arthralgia due to wind—cold—dampness, pain in the loins and knees, twisting of extremties and ankylosis.

Administration and Dosage: Taken orally. I bolus each time, once or twice daily.

Preparation Form: Honeyed bolus.

Package: 9g in each bolus.

Notes: The recipe is quoted from the book *Bei Ji Qian Jing Yao Fang* compiled by *Sun Simiao* (a famous physician) in the *Tang* Dynasty.

This bolus is efficacious for chronic arthritis and rheumatic ischialgia due to insufficiency of *Qi* and blood which is resuted from asthenia of the liver and kidney.

Wuli Bahan San

Main Ingredients:

Semen Cleomis   *Baihuacaizi*

other drugs

Actions: Expelling wind, dispersing cold, promoting blood circulation and stopping pain.

Indications: Arthratgia due to wind—cold—dampness, numbness of muscles and tendons, pain in the shoulder and back, stomach—ache due to cold, poor appetite, dysmenorrhea due to kidney—cold and leuiorrhea due to cold—dampness.

Administration and Dosage: A proper amount of *Wuli Bahan San* is mixed with egg white and warm boiled water or with breast milk into a paste. The paste is spread on a piece of wax—papper and applied to the acupoint or the affected part, or where the symptom is more severe when there are general symptoms.

Preparation Form: Powder.

Package: 16.5g of the powder in each bag.

Notes: This drug has the effects of antibiosis, anti—inflammation, analgesia and microcirculatory improvement. It is clinically efficacious for rheumatic arthritis, muscle—fiber inflammation, neuritis, hernia, nervous stomachache and menalgia.

It is normal if there appears slight pain after the paste is applied. This paste is not allowed to be applied to the umbilicus or the centre of sole. While it is used, raw or cold food should be kept off. And it is contraindicated for those under 15 years old.

The paste is removed 2—3 hours later after applied. If there appears severe pain, it should be removed earlier.

Dahuoluo Wan

Ingredients:

Agkistrodon	*Qishe*
Radix Clematidis	*Weilingxian*
Scorpio	*Quanxie*
Radix Ginseng	*Renshen*
Rhizoma Gastrodiae	*Tianma*
Radix Angelicae Sinensis	*Danggui*
Calculus Bovis man—made	*Rengongniuhuang*

Actions: Expelling wind, relaxing muscles and tendons, activating collaterals and eliminating dampness.

Indications: Arthalgia due to wind—cold—dampness marked by pain and numbness of limbs, twisting of extremities, palsy due to stroke, deviation of the eyes and mouth, hemiparalysis and alalia.

Administration and Dosage: Taken orally, 2 bolus each time, twice a day.

Preparation Form: Honeyed bolus.

Package: 3.6g in each bolus.

Notes: This bolus acts as an agent of anti—inflammation, analgesia and anti—rheumatism. With the effect of promoting blood circulation, it is clinically good for rheumatic arthritis, rheumatic muscle—fiber inflammation, neurities, hyperosteogeny, ischialgia, and cerabrovascular accident and cerebral angiospasm in the convalescence.

It is contraindicated for pregnant women.

Tianma Wan

Ingredients:

Rhizoma Gastrodiae	7.7%	Tianmanan
Rhizoma seu Radix Notopterygii	12.8%	Qianghuo
Radix Angelicae Pubescentis	12.8%	Duhuo
Rhizoma Dioscorae	7.7%	Bixie
Cortex Eucommiae	9%	Duzhong
Radix Achyranthis Bidentatae	7.7%	Niuxi
Radix Rehmanniae	20.5%	Dihuang
Radix Angelicae Sinensis	12.8%	Danggui
Radix Aconiti Praeparata	1.3%	Fuzi
Radix Scrophulariae	7.7%	Xuanshen

Actions: Expelling wind, promoting blood circulation, relaxing tendons and stopping pain.

Indications: Twisting pain of muscles, numbness of hands and feet, pain of loins and legs, deviation of the eyes and mouth and hemiparalysis due to apoplexy, all of which are dut to the attack of wind on the channels and collaterals.

Administration and Dosage: Taken orally. 1 bolus each time, 1 to 2 bolus a day.

Preparation Form: Honeyed bolus.

Package: 9g in each bolus.

Notes: This drug has the effects of anti—inflammation,

analgesia and anti—rheumatism, With the effect of improving microcirculation, it is clinically used for rheumatic arthritis, retrograde arthropathy, gouty arthritis, rheumatoid arthritis, sequelae of cerebral hemorrhage, cerebral angiospasm and senile chiropodalgia.

Xiaohuoluo Wan

Ingredients:

Arisaema cum Bile	21.2%	*Dannanxing*
Radix Aconiti	21.1%	*Chuanwu*
Radix Aconiti Kusnezoffii	21.1%	*Caowu*
Lumbricus	21.2%	*Dilong*
Resina Olibani	7.7%	*Ruxiang*
Myrrha	7.7%	*Moyao*

Actions: Expelling wind, eliminating dampness and promoting blood circulation to treat arthralgia.

Indications: Arthralgia due to wind—cold—dampness marked by pain, numbness and twisting of limbs.

Administration and Dosage: Taken orally, 1 bolus each time, twice a day.

Preparation Form: Honeyed bolus.

Package: 3g in each bolus.

Notes: The effects of this bolus are antibiosis, anti—inflammation, analgesia, antirheumatism and improvment of microcirculation. It is clinically efficacious for rheumatic arthritis, rheumatoid arthritis, muscle—fiber inflammation and hyperosteogeny.

It is contraindicated for pregnant women and it should not be taken with atropine, caffeine and aminophylline at same time.

Jiufen San

Ingredients:

Semen Strychni Powder	25%	*Maqianzifen*
Herba Ephedrae	25%	*Mahuang*
Resina Olibani	25%	*Ruxiang*
Myrrha	25%	*Mayao*

Actions: Promoting blood circulation to remove blood stasis, relieving swelling and stopping pain.

Indications: Traumatic injury, and pain due to blood stasis.

Administration and Dosage: Taken orally after meal, 0.25g each time, once a day.

Preparation Form: Powder.

Package: 2.7g in each bag.

Notes: This drug is clinically beneficial for rheumatic muscle—fiber inflammation, myoasthenia and rheumatic arthritis.

With toxicity, not more than 2.7g of it is taken each time. Any of it is not allowed to be used for pregnant women, those with hypertension or heart or kidney disease and those with bleeding injury. Whether children and weak patients can take it or not depends on the order of a physician.

Mugua Wan

Ingredients:

Fructus Chaenomelis	10.8%	*Mugua*
Radix Achranthis Bidentatae	8.2%	*Niuxi*
Rhizoma Cibotii	5.4%	*Gouji*
Caulis Piperis Kadsurae	10.8%	*Naifengteng*
Radix Clematidis	10.8%	*Weilingxian*

Caulis Spatholobi	5.4%	*Jixueteng*
Radix Angelicae Dahuricae	10.8%	*Baizhi*
Radix Aconiti Praeparata	5.4%	*Zhichuanwu*
Radix Aconiti Kusnezoffii praeparata	5.4%	*Zhicaowu*
Radix Angelicae Sinensis	10.8%	*Donggui*
Rhizoma Chuanxiong	10.8%	*Chuanxiong*
Radix Ginseng	5.4%	*Renshen*

Actions: Expelling wind, removing dampness and activating the collaterals to relieve pain.

Indications: Arthralgia due to wind—cold—dampness marked by numbness of the limbs and pantalgia.

Administration and Dosage: Taken orally. 1 bolus each time, twice a day.

Preparation Form: Honeyed bolus.

Package: 9g in each bolus.

Notes: This drug has the effects of antibiosis, anti—inflammation, antirheumatism and improvment of microcirculation. It is clinically efficacious not only for rheumatic arthritis and rheumatoid arlhritis both with prolonged course and marked by soreness of the loins and knees and ache of the muscles, but also for senile numbness of limbs or soreness of loins and knees.

Fufang Danggui Zhusheye

Ingredients:

Radix Angelicae Sinensis	18%	*Danggui*
Rhizoma Chuanxiong	41%	*Chuanxiong*
Flos Carthami	41%	*Honghua*

Actions: Promoting blood circulation to remove bood stasis.

Indications: All types of chronic and acute strain, soreness of the loins and legs, numbness of the limbs, arthralgia and dysmenorrhea.

Administration and Dosage: Given through intramuscular injection, 2 ml each time, once a day or every other day.

Preparation Form: 2ml in each ampoule.

Notes: The injection has the effects of improving microcirculatin, resisting inflammation, reducing swelling and relieving pain, It is efficacious for all types of acute and chronic muscle—fiber strain, muscle—fiber inflammation, neuritis, sciatica, dysmenorrhea, arthritis, traumatic paraplegia and poliomyelitis.

Contraindicated for pregnant women, this injection must be cautionsly used for those prone to bleed and women having profuse menstruation.

Qufeng Shujin Wan

Ingredients:

Radix Ledebouriellae	5.6%	*Fongfeng*
Ramulus Cinnamomi	5.6%	*Guizhi*
Herba Ephedrae	5.6%	*Mahuang*
Radix Clematidis	5.6%	*Weilingxian*
Radix Aconiti	5.6%	*Chuanwu*
Radix Aconiti Kusnezoffii	5.6%	*Caowu*
Rhizoma Atractylodis	5.6%	*Changzhu*
Poria	5.6%	*Fuling*
Fructus Chaenomelis	5.6%	*Mugua*
Radix Gentianae Macrophyllae	5.6%	*Qinjiao*
Rhizoma Drynariae	5.6%	*Gusuibu*
Radix Achyranthis Bidentatae	5.6%	*Niuxi*
Radix Glycyrrhizae	5.5%	*Gancao*

Caulis Piperis Kadsurae	5.5%	*Haifengteng*
Rhizoma Dioscoreae Nipponicae	5.5%	*Chuanshanlong*
Herba Erodii seu Geranii	5.5%	*Laoguancao*
Caulis Sinomenii	5.5%	*Qingfengtong*
Radix Solani Melongenae	5.5%	*Qiegen*

Actions: Expelling wind, removing cold, relaxing muscles and tendons, and activating the collaterals.

Indications: Arthralgia due to wind—cold—dampness marked by numbness of the limbs and pain in the lower back and legs.

Administration and Dosage: Taken orally, 1 bolus each time, twice a day.

Preparation Form: Honeyed bolus.

Package: 9g in each bolus

Notes: This drug has the effects of antivirus, anti—inflammation, antirheumatism and improvment of microcirculation. It is clinically used for rheumatic arthritis and muscle—fiber inflammation, and fever and headache due to common cold.

This bolus should be carefully administrated to pregnant women.

Kanlisha

Ingredients:

Herba Ephedrae	0.2%	*Mahuong*
Rhizoma seu Radix Notopterygii	0.2%	*Qianghuo*
Radix Angelicae Pubescentis	0.2%	*Duohuo*
Radix Ledebouriellae	0.2%	*Fangfeng*
Herba Schizonepetae	0.2%	*Jingjie*
Herba Impatientis	0.2%	*Tougucao*
Flos Carthami	0.2%	*Honghua*

Radix Angelicae Dahuricae	0.2%	*Baizhi*
Radix Angelicae Sinensis	0.2%	*Danggui*
Radix Achyranthis Bidentatae	0.2%	*Niuxi*
Mugwort floss	0.2%	*Shengairong*
Fructus Chaenomelis	0.2%	*Mugua*
Ramulus Cinnamomi	0.2%	*Guizhi*
Radix Aconiti Praeparata	0.2%	*Fuzi*
Rhizoma Zingiberis	0.2%	*Ganjiang*

Actions: Expelling wind, dispersing cold and promoting blood circulation to stop pain.

Indications: Pain of lower back and legs, numbness of limbs, twisting of tendons, abdominal pain due to coldness of the genitals, and herniation of small intestine.

Administration and Dosage: One bag of the drugs are mixed rapidly with 10—15g of vinegar, put into a cloth bag, covered with cotton yarn and kept still for about one hour up to the time when the drugs become hot. Then hot compress with the hot drug bag is done on the affected part.

Preparation Form: Agent for hot compress.

Package: 30g in each bag.

Notes: This drug has the effects of antibacteria, anti—inflammation and promotion of blood circulation. It is clinically efficacious for muscle—fiber inflammation, neuritis and rheumatic arthritis.

The performance is not done in wind and over—hot drug bag is not used.

Shenjiandan Jiaonang

Ingredients:

Lumbricus	25.7%	Dilong
Semen Strychni	17.9%	Maqianzi
Flos Carthami	17.9%	Honghua
Resina Olibani	7.7%	Ruxiang
Radix Stephaniae Tetrandrae	7.7%	Fangji
Myrrha	7.7%	Moyao
Cortex Periplocae	7.7%	Xiangjiapi
Rhizoma Drynariae	7.7%	Gusuibu

Actions: Relaxing muscles and tendons, activating the flow of Qi and blood in the channels and collaterals, promoting blood circulation, removing bloodstasis, relieving swelling and stopping pain.

Indications: Arthralgia due to wind—cold—dampness marked by pain of lower back and legs and numbness of limbs, sprain of tendons, and welling and pain due to blood stasis.

Administration and Dosage: Taken orally, 5 capsules each time, 3 times a day.

Preparation Form: Capsule.

Package: 0.15g in each capsule.

Notes: This drug has the effects of reducing inflammation, relieving pain and promoting local blood circulation. It is clinically efficacious for scapulohumeral periarthritis, sciatica, chronic osseous arthritis, hypertrophic spondylitis, cervical spondylopathy and fracture sequel. It is contraindicated for pregnant and breast—feeding women.

10 Antiparasitics

Wumei Wan

Ingredients:

Fructus Mume	19.9%	*Wu mei*
Pericarpium Zanthoxyli	5%	*Huajiao*
Rhizoma Coptidis	20.7%	*Huanglian*
Radix Angelicae Sinensis	12.4%	*Danggui*
Rhizoma Zingiberis	7.4%	*Ganjiang*
Cortex Phellodendri	7.4%	*Huangbai*
Ramulus Cinnamomi	7.4%	*Guizhi*
Radix Aconiti Lateralis Preparata	7.4%	*Fuzi*
Radix Ginseng	7.4%	*Renshen*
Herba Asari	7.4%	*Xixin*

Actions: Reinforcing *Qi* and warming the viscera, expelling ascaris and alleviating pain.

Indications: Colic caused by ascaris, cold intestine, stomachache, vomiting of ascaris, protracted dysentery due to insufficiency of the spleen and deadly cold hands and feet.

Administration and Dosage: Taken orallys. 1 blolus each time 3 times a day. When Children under three years old are treated, the dosage should be reduced properly.

Preparation Form: Honeyed bolus.

Package: 9 g in each bolus.

Notes: This recipe is from the book *Shang Han Lun* written

by *Zhang Zhongjing* in the *Han* Dynasty.

This drug has the effects of destroying parasites and stopping pain. It is clinically efficacious not only for biliary ascariasis, ascaris intestinal obstruction and chronic cholecystisis, but also for chronic gastroenteritis, irritable colitis, bacillary dysentery, amebic dysentery and appendicitis.

This drug shouldn't be taken together with sodium bicarbonate, aluminumbydroxide, gastropine and aminophylline.

Wumei Anwei Wan

Ingredients:

Fructus Mume	24.0%	*Wumeirou*
Rhizoma Coptidis	19.0%	*Huanglian*
Radix Aconiti Lateralis Praeparata	7.1%	*Fuzi*
Rhizoma Zingiberis	11.9%	*Ganjiang*
Ramulus Cinnamomi	7.1%	*Guizhi*
Radix Codonopsis Pilosulae	7.1%	*Dangshen*
Herba Asari	7.1%	Xixin
Radix Angelicae Sinensis	4.8%	*Danggui*
Cortex Phellodendri	7.1%	*Huangbai*
Pericarpium Zanthoxyli	4.8%	*Huajiao*

Actions: Removing ascaris to alleviate pain.

Indications: Colic caused by ascaris, interval pains of belly, deadly cold of hands and feet and vomiting of ascaris.

Administration and Dosage: Taken orally, 9 g each time, twice a day.

Preparation Form: Water—paste pill.

Package: About 2 g in every 40 pills.

Notes: This recipe is from the book *Shan Han Lun* written by

Zhang Zhongjing in the *Han* Dynasty.

The effect of the pill is to destroy parasities and stop pain. It is clinically efficacious for biliary ascariasis.

Chuanliansu Pian

Ingredients:

Cortex Meliae Toosendan   *Chuanlianpi* 100%

Actions: Destroying parasities and stopping itch.

Indications: Abdominal pain due to ascaris, whipworm and pinworm.

Administration and Dosage: Taken orally on an empty stomach, 8 to 10 tablets each fiine, once a day. The dosage for infants is based on their age. Every one year older, half tablet is added.

Preparation Form: Tablet.

Package: 0.3 g in each tablet.

Notes: This drug is a preparation extracted from *Chuanlianpi* Cortex Meliae Toosendan. It has the effect of anti–parasite and is clinically efficacious for ascaris, pinworm and other parasites harboured in the digestive tract.

It is confraindicated for those who have peptic ulcer.

Quchong Pian

Ingredients:

Radix Aucklandiae	15.5%	*Muxiang*
Semen Arecae	15.5%	*Binglang*
Fructus Quisqualis	15.5%	*Shijunzi*
Omphalia	4.5%	*Leiwan*
Alumen	4.5%	*Baifan*

Aloe	4.5%	*Luhui*
Radix et Rhizoma Rhei	15.5%	*DaHuang*
Semen Pharbitidis	15.5%	*Qianniuzi*
Realgar	4.5%	*Xionghuang*

Actions: Destroying parasites, removing food stagnancy and relaxing the bowels.

Indications: Abdominal pain due to enterositosis, anorexia, sallow complexion. and emaciation.

Administration and Dosage:

Taken orally, 8 tablets each time, twice a day. Appropriate reduction of the dosage is done for children.

Preparation Form: Table.

Package: 0.3 g in each tablet.

Notes: This drug has the effects of antiparasites and laxation. It is clinically efficacious for ascaeis and chronic digestive disease of children.

Nangchong Wan

Ingredients:

Poria	16.8%	*Fuling*
Omphalia	8.4%	*Leiwan*
Radix Aconiti	1.0%	*Chuanwu*
Semen Persicae	12.6%	*Taoren*
Hirudo	2.9%	*Shuizhi*
Radix et Rhizoma Rhei	1.0%	*Dahuang*
Flos Genkwa	4.2%	*Yuanhua*
Rhizoma Coptidis	12.6%	*Huanglian*
Bombyx Batryticatus	5.0%	*Jiangcan*
Exocarpium Citri Reticulatae	8.4%	*Juhong*

Radix Morindae Offidnalis	20.0%	*Baqitan*
Cortex Moutan Radicis		*Mudanpi*
Liquid Extract of Faeces Trogopterorum		*Wulingzhi Liujingao*

Actions: Promoting blood circulation to remove blood stasis, softening hard masses to eliminate cystis, relieving convulsion and alleviating pain.

Indications: Cystis and sore.

Administration and Dosage: Taken orally, 1 bolus each time, 2 to 3 times a day.

Preparation Form: Honeyed bolus.

Package: 5 g in each bolus.

Notes: This drug has the effects of destroying parasites and alleviating pain. It is clinically efficacious for cysticercosis cellulosae in human, cerebral cysticercosis and epilepsy caused by cerebral cysticercosis.

Shijunzi Wan

Ingredients:

Fructus Quisqualis	50%	*Shijunzi*
Rhizoma Arisaematis	25%	*Tiannanxing*
Semen Arecae	25%	*Binlang*

Actions: Removing food stagnancy and expelling parasites.

Indications: Infantile parasitic infestation marked by malnutrition, abdominal distention and pain, sallow complexion, emaciation, polyphagia and morbid crying.

Administration and Dosage: Taken orally, 9 g each time, once a day.

Preparation Form: Warter—paste pill.

Package: 3 g in every 50 pills.

Notes: This recipe is quoted from the book Zheng Zhi Zhun Sheng written by *Wang Kentang* in the *Ming* Dynasty.

This drug has the effect of antiparasites. It is clinically efficacious for ascaris pinworm.

Biejiajian Wan

Ingredients:

Colla Carapax Trionycis	*Biejiajiao*
Colla Coril Asini	*Ejiao*
Uidus Uespae	*Fengfang*
Armadillidium Vulgare	*Shufuchong*
Eupolyphaga seu Steleophaga	*Tubiechong*
Statilia Maculatae	*Tanglang*
Natrii Sulfas	*Mangxiao*
Radix Bupleuri	*Chaihu*
Radix Scutellariae	*Huangqin*
Rhizoma Pinelliae	*Banxia*
Radix Codonopsis Pilosulae	*Dangshen*
Rhizoma Zingiberis	*Ganjiang*
Cortex Magnoliae Officinalis	*Houpo*
Ramulus Cinnamomi	*Guizhi*
Radix Paeoniae Alba	*Baishao*
Rhizoma Belamcandae	*Shegan*
Semen Persicae	*Taoren*
Cortex Moutan Radicis	*Mudanpi*
Radix et Rhizoma Rhei	*Dahuang*
Flos Campsis	*Lingxiaohua*
Semen Lepidii	*Tinglizi*
Herba Pyrrosiae	*Shiwei*

Herba Dianthi   *Qumai*

Actions: Promoting blood circulation to remove blood stasis, removing food staguancy and treating malaria.

Indications: Prolonged malaria, fullness in the hypochondrium and mass in the epigastric area, and rigidity.

Administration and Dosage: Taken orally, 2 boluses each time, 2 to 3 times a day.

Preparation Form: Honeyed bolus.

Package: 3 g in each bolus.

Notes: This recipe is found in the book *Jin Gui Yao Lue* written by Zhang Zhongjing in the Han Dynasty.

This drug has the antimalarial effect. It is clinically efficacious for malaria, black sickness, chronic hepatitis and schistosomiasis.

Huachong Wan

Ingredients:

Fructus Carpesii	20%	*Heshi*
Semen Arecae	10%	*Binglang*
Cortex Meliae	10%	*Kulianpi*
Fructus Quisqualis	10%	*Shijunzi*
Omphalia	10%	*Leiwan*
Radix et Rhizoma Rhei	10%	*Dahuang*
Semen Pharbitidis	10%	*Qianniuzi*
Natrii Salfas Exsiccatus	20%	*Xuanmingfen*

Actions: Expelling parasites and removing food stagnancy.

Indications: Intestinal enterositiosis, abdominal pain and pruritus ani.

Adminstration and Dosage: Taken orally, 6 to 9 g each time

1 or 2 times a day. The dosage should be reduced properly for children below 3 years old.

Preparation Form: Water—paste pill.

Package: About 1 g in every 30 pills.

Notes: This recipe is quoted from the book Tai Ping Hui Min He Ji Ju Fang written by Chen Shiwen in the Song Dynasty. This drug has the parasiticide effect. It is clinically efficaci-ous for intestinal parasitic diseases such as ascariasis, ancylostomiasis, taeniasis, fasciolopsiasis and oxyuriasis. This drug should be cau-tiously used for infants and those infirm with age.

Meidijing Pian

Ingredients:

Herba Erodii seu Geranii	Laoguancao
Boric Acid	Pengsuan
Realgar	Xionghuang
Fructus Cnidii	Shechuangzi
Indigo Naturalis	Qingdai
Natrii Sulfas Exsiccatus	Xuanmingfen
Camphora	Zhangnao
Borneolum Syntheticum	Bingpian

Actions: Removing dampness and destroying parasites.

Indications: Downward flow of damp—heat marked by itch and pain in the vulvae and leukorrhea with reddish discharge.

Administration and Dosage: In the evening, the pudendum is washed, then, one tablet is taken and pushed deep into the vagina, 12 times of doing this is 1 course of treatment.

Preparation Form: Tablet

Package: 0.5 g in each tablet.

Notes: This drug has the effects of resisting bacteria, reducing inflammation and destroying parasites. It is clinically used for colpitis mycotica, trichomonal vaginitis and cervicitis.

Contraindicated for women in the period, this drug is cautiously considered]when patients to be treated are pregnant women.

11 Antineoplastics

Xihuang Wan

Main Ingredients:

Resina Olibani   *Ruxiang*

Myrrha   *Moyao*

Calculus Bovis(man-made)   *Rengongniuhuang*

Actions: Removing toxic materials, resolving mass, reducing swelling and alleviating pain.

Indications: Carbuncle, scrofula, subcutaneous nodule and multiple abscess.

Administration and Dosage: Taken orally. 3 g each time, twice a day.

Preparation Form: Water—paste pill.

Package: 1 g in every 20 Pills.

Notes: This drug is clinically efficacious for many kinds of tumours, initial angitis, multiple abscesses, lymphnoditis, acute phlegmon, appendiceal abscess, osteomyelitis, pulmonary abscess and hepatic abscess, with special curative effects when used to treat mammary cancer. It is contraindicated for pregnant women.

Pianzihuang

Main Ingredients:

Calculus Bovis   *Niuhuang*

Fel Serpentis   *Shedan*

Radix Notoginseng   *Sanqi*

Actions: Clearing away heat, removing toxic materials, reducing swelling and alleviating pain.

Indications: Swelling and pain due to toxic heat, furunculosis and tonsillitis.

Administration and Dosage: Taken orally, 0.15 g to 0.3 g each time for those under 8 years old, 0.6 g each time for those above 8 years old. 2 to 3 times a day.

Used externally, mixed with cold—boiled water and applied to the affected part, several times a day.

Preparation Form: Fermented cake and capsule.

Package: 3 g in each cake or 0.3 g in each capsule.

Notes: This drug is clinically efficacious for acute or chronic hepatitis, otitis, ophthalmitis, tonsillitis, swelling and pain of gum, aphtha, tumour, scald and burn.

It is contraindicated for pregnant women.

Xinhuan Pian

Ingredients:

Calculus Bovis   *Niuhuang*

Radix Notoginseng   *Sanqi*

Actions: Clearing away heat, removing toxic materials and dispersing blood stasis and reducing swelling.

Indications: Tumour and furunculosis due to toxic heat.

Administration and Dosage: Taken orally, 2 to 4 tablets each time, 3 times a day. For children, the dosage should be reduced appropriately. When used externally, it is mixed with water and spread on the affected part.

Preparation Form: Sugar—coated tablet.

Package: 0.32 g in each tablet.

Notes: This drug is clinically efficacious for esophageal cancer, cardiac cancer, acute icterohepatitis, cholecystitis, rheumatic arthritis, hemorrhoid, surgical infection, and various kinds of tumours.

Caution is needed when such patients are treated with this drug as pregnant women and those with gastroduodenal ulcer or renal dysfunction. Using it to treat those with hemorrhage of digestive tract is not allowed.

Yadanziru Zhusheye

Ingredients:

Fructus Bruceae   100%   *Yadanzi*

Actions: Clearing away heat, removing toxic materials, resolving mass and reducing swelling.

Indications: Carbuncle, cellulitis, scrofula and mass in the abdomen, all due to accumuation of toxic heat.

Administration and Dosage: Civen through intravenous injection, 5 to 10 ml each time, once a day. A course of treatment involves 4 months. The dosage can be increased to 10—30 ml each time according to disease condition. It is diluted before injected with 250—500 ml of 5—50% glucose injection or normal saline.

Preparation Form: Emulsion for intravenous injection.

Package: 2 ml in each ampoule. This injection contains 10% *Yadanzi* Fructus Bruceae

Notes: This drug is clinically efficacious for carcinomas of the digestive system such as esophageal cancer, gastric carcinoma and rectal carcinoma, and pulmonary carcinoma. as well.

A few of patients can have such reactions of the digestive

tract as aversion to greasy food, nausea and anorexia, which can be relieved through expectant treatment.

Gongjingai Pian

Ingredients:

Rhizoma Pinelliae   100%   *Zhangyebanxia*

Actions: Removing toxic material, resolving mass, reducing swelling and alleviating pain.

Indications: Scrifula and multiple abscess due to downward flow of damp—heat.

Administration and Dosage: Taken orally, 2 to 3 tablets each time, 3 times a day.

Preparation Form: Sugar—coated tablet.

Package: 0.3 g of alcohol—soluble extract in each tablet.

Notes: This drug is against tumors. It is clinically efficacious for carcinoma of uterine cervix and precancerous condition of the uterine cervix.

Hekui Zhusheye

Ingredients:

Ramulus Persicae   91%   *Hetaozhi*

Herba Solani Nigri   9%   *Longkui*

Actions: Removing dampness and reducing swelling Indications: Distention and fullness of the epigastric region due to accumulation of damp—heat caused by deficiency of both the spleen and kidney.

Administration and Dosage: Given through intramuscular injection, 2 to 4ml each time, once or twice a day. A course of treatment involves two months. Injected into tumour body (injection of the body of cervical cancer): 4—8 ml each time, once a day.

Preparation Form. Injection.

Package: 2 ml in each ampoule.

Notes: This drug is clinically efficacious for hydrothorax, ascites, pain and cervical bleeding resulting from various kinds of tumors. It can inhibit the growth of lung or cervical cancer, and shrink cervical cancer in some patients.

12　Drugs used in Surgery

12.1　Drugs used in Traumatology Department

Dieda Wan

Ingrediants:

Radix Notoginseng	5.2%	Sanqi
Radix Angelicae Sinensis	2.6%	Dang gui
Radix Paeoniae Alba	3.9%	Baishao
Radix Paeoniae Rubra	5.2%	Chishao
Semen Persicae	2.6%	Taoren
Flos Carthami	3.9%	Honghua
Resina Draconis	3.9%	Xuejie
Herba Artemisiae Anomalae	2.6%	Liujinu
Rhizoma Drynariae	2.6%	Gusuibu
Radix Dipsaci	25.8%	Xuduan
Lignum Sappan	3.9%	Sumu
Cortex Moutan	2.6%	Mudanpi
Resina Olibani	3.9%	Ruxiang
Myrrha	3.9%	Moyao
Rhizoma Curcumae Longae	1.9%	Jianghuang
Semen Melo	2.6%	Tianguazi
Radix Ledebouriellae	2.5%	Fangfeng
Fructus Aurantii Immaturus	2.5%	Zhishi
Radix Platycodi	2.5%	Jiegeng

Radix Glycyrrhizae	3.9%	*Gancao*
Caulis Clematidis Armandii	2.5%	*Chuan Mutong*
Pyritum	2.6%	*Zirantong*
Eupolyphaga seu Steleophaga	2.5%	*Tubiechong*
Rhizoma Sparganii	3.9%	*Sanleng*

Action: Activating blood flow to remove blood stasis, promoting the subsidence of swelling to alleviate pain, expelling wind to dredge the channels.

Indications: Traumatic injury, painful swelling due to blood stasis, sudden sprain of the lumbar and a pain in the chest occurring when breathing.

Administration and Dosage: Taken orally, one bolus each time, twice daily.

Preparation Form: Honeyed bolus.

Package: 3 g in each bolus.

Notes: This drug has the actions of reducing inflammation, arresting pain and promoting blood circulation. It is clinically efficacious for various sort of fracture, and damage of joints, ligaments and back muscles. It is contraindicated for pregnant women.

Zhonghua Dieda Wan

Main Ingredients:

Radix Stephaniae	*Jinbuhuan*
Herba Lobeliae Radicantis	*BanbianLian*
Herba Centipedae	*Ebushicao*
Cortex Eucommiae	*Duzhong*
Herba Hyperici Japonici	*Tianjihuang*
Radix Belladonnae	*Dianqiegeng*

Actions: Reducing swelling, alleviating pain, relaxing rigidity of muscles, activating collaterals arresting bleeding and promoting tissue regeneration.

Indications: Contusion of muscles, injury, and pain or numbness due to wind—wetness.

Administrationg and Dosage: Taken orally, one bolus each time, 2—3 times a day. Mixed with alcohol and put on affected part for external use.

Preparation Form: Honeyed bolus.

Package: 6 g in each bolus.

Notes: This drug is clinically efficacious for various surgical traumas, sprain, injury, cut, rheumatic arthritis, etc.

Algefacient may be drunk if dry throat or bitter taste occurs after the bolus is taken. Administration of this drug should be stopped whenever there appear fever, cough or thick sputum due to exogenous factors.

Qiti San

Main Ingredients:

Resina Draconis	Xue jie
Resina Olibani	Ruxiang
Myrrha	Moyao
Flos Carthami	Honghua
Catechu	Ercha
Borneolum Syntheticum	Bingpian
Cinnabaris	Zhusha

Actions: Removing blood stasis, reducing swelling, alleviating pain and arreting bleeding.

Indications: Traumatic injury, pain due to blood stasis and

traumatic bleeding.

Administration and Dosage: Taken orally, 1—1.5 g each time.1—3 times daily.

Preparation Form: Powder.

Package: 1.5 g in a bottle

Notes: This drug has the effects of allaying inflammation, alleviating pain, arresting bleeding and promoting local blood circulation. It is clinically efficacious for various traumatic bleeding, sprain, contusion, fracture, soft tissue injury, ligament strain, etc.; for toxic myocarditis, hepatitis, cornary heart disease and angina pectoris; and for all kinds of innominatal toxic swelling, burn, scalds and shingles.

It shouldn't be taken together with potassium bromide, sodium bromide, or sodium iodide.

Guzhe Cuoshang San

Main Ingredients:

Resina Olibani	*Ruxiang*
Myrrha	*Moyao*
Radix et Rhizoma Draconis	*Dahuang*
Flos Carthami	*Honghua*
Eupolyphaga seu Steleophaga	*Biechong*

Actions: Relaxing musucles and tendons to promote blood circulation, benefiting bone—knitting, alleviating pain, dissipating blood stasis and eliminating swelling.

Indications: Traumatic injury, painful swelling due to blood stasis, pain or numbness due to wind—wetness.

Preparation and Dosage: Taken orally, 9 pills each time, 2 times daily.

Preparation Form: Capsule.

Package: 0.4 g in each capsule.

Notes: This drug has the effects of allaying inflammation, promoting local blood circulation and accelerating fracture union. It is clinically efficacious for various contusion, sprain of ligament, rheumatic arthritis, etc.

Sanqi Shanyao Pian

Ingredients:

Radix Notogingseng	3.1%	Sanqi
Radix Aconiti Kusnezoffii	3.1%	Caowu
Borneolum Syntheticum	0.06%	Bingpian
Radix Aconiti Brachypodi	3.1%	Xueshangyizhihao
Rhizoma Drynariae	29.2%	Gusuibu
Caulis Sambuci	46.8%	Jiegumu
Flos Carthami	9.4%	Honghua
Radix Paeoniae Rubra	5.2%	Chishao

Actions: Relaxing musucles and tendons to promote blood circulation, dissipating blood stasis and alleviating pain.

Indications: Contusion, sprain and traumatic injury.

Administration and Dosage: Taken orally, 3 tablets each time, 3 times daily.

Preparation Form: Sugar—coated tablet.

Package: 0.33 g in each tablet.

Notes: This drug has the effects of allaying inflammation and arresting pain. It is clinically efficacious for various trauma, arthralgia, neuralgia and soft tissue injury.

Dieda Yaojing

Ingredients:

Flos Carthami	*Hong hua*
Catechu	*Ercha*
Radix Angelicae Sinensis	*Danggui*
Benzoinum	*Anxixiang*
Resina Olibani	*Ruxiang*
Myrrha	*Moyao*

Actions: Dissipating blood stasis and reducing swelling, activating the colaterals and alleviating pain.

Indications: Injury from fall, sprain of muscles and joints, and painful swelling due to blood stasis.

Administration and Dosage: Taken orally, 5—10 ml each time or put on the affected part for external use.

Preparation Form: Tinctura.

Package: 50 g in each bottle.

Notes: This drug has the action of allaying inflammation, arresting pain and promoting local blood circulation. It is clinically efficacious for various swelling and pain seen in the department of traumatology.

Yili Zhitong Dan

Ingredients: (omitted)

Actions: Activating blood flow, dissipating blood stasis, promoting the subsidence of swelling and alleviating pain.

Indications: Traumatic injury,. painful swelling due to blood stasis and menstrual pain.

Administration and Dosage: Taken orally, 1 pill each time,

2—3 times daily.

Preparation Form: Pill.

Package: 1 g in every 10 pills.

Notes: With the remarkable action of analgesia, this drug can allay inflammation and eliminate swelling. It is clinically efficatious for local pain due to knife trauma, traumatic injury and dysmenorrhea, and for pain due to some kinds of advanced cancer.

Jiegu San

Ingredients:

Herba Ephedrae	16.7%	*Mahuang*
Eupolyphaga seu Steleophaga	16.7%	*Tubiechong*
Resina Olibani	16.7%	*Ruxiang*
Myrrha	16.7%	*Mo yao*
Lumbricus	16.6%	*Dilong*
Pyritum	16.6%	*Zirantong*

Actions: Activating blood flow, alleviating pain and promoting reunion of broken bones.

Indications: Injury of the muscles, tendons and bones, and swelling, and pain due to blood stasis.

Administration and Dosage: Taken orally, 1 / 3—1 bag each time, 1—2 times daily. or mixed with alcohol and put on the affected part for external use.

Preparation Form: Powder.

Package: 9 g in each bag.

Notes: This drug has the actions of relieving pain and accelerating the grow of granulation tissue. It is clinically efficatious for various swelling and pain seen in the department of traumatology.

Wuhu San

Ingredients:

Radix Angelicae Sinensis	21.3%	*Danggui*
Flos Carthami	21.3%	*Honghua*
Radix Ledebouriellae	21.3%	*Fangfeng*
Rhizoma Arisaematis	21.3%	*Tiannanxing*
Radix Angelicae Dahuricae	14.6%	*Baizhi*

Actions: Activating blood flow, dissipating blood stasis, reducing swelling and alleviating pain.

Indications: Traumatic injury and red—painful swelling or black and purple skin due to blood stasis.

Administration and Dosage: Taken orally, 6 g each time, twice daily. For external use, proper amount of the powder is mixed with alcohol and put on the affected part.

Preparation Form: Powder.

Package: 6 g in each bag.

Notes: This drug has the actions of promoting blood circulation and arrestig pain. It is clinically efficacious for injury from fall, sprain and rheumatic arthritis.

It is contraindicated for pregnant women.

Zhenggu Shui

Main Ingredients:

Fructus Arctii	*Dalizi*
Herba Asari	*Xixin*
Mentholum	*Bohenao*
Rhizoma Lophantheri	*Suigushui*

Actions: Relaxing muscles and tendons, activating collaterals, promoting blood circulation and alleviating pain.

Indications: Traumatic injury, pain of muscles and joints.

Administration and Dosage: Used to coat the affected part; or to do wet dressing with a cotton ball on the severe affected part, for one hour if the part is on the upper limb, for one and a half hour if on the lower limb; 2—3 times daily.

Preparation Form: Tincture.

Package: 30 ml in each bottle.

Notes: This drug has the action of promoting local blood circulation and relieving pain. It is clinically efficacious for various fractures, contusion, swelling due to luxation.

It is conrtraindicated for pregnant women.

Hongyao Pian

Main Ingredients:

Radix Notogingseng	5.2%	*Sanqi*
Eupolyphaga seu Steleophaga	10.8%	*Tubiechong*
Radix Angelicae Sinensis	10.8%	*Danggui*
Radix Angelicae Dahuricae	10.8%	*Baizhi*
Rhizoma Ligustici	10.8%	*Gaoben*
Flos Carthami	10.8%	*Honghua*

Actions: Activating blood flow, alleviating pain and removing blood stasis.

Indications: Traumatic injury, swelling and pain of muscles and joints, and pain or numbness due to wind-wetness.

Administration and Dosage: Taken orally, 2 tablets each time, twice daily.

Preparation Form: Surgar—coated tablet.

Package: 0.25 g in each tablet.

Notes: This drug has the effects of allaying inflammation, arresting pain and promoting blood circulation. It is clinically efficacious for various kinds of fractures and soft tissue injures.

Dieda Sunshang Wan

Ingreduents:

Herba Ephedrae	20%	*Mahuang*
Semen Strychni	10%	*Maqianzi*
Eupolyphaga seu Steleophaga	20%	*Tubiechong*
Radix Angelicae Sinensis	20%	*Danggui*
Flos Carthami	20%	*Honghua*
Pyretum	10%	*Zirantong*

Actions: Activating blood flow to remove blood stasis, reducing swelling to alleviate pain.

Indications: Traumatic injury, sudden sprain of the lumbar, pain in the chest occurring in breathing, injury of muscles, and tendons and bones, and pain and swelling due to blood stasis.

Administration and Dosage: Taken orally, 1 / 2 bolus each time in the beginning, twice daily; then, another 1 / 2 bolus is added if there didn't occur side effects such as numbness of the lips. Mild diaphoresis should be induced just after the bolus is taken.

Preparation Form: Honeyed bolus.

Package: 3 g in each bolus.

Notes: This drug has the effects of allaying inflammation, arresting pain, and promoting blood circulation. It is clinically efficacious for various surgical damages, swelling and pain.

It is contraindicated for those with heart disease, pregnant women and children.

Dieda Huoxue San

Ingreduents:

Flos Carthami	2.6%	Honghua
Radix Angelicae Sinensis	12.8%	Danggui
Resina Draconis	3.0%	Xuejie
Rhizoma Drynariae	12.8%	Gusuibu
Radix Notogingseng	5.2%	Sanqi
Radix Dipsaci	12.8%	Xuduan
Resina Olibani	12.8%	Ruxiang
Myrrha	12.8%	Moyao
Catechu	8.4%	Ercha
Radix et Rhizoma Rhei	8.4%	Dahuang
Borneolum Syntheticum	0.9%	Bingpian
Eupolyphaga seu Steleophaga	8.4%	Tubiechong

Actions: Relaxing musucles and tendons, activating blood flow, dissipating blood stasis and alleviating pain.

Indications: Traumatic injury, pain and swelling due to blood stasis , sudden sprain of the lumbar and pain in the chest occurring in breathing.

Administration and Dosage: Taken orally, 3 g each time, twice daily. Or mixed with vinegar or yellow wine and put on the affected part for external use.

Preparation Form: Powder.

Package: 3 g in each bag.

Notes: This drug has the effect of improving microcirculation, reducing swelling and arresting pain. It is clinically efficacious for various injuries from fall, swelling and pain due to sprain.

It is contraindicated for pregnant women.

Yaotong Wan

Main Ingredients:

Herba Reineckeae Carneae	15%	*Jixiangcao*
Rhizoma Dioscoreae	30%	*Shanyao*
Fructus Psorale ae	30%	*Buguzhi*
Radix Achyranthis Bidentatae	7.5%	*Huainiuxi*
Radix Dipsaci	10%	*Xuduan*

Actions: Promoting the flow of Qi to activate blood circulation, dissipating blood stasis to alleviate pain.

Indications: Sudden sprain, and swelling and pain due to blood stasis.

Administration and Dosage. Taken orally, 1—2 bolus each time, twice daily.

Preparation Form: Honeyed bolus.

Package: 9 g in each bolus

Notes: This drug has the effects of anti—inflammation and analgesia. It clinically efficacious for various swelling and pain seen in the traumatic department, lumbago and acute lumbar muscle strain.

Yaoaitiao

Ingredients:

Folium Artemisiae Argyi	74.0%	*Aiye*
Ramulus Cinnamomi	3.9%	*Guizhi*
Lignum Dalbergiae Odoriferae	5.4%	*Jiangxiang*
Rhizoma Alpiniae Officinarum	3.9%	*Gaoliangjiang*
Herba Pogostemonis	1.6%	*Guanghuoxiang*

Rhizoma Cyperi	1.6%	*Xiangfu*
Radix Salviae Miltiorrhizae	1.6%	*Dan shen*
Radix Angeliae Dahuricae	3.1%	*Baizhi*
Pericicarpium citri Reticulatae	1.6%	*Chenpi*
Radix Aconiti	2.3%	*Shengchuanwu*
Realgar	0.4%	*Xionghuang*

Actions: Promoting the circulation of *Qi* and blood, and dispelling cold and dampness.

Indications: Pain and numbness due to wind—wetness, aching and numbness of muscles, pain of joints and limbs, and abdominal cold—pain.

Administration and Dosage: Moxibustion is done with this moxa—cone on the affected part until the skin becomes light red, twice daily.

Preparation Form: Moxa—cone.

Package: 29. 6 g in each moxa—cone.

Notes: This drug has the effects of anti—inflammation and analgesia. It is clinically efficacious for aching and numbness of muscles and pain due to chronic rheumatic arthritis.

12.2 Drugs Used in Surgery

Meihua Dianshe Dan

Main Ingredients:

Margarita	*Zhenzhu*
Venenum Bufonis	*Chansu*
Realgar	*Xionghuang*
Cinnabaris	*Zhusha*
Borax	*Pengsha*

Semon Lepidii seu Descurainiae	*Tinglizi*
Resina Olibani	*Ruxiang*
Myrrha	*Moyao*
Resina Draconis	*Xuejie*
Lignum Aquilariae Resinatum	*Chenxiang*
Borneolum Syntheticum	*Bingpian*

Actions: Clearing away heat, removing toxic materials, reducing swelling and alleviating pain.

Indications: Furuncle and carbuncle at the primary stage, swelling and pain of throat and gum, and sore on the tongue and oral cavity.

Administrationg and Dosage: Taken orally, 3 pills each time 1—2 times, or mixed with vinegar and put on the affected part.

Preparation Form: Water—paste pill.

Package: 1 g in every 10 pills.

Notes: This drug has the effects of resisting bacteria and inflammation, and arresting pain. It is clinically efficacious for parotitis, mastitis, acute lymphadenitis, pyosepticemia, tonsillitis, periodontitis, pharyngitis and innominate pyogenic infections.

Zijinding

Main Ingredients:

Bulbus Cremastrae	*Shancigu*
Radix Knoxiae	*Hongdaji*
Semen Euphorbiae Lathyridis / Pulveratum	*Qianjinzishuang*
Fructus Schisandrae	*Wubeizi*

Actions: Getting rid of filth and turbity, clearing away heat, removing toxic materials, activating blood flow and reducing swelling.

Indications: Sunstroke, swelling pain in the gastric cavity, nausea, vomiting, diarrhea. or boils, furuncle, mumpus, erysipelas and acute throat trouble.

Administration and Dosage: Taken orally, 0.6—1.5 g each time, twice daily. Or, mixed with vinegar and put on the affected part for external use.

Preparation Form: Pastille.

Package: 0.3 g in each pastille.

Notes: This drug is clinically efficacious for enterogastric—type common cold in summer, acute cholecystitis, parotitis, lymphadenitis, furuncle, insect—bite and snake—bite, innominate pyogenic infection, etc.

Xiaojin Wan

Main Ingredients:

Semen Momordicae	Mubiezi
Radix Aconiti Kusnezoffii	Caowu
Resina Liquidambaris	Fengxiangzhi
Resina Olibani	Ruxiang
Myrrha	Mo yao
Faeces Trogoterorum	Wulingzhi
Radix Angelicae Sinensis	Danggui
Lubricus Dilong	Donggui
Xiangmo	China ink stick

Actions: Dissipating blood stasis, promoting the subsidence of swelling, activating blood flow and alleviating pain.

Indications: Deep—rooted carbuncle of *Yin* type at the primary stage which is hard and painful, skin and external diseases, subcutaneous nodule and goiter.

Administration and Dosage: Taken orally after broken into pieces, 1.5 g each time, twice daily. The dosage for children should be decreased properly.

Preparation Form: Paste pill or water—paste pill.

Package: 0.6 g in each pill, 3 g in every 50 water—paste pills.

Notes: This drug has the actions of resisting inflammation and bacteria, arresting pain and treating tuberculosis. It is clinically efficacious for multiple abscesses, bone tuberculosis, tuberculosis mesenteric lymphadenitis, thyroma, lymphadenitis, mastitis, mammary cancer, etc.

It is contraindicated for pregnant women.

Ruyi Jinhuang San

Ingredients:

Rhizoma Curcumae Longae	12.5%	Jianghuang
Radix et Rhizoma Rhei	12.5%	Dahuang
Cortex Phellodendri	12.5%	Huangbai
Rhizoma Atractylodis	5%	Cangzhu
Cortex Magnoliae Officinalis	5%	Houpo
Pericarpium Citri Reticulatae	5%	Chenpi
Radix Glycyrrhizae	5%	Gancao
Rhizoma Arisaematis	5%	Tiannanxing
Radix Angelicae Dahuricae	12.5%	Baizhi
Radix Trichosanthis	25%	Tianhuafen

Actions: Removing toxic substances, reducing swelling and alleviating pain.

Indications: New—born boils, primary pyogenic infections, local hardness and red swelling with burning pain.

Administration and Dosage: Mixed with liquid for external application, several times a day.

Preparation Form: Powder.

Package: 15 g in each bag.

Notes: This prescription is from the book *Wai Ke Zheng Zong* written by Chen Shigong in the Ming Dynasty.

This drug has the actions of antisepsis and anti–inflammation. It is clinically efficacious for surgical acute pyogenic infection, acute phelgmon, and acute body surface inflammation, acute lymphadenitis, parotitis, mastitis, folliculitis, eczema and erysipelas due to hemolytic streptococcus infection, and traumatic swelling pain as well.

Xingxiao Wan

Main Ingredients:

Reaglar	*Xionghuang*
Resina Olibani	*Ruxiang*
Myrrha	*Moyao*

Actions: Activating blood flow to remove blood stasis, reducing swelling to alleviate pain.

Indications: Boils, pyogenic infections red swelling and burning pain.

Administration and Dosage: Taken orally, 1.5–3 g each time twice daily.

Preparation Form: Water–paste pill.

Package: 1 g in every 20 pills.

Notes: This drug has the effects of resisting bacteria and inflammation and reducing swelling. It is clinically efficacious for erysipelas, pyosepticemia, scrofula, mastitis, erythema, induratum, tumor, etc. It is contraindicated for pregnant women.

Yanghe Wan

Ingredients:

Rhizoma Rehmanniae Praeparatae	55.6%	Shudihuang
Colla Cornus Cervi	16.7%	Lujiaojiao
Cortex Cinnamomi	5.6%	Rougui
Rhizoma Zingiberis Praepartae	2.8%	Paojiang
Herba Ephedrae	2.8%	Mahuang
Semen Sinapis Albae	11.1%	Baijiezi
Radix Glycyrrhizae	5.6%	Gancao

Actions: Warming Yang, enriching the blood, expelling cold and resolving phelgm.

Indications: Syndrome of local diffuse swelling with unchanged skin such as various deep—rooted carbuncle of Yin type, pyogenic infection of bone, gravity abscess, arthroncus of knee, etc.

Administration and Dosage: Taken orally, 3 g each time, twice daily.

Preparation Form: Water—paste pill.

Package: 1 g in every 30 pills.

Notes: The recipe is from the book Wai Ke Zheng Zhi Quan Sheng Ji written by Wan Hongxu in the Qing Dynasty.

This drug has the effects of resisting bacteria and inflammation, and treating turberculosis. It is clinically efficacious for bone tuberculosis, tuberculosis of peritoneum, scrofula, thrombvagitis obliterans, osteomyelitis, chronic deep abscess, chronic bronchitis, dysmenorrhea, chronic arthritis, prolapes of lumbar intervertebral disc, lumb sacral enlargement, etc.

It is contraindicated for persons with fester carbuncle or deep—rooted carbuncle.

Badu Gao

Main Ingredients:

Lithargyrum	0.97%	Mituoseng
Semen Momordicae	0.97%	Mubiezi
Rhizoma Bletillae	0.5%	Baiji
Radix Ampelopsis	0.5%	Bailian
Spica Prunellae	1.9%	Xiakucao
Fructus Xanthii	0.97%	Cangerzi
Fructus Gleditsiae Abnormalis	0.97%	Zhuyazao
Radix Arnebiae seu Lithospermi	0.5%	Zicao
Herba Violae	0.5%	Diding
Bulbus Cremastrae	0.5%	Shancigu
Semen Hydnocarpi	0.5%	Dafengzi
Fructus Cnidii	0.5%	Shechuangzi
Herba Leonuri	0.96%	Yimucao
Fructus Forsythiae	0.96%	Lianqiao
Resina Draconis	0.5%	Xuejie
Myrrha	0.5%	Moyao
Resina Olibani	0.5%	Ruxiang
Catechu	0.5%	Ercha
Borneolum Syntheticum	0.5%	Bingpian
Alumen	0.5%	Baifan
Cera Flava	3.9%	Huangla
Calomelas	19.4%	Qingfen
Oleum Plantae	62.5%	Zhiwuyou

Actions: Removing toxic substances, alleviating pain, eliminating rotteness and promoting regeneration of tissue.

Indications: All external skin diseases with ulceration, swelling and pain, injury infliction caused by insect or animal bite, and innominate pyogenic infection.

Administration and Dosage: Stuck to the affected part.

Preparation Form: Plaster

Package: 0.125 g in each piece of plaster.

Notes: This drug has the effects of resisting bacteria, reducing inflammation, and promoting healing of trauma. It is clinically efficacious for furuncle, carbuncle, pyogenic infections, phelgmon, infection of scorpion venom, etc.

Chansu Wan

Main Ingredients:

Venenum Bufonis	Chansu
Realgar	Xionghuang
Calomelas	Qingfen
Alumen Exsiccatum	Kufan
Calcitum	Hanshuishi
Verdigris	Tonglu
Resina Olibani	Ruxiang
Myrrha	Moyao
Chalcanthitum	Danfan
Cathaica Fasciola	Woniu

Actions: Clearing away heat, removing toxic materials, reducing swelling and alleviating pain.

Indications: Malignant boils such as furuncle, lumbodorsal carbuncle, acute mastitis, etc.

Administration and Dosage: Taken orally, 5—15 pills each

time, 1—2 times daily.

Mixed with vinegar and put on the affected part. for external use.

Preparation Form: Water—paste pill.

Package: 1 g in every 30 pills.

Notes: This product has the effects of antisepsis, anti—inflammation and analgesia. It is clinically efficacious for various pyogenic infection, furuncle, carbuncle, phlegmon and pygenic lymphadenitis.

It is contraindicated pregnant women and festered sore.

Zicao Gao

Ingredients:

Radix Arnebiae	35.8%	Zicao
Radix Angelicae Dahuricae	10.7%	Baizhi
Radix Ledebouriellae	10.7%	Fangfeng
Resina Olibani	10.7%	Ruxiang
Myrrha	10.7%	Moyao
Radix Angelicae Sinensis	10.7%	Danggui
Radix Rehmanniae	10.7%	Dihuang

Actions: Removing putridity, promoting regeneration of tissues, reducing swelling and alleviating pain.

Indications: Unhealing ulcerated ulcer with incessant pain.

Administration and Dosage: Applied to the affected part with dressing change done every 2 or 3 days.

Preparation Form: Oinment.

Package: 15 g in each box.

Notes: The recipe is from the book *Yang Yi Da Quan* written by *Gu Shicheng* in the Qing Dynasty.

This drug has the effects of relieving inflammation, stopping pain, and promoting wound—healing. It is clinically efficacious for various pyogenic infections with diabrosis, pus and blood, ulceration of chickenpox, cold injury, burn and scald.

Neixiao Luoli Pian

Ingredients:

Spica Prunellae	26.18%	Xiakucao
Bulbus Fritillariae Thunbergii	3.2%	Zhebeimu
Sargassum	3.2%	Haizao
Radix Ampelopsis	3.2%	Bailian
Radix Trichosanthis	3.2%	Tianhuafen
Fructus Forsythiae	3.2%	Lianqiao
Radix et Rhizoma Rhei	3.2%	Shudahuang
Natrii Sulfas Exsiccatus	3.2%	Xuanmingfen
Concha Meretricis seu Cyclinae	3.2%	Geqiao
Halitum	16.1%	Daqingyan
Fructus Aurantii	3.2%	Zhiqiao
Radix Platycodi	3.2%	Jiegeng
Mentholum	0.02%	Bohebing
Radix Angelicae Sinensis	3.2%	Danggui
Radix Rehmanniae	3.2%	Dihuang
Radix Scrophulariae	16.1%	Xuanshen
Radix Glycyrrhizae	3.2%	Gancao

Actions: Softening and resolving hard mass, removing toxic materials and reducing swelling.

Indications: Scrofula and subcutaneous nodule, goiter and tumor on the neck due to stagnation of phelgm and Qi.

Administration and dosage: Taken orally, 4—8 tablets each

time, 1—2 times daily.

Preparation Form: Tablet.

Package: 0.6 g in each tablet.

Notes: This recipe is from the book *Yang Yi Da Quan* written by *Gu Shicheng* in the *Qing* Dynasty.

This drug has the effects of antisepsis, antituberculosis and analgesia. It is clinically efficacious for chronic lymphadenitis, scrofula and thyroid enlargement.

Zhizi Jinhua Wan

Ingredients:

Fructus Gardeniae	*Zhizi*
Rhizoma Coptidis	*Huang Lian*
Radix Scutellariae	*Huangqin*
Cortex Phellodendri	*Huangbai*
Radix et Rhizoma Rhei	*Dahuang*
Flos Lonicerae	*Jinyinhua*
Rhizoma Anemarrhenae	*Zhimu*
Radix Trichosanthis	*Tianhuafen*

Actions: Clearing away heat and purging fire to cool blood and remove toxic materials.

Indications: Excessive heat in the lung and stomach, marked by sore on the tongue and oral cavity, swelling and pain of the gum, conjunctival congestion, dizziness, sore and swollen throat and constipation.

Administration and Dosage: Taken orally, 9 g each time, once a day.

Preparation Form: Water—paste pill or honeyed bolus.

Package: 3 g in every 50 pills, 9 g in each bolus.

Notes: This recipe is from the book *Xuan Ming Lun Fang* written by *Liu Wansu* in the Jin Dynasty.

This drug has the effects of antisepsis and anti-inflammation. It is clinically efficacious for chronic pharyngitis, periodontitis, aphthae, erysipelas, phelgmon, anorectal infection and nosebleeding.

It is contraindicated for pregnant women.

Jingfang Baidu Wan

Ingredients:

Herba Schizonepetae	11.4%	Jingjie
Radix Ledebouriellae	11.4%	Fangfeng
Poria	11.3%	Fuling
Radix Peucedani	11.3%	Qianhu
Radix Platycodi	11.3%	Jiegeng
Rhizoma seu Radix Notopterygii	7.5%	Qianghuo
Radix Angelicae Pubescentis	7.5%	Duhuo
Radix Bupleuri	7.5%	Chaihu
Rhizoma Chuanxiong	7.5%	Chuanxiong
Fructus Aurantii	7.5%	Zhiqiao
Radix Glycyrrhizae	3.9%	Gancao
Herba Menthae	1.9%	Bohe

Actions: Clearing away heat, removing toxic materials, dispelling wind and resolving masses.

Indications: Newborn sores with burning sensation, swelling and pain, and disorders due to exogenous wind-cold.

Administration and Dosage: Taken orally, 6 g each time, 3 times daily.

Preparation Form: Water-paste pill.

Package: 1 g in every 20 pills.

Notes: This recipe is from the book *She Sheng Zong Miao Fang*. This drug has the effects of antisepsis, anti-inflammation and antivirus. It is clinically efficacious for skin diseases such as sarcoptidosis, tinea, and eczema, and urticaria, nail-like boil, mastitis, influenza and epidemic parotitis.

Lanwei Xiaoyan Pian

Ingredients:

Flos Lonicerae	14.3%	*Jinyinhua*
Folium Isatidis	14.3%	*Daqingye*
Herba Patriniae	14.3%	*Baijiangcao*
Herba Taraxaci	14.3%	*Pugongying*
Caulis Sargentodoxae	14.3%	*Daxueteng*
Fructus Toosendan	2.9%	*Chuanlianzi*
Radix et Rhizoma Rhei	4.3%	*Dahuang*
Radix Aucklandiae	4.3%	*Muxiang*
Semen Benincasae	4.3%	*Dongguazi*
Semen Persicae	2.9%	*Taoren*
Radix Paeoniae Rubra	5.5%	*Chishao*
Radix Scutellariae	4.3%	*Huangqin*

Actions: Activating blood flow, dissipating blood stasis, reducing swelling and alleviating pain.

Indications: Periappendicular abscess, distension and fullness in the stomach, and epigastralgia aggravated by pressure.

Administration and Dosage: Taken orally, 10-15 tablets each time, 3 times daily.

Preparation Form: Surgar-coated tablet.

Package: 0.25 g in each tablet.

Notes: This drug has the effects of antisepsis and anti—inflammation. It is clinically efficacious for acute and chronic appendicitis.

Saixianyan Pian

Ingredients:

Folium Polygoni Tinctorri	21.4%	*Liaodaqingye*
Radix Isatidis	21.4%	*BanLangen*
Fructus Forsythiae	21.4%	*Lianqiao*
Herba Taraxaci	21.4%	*Pugongying*
Spica Prunellae	14.26%	*Xiakucao*
Calculus Bovis man-made	0.14%	*Rengongniuhuang*

Actions: Clearing away heat, removing toxic materials, reducing swelling and resolving hard mass.

Indications: Mass, and swelling and pain due to boils.

Administration and Dosage: Taken orally, 6 tablets each time, 3 time daily.

Preparation Form: Tablet.

Package: 0.3 g in each tablet.

Notes: This drug has the effects of antivirus and anti—inflammation. It is clinically efficacious for epidemic parotitis.

12.3 Drugs For Treating Hyperosteogeny

Guci Pian

Ingredients:

Radix Rehmanniae	20%	*Dihuang*
Caulis Spatholobi	15%	*Jixueteng*

Radix Clematidis	12.5%	*Weilingxian*
Herba Epimedii	12.5%	*Yinyanghuo*
Herba Cistanchis	7.5%	*Roucongrong*
Herb Pyrolae	12.5%	*Luxiancao*
Rhizoma Drynariae	12.5%	*Gusuibu*
Semen Raphani	7.5%	*Laifuzi*

Actions: Tonifying the kidney, activating blood flow, expelling wind and softening hard masses.

Indications: Stiff and sore neck with distending pain, numbness of arms and pain in the loins and legs.

Administration and Dosage: Taken orally, 5 tablets each time, 3 times daily.

Preparation Form: Surgar—coated tablet.

Package: 0.3 g in each tablet.

Notes: This drug has the effects of improving blood microcirculation, diminishing inflammation and arresting pain. It is clinically efficacious for cervical vertebrae hypertrophy, lumbar vertebrae hypertrophy and thoracic hypertrophy due to hyperosteogeny, and proliferation of four—limb joints as well.

Slight reactions of the digestive canal may appear in some patients just after this drug is taken. but they can spontaneously disappear.

Guzhi Zengsheng Wan

Ingredients:

Rhizoma Rehmanniae Preaeparatae	21.4%	*Shudihuang*
Herba Cistanchis	14.3%	*Roucongrong*
Rhizoma Drynariae	14.3%	*Gusuibu*
Herba Epimedii	14.3%	*Yinyanghuo*

Caulis Spatholobi	14.3%	*Jixueteng*
Semen Raphani	7.1%	*Laifuzi*
Herba Pyrolae	14.3%	*Luxiancao*

Actions: Tonifying the kidney, strengthening the bones and muscles, promoting circulation of *Qi* and blood, and alleviating pain.

Indications: Weak loins and knees, stiff neck, and painful limbs with difficulty in moving.

Administration and Dosage: Taken orally, one bolus or 10—15 pills each time, 2—3 times daily.

Preparation Form: Honeyed bolus or concentrated pill.

Package: 3 g in each bolus, 1 g in every 8 pills.

Notes: This drug has the effects of promoting blood microcirculation, diminishing inflammation and arresting pain. It is clinically efficacious for hypertrophic spondylitis, cervical spondylasis, hypertrophy of lumbar and thoracic vertebrae, calcaneal spur, osteoarthrosis deformans endemica and hyperplastic arthritis.

Guci Wan

Ingredients:

Rhizoma Dioscoreae Nipponicae	*Cuanshanlong*
Radix Cynanchi Paniculati	*Xuchangqing*
Semen Strychni Praeparata	*Zhimaqianzi*
Caulis Millettiae Reliculatae	*Ji xueteng*

Actions: Clearing and activating the channels and collaterals, eliminating dampness, stopping pain, and softening and resolving hard mass.

Indications: Syndrome due to wind—cold—damp marked by

stiffness and soreness or distending pain of the neck and ache of the loins and legs.

Administration and Dosage: Taken orally, one bolus each time, 2—3 times daily.

Preparation Form: Honeyed bolus.

Package: 6 g in each bolus.

Notes: This drug has the effects of improving blood microcirculation, diminishing inflammation and arresting pain. It is clinically efficacious for hyperosteogeny, rheumatic arthritis, rheumatoid arthritis, rheumatism, etc.

Guxian Pian

Ingredients:

Rhizoma Drynariae	Gusuibu
Radix Stephaniae Tetrandrae	Fengfangji
Radix Rehmanniae Praeparatae	Shudihuang
Semen Sojae Nigrum	Heidou
Semen Cuscutae	Tusizi

Actions: Replenishing essence, invigorating the kidney, relaxing musucles and tendons and activating the flow of Qi and blood in the channels and collaterals.

Indications: Numbness of the extremities, soreness of the loins and legs, and stiffness of the neck.

Administration and Dosage: Taken orally, 4—6 tablets each time, 3 times daily. 30 to 50 days of treatment with the drug is a course.

Preparation Form: Surgar—coated tablet.

Package: 0.5 g in each tablet.

Notes: This drug has the effects of improving blood

microcirculation, allaying inflammation and arresting pain. It is clinically efficacious for hyperosteogeny, such as heel bone proliferation, knee joint proliferation, cervical vertebrae proliferation, and proliferation of lumbar and thoracic vertebrae.

It is contraindicated for patients with fever due to common cold.

Guci Xiaotong Ye

Ingredients:

Radix Aconiti	*Chuanwu*
Fructus Chaenomelis	*Mugua*
Radix Clematidis	*Weilingxian*
Fructus Mume	*Wumei*
Radix Achyranthis Bidentatae	*Huainiuxi*
Ramulus Cinnamomi	*Guizhi*

Actions: Activating blood flow, removing dampness and alleviating pain.

Indications: Stiff neck with soreness, numbness of the extremities and pain of the loins and legs due to the combination of wind, cold and dampness as well as the accumulation of dampness and heat.

Administration and Dosage: Taken orally, 10—15ml each time, twice daily.

Preparation Form: Tincture.

Package: 30 ml in each bottle.

Notes: This drug has the effects of improving blood microcirculation, allaying inflammation and arresting pain. It is clinically efficacious for of lumbar and thoracic vertebrae, cervical spondylosis, rheumatic arthritis and rheumatoid arthritis.

It is not to be taken with aspirin and sollium salicylate.

12.4 Drugs For Treating Hemorrhoid Complicated By Anal Fistula

Zhilou Wan

Main Ingredients:

Radix et Rhizoma Rhei	*Dahuang*
Rhizoma Picrorhizae	*Huhuanglian*
Natrii Sulphas	*Mangxiao*
Semen Pruni	*Yuliren*
Flos Sophorae	*Huaihua*
Radix Sanguisorbae	*Diyu*
Semen Persicae	*Taoren*
Resina Olibani	*Ruxiang*
Myrrha	*Moyao*
bits of elephant tusk	*Xiangyaxiao*
Talcum	*Huashi*
Realgar	*Xionghuang*
Spica Schizonepetae	*Jingjiesui*
Concha Haliotidis	*Shijueming*
Radix Angelicae Sinensis	*Danggui*

Actions: Clearing away heat, removing toxic materials, reducing swelling, relaxing the bowels, resolving hemorrhoid and mass.

Indications: Hemorrhoid with swelling and pain and anal fistula with bleeding both due to downward flow of damp–heat and heat in the blood.

Administration and Dosage: Taken orally, 9 g each time,

twice daily.

Preparation Form: Honeyed bolus.

Package: 9 g in each bolus.

Notes: This drug has the effects of allaying inflammation and arresting bleeding. It is clinically efficacious for internal or external hemorrhoid, bleeding of combined hemorrhoid, anal fissure and proctoptosis.

Huaijiao Wan

Ingredients:

Fructus Sophorae	28.5%	Huaijiao
Radix Sanguisorbae	14.3%	Diyu
Radix Scutellariae	14.3%	Huangqin
Fructus Aurantii	14.3%	Zhiqiao
Radix Angelicae Sinensis	14.3%	Danggui
Radix Ledebouriellae	14.3%	Fangfeng

Actions: Clearing the bowels, dispelling wind, removing heat from blood and stopping bleeding.

Indications: Syndrome due to excessive heat in the large intestines marked by hemorrhoid with swelling and pain, and blood in stools.

Administration and Dosage: Taken orally, one bolus each time, twice daily.

Preparation Form: Honeyed bolus.

Package: 9 g in each bolus.

Notes: The recipe is from the book *Xi Shi Zun Sheng Shu*.

This drug has the effects of allaying inflammation and arresting bleeding. It is clinically efficacious for internal or external hemorrhoid, mixed hemorrhoid, anal fissure with hemorrhage, hematochezia, etc.

Xiaozhiling Pian

Ingredients:

Fructus Schisandrae	4.8%	*Wu wei zi*
Radix Ampelopsis	23.5%	*BaiLian*
Herba Selaginellae	23.5%	*Juanbai*
Radix Sanguisorbae	23.5%	*Diyu*
Flos Sophorae	23.5%	*Huaihua*
ointment made from bile of cattle and sheep	1.2%	*Niuyang Dangao*

Actions: Clearing away heat from blood, reducing swelling and removing toxic materials.

Indications: Swelling, pain and hematochezia due to hemorrhoid complicated by anal fistula.

Administration and Dosage: Taken orally, 3—5 tablets each time, 3 times daily.

Preparation Form: Sugar—coated tablet.

Package: 0.3 g in each tablet.

Notes: This drug has the effects of allaying inflammation, arresting bleeding and promoting wound—healing. It is clinically efficacious for internal, external, or mixed hemorrhoid or anal fissure with hemorrhage.

Huazhiling Pian

Ingredients:

Rhizoma Coptidis	1.5%	*Huanglian*
Succinum	1.5%	*Hupo*
Radix Notoginseng	3.8%	*Sanqi*

Galla Chinensis	30%	*Wubeizi*
Pericarpium Granati	30%	*Shiliupi*
Alumen Exsiccatum	17.4%	*Kufan*
Realgar	6.3%	*Xionghuang*
Flos Sophorae	3.2%	*Huaihua*
Fructus Mume	3.1%	*Wumei*
Fructus Chebulae	3.2%	*Kezi*

Actions: Removing heat from blood and astringing.

Indications: Swelling, and hematochezia due to hemorrhoid complicated by anal fistula.

Administration and Dosage: Taken orally, 4-6 tablets each time, 3 times daily.

Preparation Form: Sugar-coated tablet.

Package: 0.3 g in each tablet.

Notes: This drug has the effects of resisting bacteria, allaying inflammation and promoting wound-healing. It is clinically efficacious for internal, external or mixed hemorrhoid and anal fissure with hemorrhage.

12.5 Drugs For Treating Burn And Scald

Jingwanhong Tangshang Yaogao

Main Ingredients:

Radix Sanguisorbae	*Diyu*
Fructus Gardeniae	*Zhizi*
Radix et Rhizoma Rhei	*Dahuang*
Borneolum Syntheticum	*Bingpian*

Actions: Reducing swelling, alleviating pain. resolving putridity and promoting regeneration of tissues.

Indications: Burn, scald and ulceration of purulent sore.

Administration and Dosage: Applied to the affected part.

Preparation Form: Ointment.

Package: 30 g in each bottle.

Notes: This drug has the effects of resisting bacteria, allaying inflammation, arresting pain and promoting wound—healing. It is clinially efficacious for burn or scald of 1 or 2 degree, internal or external hemorrhoid and bed—sore.

Huanyou

Ingredients:

Meles Fat	97%	*Huanyou*
Borneolum Syntheticum	3%	*Bingpian*

Actions: Moistening the skin, promoting regeneration of tissues, reducing swelling and alleviating pain.

Indications: Scald due to hot water and burn due to fire marked by the skin with swelling, blisters and ulcer.

Administration and Dosage: Applied to the affected part.

Preparation Form: Ointment.

Package: 15 g in each bottle.

Notes: This drug has the effects of allaying inflammation, arresting pain and protecting the skin. It is clinically efficacious for mild burn and scald with blisters and ulcer on the skin, hemorrhoid, sore and tinea.

Shaoshang Qiwuji

Ingredients:

Galla Chinensis	*Wubeizi*
Fructus Chebulae	*Kezi*

Actions: Clearing away heat, removing toxic materials, dispelling dampness and astringing.

Indications: Burn and scald with swelling, pain and ulcer.

Administration and Dosage: Nebulizied on the affected part, 3–4 times daily.

Preparation Form: Aerosol.

Package: 20 ml in each bottle.

Notes: This drug has the effects of resisting bacteria and promoting wound–healing. It is clinically efficacious for scald, and various burns.

12.6 Drugs For Treating Snake–bite

Yunnan Sheyao

Ingredients: (omitted)

Actions: Removing toxic materials, reducing swelling, arresting bleeding and alleviating pain.

Indications: Bites of poisonous snakes.

Administration and Dosage: Applied to the affected part.

Preparation Form: Tincture.

Package: 200 ml in each bottle.

Notes: This drug has the effects of allaying inflammation, removing toxic materials and arresting bleeding. It is clinically efficacious for various kinds of bite of poisonous snakes.

Jidesheng Sheyao Pian

Ingredients: (omitted)

Actions: Removing toxic materials, reducing swelling, arresting bleeding and alleviating pain.

Indications: Bites of poisonous snakes and insects.

Administration and Dosage: Taken orally, 1 tablet each time, 3 times daily.

Preparation Form: Tablet.

Package: 0.3 g in each tablet.

Notes: This drug has the effects of removing toxic materials and arresting pain. It is mainly used for bites of poisonous snakes and insects.

13 Drugs used in Departments of Obstetrics and Gynecology

13.1 Drugs for Treating Menoxenia

Aifu Nuangong Wan

Ingredients:

Folium Artemisiae Argyi	13.2%	Aiye
Cortex Cinnamomi	2.2%	Rougui
Rhizoma Cyperi	26.0%	Xiangfu
Radix Angelicae Sinensis	13.0%	Danggui
Fructus Evodiae	8.7%	Wuzhuyu
Rhizoma Chuanxiong	8.7%	Chuanxiong
Radix Paeoniae Alba	8.7%	Baishao
Radix Rehmanniae	4.3%	Dihuang
Radix Astragali	8.7%	Huangqi
Radix Dipsaci	6.5%	Xuduan

Actions: Regulating and invigorationg Qi, warming the womb and normalizing menstruation.

Indications: Womb—cold of insufficiency type, irregular menstruation, dysmenorrhea, soreness of the waist, and whites.

Administration and Dosage: Taken orally, 1 pill each time, twice daily.

Preparation Form: Honeyed bolus.

Package: 9 g in each bolus.

Notes: The prescription originates from the book *Shou Shi Bao Yuan* compiled by Gong Tingxian in the Ming Dynasty. This drug has the effects of arresting pain. regulating the function of the womb and nourishing and strengthening the body. It can be used to treat acyesis, irregular menstruation, dysmenorrhea and leukorrhagia.

Wuji Baifeng Wan

Ingredients:

Blackchicken	25.1%	Wuji
Colla Cormus Cervi	5.0%	Lujiaojiao
Carapax Trionycis	2.5%	Beijia
Cotheca Mantidis	1.9%	Sangpiaoxiao
Concha Ostreae	1.9%	Muli
Radix Ginseng	5.0%	Renshen
Radix Astragali	1.3%	Huangqi
Radix Angelicae Sinensis	5.6%	Danggui
Rhizoma Cyperi	5.0%	Xiangfu
Radix Paeoniae Alba	5.0%	Baishao
Radix Asparagi	2.5%	Tiandong
Radix Glycyrrhizae	1.3%	Gancao
Radix Rehmanniae Praeparata	10.0%	Shudihuang
Radix Rehmanniae	10.0%	Dihuang
Radix Stellariae	1.0%	Yinchaihu
Rhizoma Chuanxiong	2.5%	Chuanxiong
Semen Euryales	2.5%	Qianshi
Radix Salviae Miltiorrhizae	5.0%	Danshen
Cornu Ceriv Degelatinatum	1.9%	Lujiaoshuang
Rhizoma Dioscoreae	5.0%	Shanyao

Actions: Invigorating *Qi,* nourishing blood, regulating menstruation and arresting leukorrhagia.

Indications: Deficiency of both *Qi* and blood marked by thin and weak body, lassitude of the loins and legs, irregular menstruation, metrorrhagia and metrastaxis.

Administration and Dosage: Taken orally, 1 bolus each time, twice daily.

Preparation Form: Honeyed bolus.

Package: 9 g in each bolus.

Notes: With strengthening and astringing effects. This drug can regulate the womb. It can be clinically used to treat irregular menstruation, functional uterine bleeding, inflammation of female genital organ and leukorrhagia.

Nüjin Dan

Ingredients:

Radix Angelicae Sinensis	7.0%	*Danggui*
Radix Paeoniae Alba	3.5%	*Baishao*
Radix Rehmanniae Praeparata	3.5%	*Shudihuang*
Rhizoma Chuanxiong	3.5%	*Chuanxiong*
Radix Codonopsis Pilosulae	2.5%	*Dangshen*
Rhizoma Atractylodis Macrocephalae	3.5%	*Baizhu*
Herba Leonuri	10.0%	*Yimucao*
Poria	3.5%	*Fuling*
Cortex Moutan	3.5%	*Mudanpi*
Radix Glycyrrhizae	3.5%	*Gancao*
Myrrha	3.5%	*Moyao*
Cortex Cinnamomi	3.5%	*Rougui*
Rhizoma Corydalis	3.5%	*Yanhusuo*

Rhizoma Ligustici	3.5%	Gaoben
Radix Angelicae Dahuricae	3.5%	Baizhi
Radix Scutellariae	3.5%	Huangqin
Rhizoma Cyperi	7.5%	Xiangfu
Radix Cynanchi Atrati	3.5%	Baiwei
Halloysitum Rubrum	3.5%	Chishizhi
Fructus Amomi	2.5%	Sharen
Comu Cervi Degelatinatum	7.5%	Lujiaoshuang
Pericarpium Citri Reticulates	7.0%	Chenpi
Colla Cori Asini	3.5%	Ejiao

Actions: Nourishing blood to restore normal menstruation, regulating the flow of *Qi* to alleviate pain.

Indications: Irregular menstruation, dysmenorrhea, lassitude and pain of loins and legs and myasthenia of the extremities, all due to stagnation of *Qi* and blood stasis.

Administration and Dosage: Taken orally, 1 bolus each time, twice daily.

Preparation Form: Honeyed bolus.

Package: 9 g in each bolus.

Notes: The prescription originats from the book *Jin Dan Fang* complied by Han Maosheng in the Ming Dynasty.

With strengthening and tonic effects, this drug can regulate the womb and arrest pain. It can be clinically used to treat irregular menstruation, dysmenorrhea, functional uterine bleeding, inflammation of female genital organ and leukorrhagia.

It is to be used for pregnant women with caution.

Fuke Tiaojing Pian

Ingredients:

Rhizoma Cyperi	51.4%	*Xiangfu*
Radix Angelicae Sinensis	18.5%	*Danggui*
Fructus Jujubae	10.3%	*Dazao*
Radix Paeoniae Rubra	1.5%	*Chishao*
Radix Rehmanniae Praeparata	6.2%	*Shudihuang*
Rhizoma Atractylodis Macrocephalae	3.0%	*Baizhu*
Rhizoma Corydalis	4.1%	*Yanhusuo*
Rhizoma Chuanxiong	2.1%	*Chuanxiong*
Radix Paeoniae Alba	1.5%	*Baishao*
Radix Glycyrrhizae	1.4%	*Gancao*

Actions: Enriching blood, invigorating *Qi* and regulating menstruation.

Indications: Irregular menstruation, dysmenorrhea, redcced quantity of watery menstruation with light colour, dizziness, pale complexion and continuous pain in the lower abdomen which can be relieved by pressure.

Administratin and Dosage: Taken orally, 4 tablets each time, 3 times daily.

Preparation Form: Tablet.

Package: 0.3 g in each tablet.

Notes: With strengthening and tonic effects, this drug can regulate the function of the womb and arrest pain. It can be clinically used to treat irregular menstruation and dysmenorrhea.

Fuke Shiwei Pian

ingredients:

Radix Codonopsis Pilosulae	2.2%	*Dangshen*
Rhizoma Cyperi	76.8%	*Xiangfu*
Rhizoma Atractylodis Marcrocephalae	2.2%	*Baizhu*

Poria	2.2%	*Fuling*
Radix Glycyrrhizae	1.1%	*Gancao*
Fructus Jujubae	7.7%	*Dazao*
Radix Rehmanniae Praeparata	3.1%	*Shudihuang*
Radix Angelicae Sinensis	3.1%	*Danggui*
Radix Paeoniae Alba	0.8%	*Baishao*
Rhizoma Chuanxiong	0.8%	*Chuanxiong*

Actions: Invigorating *Qi*, nourishing blood, regulating menstruation and alleviating pain.

Indications: Irregular menstruation and dysmenorrhea.

Administration and Dosage: Taken orally, 4 tablets each time, 3 times daily.

Preparation Form: Tablet

Package: 0.25 g in each tablet.

Notes: This drug has tonic and strengthening effects and can regulate the function of the womb. It can be clinically used to treat irregular menstruation and dysmenorrhea.

Fuke Tongjing Wan

Ingredients:

Fructus Crotonis	*Badou*
Flos Carthami	*Honghua*
Lignum Aquilariae Resinatum	*Chenxiang*
Rhizoma Cyperi	*Xiangfu*
Radix et Rhizoma Rhei	*Dahuang*
Radix Curcumae	*Yujin*
Rhizoma Sparganii	*Sanleng*
Folium Artemisiae Argyi	*Aiye*
Carapax Trionycis	*Biejia*

Rhizoma Curcumae	Ezhu
Radix Scutellariae	Huangqin
Resina Toxicodendri	Ganqi
Radix Aucklandiae	Muxiang
Sal Ammoniac	Naosha

Actions: Eliminating blood stasis, normalizing menstruation, relieving depression and alleviating pain.

Indications: Dysmenorrhea, amenorrhea, oppressed feeling in the chest and distending pain in the loins and abdomen.

Administration and Dosage: Taken orally with millet gruel or millet wine on an empty stomach in the morning, 30 pills each time, once a day.

Preparation Form: Water—paste pill.

Package: 1 g in every 30 pills, 3 g in each bag.

Notes: With the effects of dilating blood vessels, improving blood circulation, removing blood stasis and regulating the function of the womb, this drug can be clinically used to treat dysmenorrhea and amenorrhea.

It is contraindicated for pregnant women and patients with diarrhea. In administration, raw or cold, pungent food or food from powdered buckweatea should be abstained from.

Xiaoyao Wan

Ingredients:

Radix Angelicae Sinensis	16.7%	Danggui
Radix Bupleuri	16.7%	Chaihu
Radix Paeoniae Alba	16.7%	Baishao
Rhizoma Atractylodis Macrocephalae	16.7%	Baizhu
Poria	16.7%	Fuling

| Radix Glycyrrhizae | 13.4% | *Gancao* |
| Herba Menthae | 3.1% | *Bohe* |

Actions: Dispersing the depressed liver—*Qi*, regulating the stomach, nourishing blood and normalizing menstruation.

Indications: Stagnation of liver—*Qi* and deficiency of the blood marked by distending pain in the chest and hypochondrium, irregular menstruation and mammary swelling.

Administration and Dosage: Taken orally, 6—9 g each time, 1—2 time daily.

Preparation Form: Water—paste pill.

Package: 1 g in every 10 pills.

Notes: The prescription originats from the book *Tai Ping Hui Min He Ji Ju Fang* compiled by Chen Shiwen in the Song Dynasty.

With analgestic and antiphlogistic effects, this drug can regulate the womb function. It is clinically used for irregular menstruation, chronic hepatitis and gastritis, neurosism and pleurisy.

Babao Kunshun Wan

Ingredients:

Radix Rehmanniae Praeparata	7.9%	*Shudihuang*
Radix Rehmanniae	7.9%	*Dihuang*
Radix Paeoniae Alba	7.9%	*Baishao*
Radix Angelicae Sinensis	7.9%	*Danggui*
Rhizoma Chuanxiong	7.9%	*Chuanxiong*
Radix Ginseng	3.9%	*Renshen*
Rhizoma Atractylodis Macrocephalae	7.9%	*Baizhu*
Poria	7.9%	*Fuling*

Radix Glycyrrhizae	3.9%	Gancao
Radix Scutellariae	7.9%	Huangqin
Herba Leonuri	3.9%	Yimucao
Radix Achyranthis Bidentatae	3.9%	Niuxi
Exocarpium Citri Rubrum	7.9%	Juhong
Lignum Aquilariae Resinatum	3.9%	Chenxiang
Radix Aucklandiae	1.6%	Muxiang
Fructus Amomi	3.9%	Sharen
Succinum	3.9%	Hupo

Actions: Nourishing blood to normalize menstruation.

Indications: Deficiency of both *Qi* and blood, marked by irregular menstruation, dysmenorrhea, soreness and pain the loins and legs and edema in the dorsum of the foot.

Administration and Dosage: Taken orally, 1 bolus each time, twice daily.

Preparation Form: Honeyed bolus.

Package: 9 g in each bolus.

Notes: With tonic, strengthening and antiphlogisitic effects, this drug can regulate the womb function. It can be used to treat irregular menstruation and dysmenorrhea.

Xuefu Zhuyu Wan

Ingredients:

Flos Carthami	12.0%	Honghua
Semen Persicae	16.8%	Taoren
Rhizoma Chuanxiong	6.0%	Chuanxiong
Radix Angelicae Sinensis	12.0%	Danggui
Radix Achranthis Bidentatae	12.0%	Niuxi
Radix Paeoniae Rubra	8.0%	Chishao

Fructus Aurantii	8.0%	*Zhiqiao*
Radix Rehmanniae	12.0%	*Shengdihuang*
Radix Platycodi	6.0%	*Jiegeng*
Radix Glycyrrhizae	4.0%	*Gancao*
Radix Bupleuri	4.0%	*Chaihu*

Actions: Promoting blood circulation to remove blood stasis and regulating the flow of *Qi* to alleviate pain.

Indications: Protracted hiccup, or dysphoria due to internal heat, palpitation, insomnia, gradual appearing of fever in the evening, amenia due to blood stasis, headache, prolonged, fixed and pricking chest—pain due to blood stasis in chest, and non—smooth circulation of blood.

Administration and Dosge: Taken orally, 1 bolus each time, twice daily.

Preparation Form: Honeyed bolus.

Package: 9 g in each bolus.

Notes: The prescription originates from the book *Yi Lin Gai Cuo* compiled by Wang Qingren in the Qing Dynasty.

This drug is clinically indicated for angina pectoris due to cornary arteriosclerotic heart disease, rheumatic heart disease, chest pain due to contusion in the chest and costal chondritis, headche and dizziness due to postconcussional syndrome, mental depression, insomnia and forgetfulness, amenorrhea and dysmenorrhea.

It is contraindicated for pregnant women.

Wenjing Wan

Ingredients:

| Radix Codonopsis Pilosulae | 18.5% | *Dangshen* |

Poria	11.1%	*Fuling*
Rhizoma Atractylodis Macrocephalae	18.5%	*Baizhu*
Radix Aconiti Lateralis Preparata	3.7%	*Fuzi*
Radix Astragali	7.4%	*Huangqi*
Cortex Cinnamomi	11.2%	*Rougui*
Fructus Evodiae	7.4%	*Wuzhuyu*
Rhizoma Zingiberis	7.4%	*Ganjiang*
Cortex Magnoliae Officinalis	3.7%	*Houpo*
Lignum Aquilarae Resinatum	3.7%	*Canxiang*
Radix Curcumae	7.4%	*Yujin*

Actions: Expelling cold from the channels, strengthening the spleen and regulating the flow of *Qi*.

Indications: Syndrome in women due to insufficiency of the spleen and cold of blood marked by dysmenorrhea, irregular menstruation, whites caused by cold—dampness, lassitude of the loins and legs, cold extremities, inappetence and acratia.

Administration and Dosage: Taken orally, 1 bolus each time, twice daily.

Preparation Form: Honeyed bolus.

Package: 9 g in each bolus.

Notes: This drug is clinically indicated for dysmenorrhea, irregular menstruation, whites and pain in the epigastrium.

Tongjing Wan

Ingredients:

Radix Angelicae Sinensis	7.6%	*Danggui*
Radix Paeoniae Alba	5.1%	*Baishao*
Radix Rehmanniae Preparata	10.0%	*Shudihuang*
Rhizoma Chuanxiong	3.8%	*Chuanxiong*

Rhizoma Cyperi	7.6%	Xiangfu
Radix Aucklandiae	1.3%	Muxiang
Fructus Crataegi	7.6%	Shanzha
Pericarpium Citri Reticulatae Viride	1.3%	Qingpi
Rhizoma Corydalis	5.1%	Yanhusuo
Rhizoma Zingiberis Praeparata	1.3%	Paojiang
Fructus Leonuri	2.5%	Chongweizi
Cortex Cinnamomi	1.3%	Rouqui
Herba Leonuri	30.4%	Yimucao
Radix Salviae Miltiorrhizae	7.6%	Danshen
Faeces Trogopterori	5.0%	Wulingzhi
Flos Carthami	2.5%	Honghua

Actions: Promoting blood circulation to remove cold, regulating menstruation to alleviate pain.

Indications: Syndrome of stagnation of blood due to cold, marked by dysmenorrhea, cold—pain in the lower abdomen reduced by warmth and smaller quantity of black menstruation with lumps.

Administration and Dosage: Taken orally before menstruation, 6—9 g each time, 1—2 times daily.

Preparation Form: Water—paste pill.

Package: 6 g in each bag.

Notes: The drug has the actions of dilating blood vessels, regulating the womb's function and arresting pain. It is clinically indicated for dysmenorrhea.

Fukangning Pian

Ingredients:

Radix Paeoniae Alba	39.3%	Baishao

Radix Angelicae Sinensis	4.9%	Danggui
Radix Ophiopogonis	9.8%	Maimendong
Radix Codonopsis Pilosulae	5.9%	Dangshen
Rhizoma Cyperi	5.9%	Xiangfu
Radix Notoginseng	3.9%	Sanqi
Herba Leonuri	29.5%	Yimucao
Folium Artemisiae Argyi Praeparata	0.8%	Aiyetan

Actions: Nourishing blood to normalize menstruation, regulating the flow of *Qi* to alleviate pain.

Indications: Syndrome in women of deficiency of both *Qi* and blood marked by irregular menstruation, dysmenorrhea, pale complexion, dizziness, shortness of breath, lanqor, weakness, and pale lips and nails.

Administration and Dosage: Taken orally regularly or from the 4—5 th day befort menstruation, 4 tablets each time, 2—3 times daily.

Preparation Form: Tablet.

Package: 0.5 g in each tablet.

Notes: With strengthening, tonic and analgestic effects, this drug can regulate the womb's function. It can be clinically used to treat irregular menstruation and dysmenorrhea.

Danggui Yangxue Wan

Ingredients:

Herba Leonuri	18.0%	Yimucao
Radix Chuanxiong	4.5%	Chuanxiong
Herba Lycopi	9.0%	Zelang
Cortex Cinnamomi	1.8%	Rougui
Radix Angelicae Sinensis	18.1%	Danggui

Radix Aucklandiae	4.5%	*Muxiang*
Cortex Magoliae Officinalis	9.0%	*Houpo*
Rhizoma Cyperi	9.0%	*Xiangfu*
Radix Paeoniae Rubra	9.0%	*Chishao*
Fructus Aurantii Immaturus	7.2%	*Zhishi*
Rhizoma Sparganii	1.8%	*Sanleng*
Flos Carthami	2.7%	*Honghua*
Fructus Foeniculi	2.7%	*Huixiang*
Rhizoma Curcumae	2.7%	*Ezhu*

Actions: Promoting blood flow by warming the channels.

Indications: Syndrome in women due to cold marked by irregular menstruation and abdominal pain caused by blood stasis or by postpartum blood–cold.

Administration and Dosage: Taken orally with boiled water before sleep, 60 pills each time.

Preparation Form: Water–paste pill.

Package: 1 g in every 20 pills.

Notes: With the effects of dilating blood vessels, removing blood stasis and regulating the womb's function, this drug can be clinically used to treat irregular menstruation, dysmenorrhea, amenorrhea and postpartum pain in the lower abdomen.

It is contraindicated for pregnant women and patients with fever due to *Yin* deficiency.

Danggui Jingao Pian

Ingredient:

Radix Angelicae Sinensis	100%	*Dang gui*

Actions: Promoting blood flow to regulate menstruation.

Indications: Irregular menstruation and dysmenorrhea.

Administration and Dosage: Taken orally, 4–6 tablets each time, 3 times daily.

Preparation Form: Tablet.

Package: 0.5 g in each tablet.

Notes: The drug has the actions of arresting pain and regulating the womb's function. It is clinically indicated for irregular menstruation and dysmenorrhea.

Qizhi Xiangfu Wan

Ingredients:

Rhizoma Cyperi	25.0%	Xiangfu
Radix Angelicae Sinensis	7.1%	Danggui
Rhizoma Sparganii	3.6%	Sanleng
Radix Paeoniae Rubra	7.1%	Chishao
Rhizoma Curcumae	3.6%	Ezhu
Rhizoma Chuanxiong	7.1%	Chuanxiong
Rhizoma Corydalis	3.6%	Yanhusuo
Radix Rehmanniae	7.1%	Dihuang
Pericarpium Citri Reticulatae Viride	3.6%	Qingpi
Radix Linderae	3.6%	Wuyao
Herba Leonuri	14.2%	Yimucao
Semen Persicae	2.7%	Taoren
Cortex Lycii	2.7%	Digupi
Pollen Typhae	3.6%	Puhuang
Flos Carthami	3.6%	Honghua
Radix Aucklandiae	1.8%	Muxiang

Actions: Regulating the flow of Qi to relieve stasis and promoting blood circulation to stop pain.

Indications: Stagnancy of Qi and blood marked by distending pain in the hypochondrium, irregular menstruation and dysmenorrhea.

Administration and Dosage: Taken orally, 6 g each time, 2—3 times daily.

Preparation Form: Water—paste pill.

Package: 1 g in every 20 pills.

Notes: The drug has the actions of dilating blood vessels, arresting pain and regulating the womb. It is clinically indicated for irregular menstruation and dysmenorrhea.

Yimu Wan

Ingredients:

Herba Leonuri	54.2%	*Yimucao*
Radix Angelicae Sinensis	27.1%	*Danggui*
Rhizoma Chuanxiong	13.6%	*Chuanxiong*
Radix Aucklandiae	5.1%	*Muxiang*

Actions: Promoting blood flow to regulate menstruation and promoting circulation of *Qi* to relieve pain.

Indications: Stagnancy of *Qi* and blood stasis marked by irregular menstruation, dysmenorrhea, and postpartum abdominal pain due to blood stasis.

Administration and Dosage: Taken orally, 1 bolus each time, twice daily.

Preparation Form: Honeyed bolus.

Package: 9 g in each bolus.

Notes: with the effects of dilating blood vessels, improving blood circulation, arresting pain and regulating the womb, this drug can be clinically used to treat irregular menstruation, dysmenorrhea, and postpartum abdominal pain.

It is contraindicated for pregnant women and menorrhagia.

Yimucao Gao

Ingredient:

| Herba Leonuri | 100% | Yimucao |

Actions: Promoting blood flow to regulate menstruation.

Indications: Amenorrhea, dysmenorrhea and abdominal pain due to blood stasis taking place after childbirth.

Administration and Dosage: Taken orally, 10 g each time, 1-2 times daily.

Preparation Form: Medicinal extract.

Package: 100 g in each bottle.

Notes: The drug has the effects of strengthening uterine contraction and tonicity. It is efficacious for amenorrhea, dysmenorrhea and postpartum pain in the lower abdomen.

It is contraindicated for pregnant women.

13.2   Drugs for Treating Leucorrhea

Guijing Wan

Ingredients:

Cortex Phellodendri	20%	Huangbai
Radix Paeoniae Alba	20%	Baishao
Radix Scutellariae	13%	Huangqin
Cortex Ailanthi	10%	Chunpli
Rhizoma Cyperi	10%	Xiangfu
Plastrum Testudinis	27%	Guiban

Actions: Nourishing Yin and reducing fever. maintaining normal menstruation and relieving leukorrhagia.

Indications: Syndrome of blood—heat due to *Yin* deficiency marked by preceded menstrual cycle, menorrhagia with dark colour and larger quantity and leukorrhea with reddish discharge.

Administration and Dosage: Taken orally, 6 g each time, twice daily.

Preparation Form: Water—paste pill.

Package: 1 g in every 20 pills.

Notes: The prescription originates from the book *Fu Ren Liang Fang Da Quan* compiled by Chen Ziming in the Song Dynasty.

The drug has the effects of regulating the womb, and inducing diuresis. It is clinically indicated for preceded menstrual cycle, and leukorrhea. It is also efficacious for male neurosism, emission, enuresis, insomnia, etc.

It is contraindicated for pregnant women.

Qianjin Zhidai Wan

Ingredients:

Rhizoma Atractylodis Marcrocephalae	3.6%	*Baizhu*
Radix Codonopsis Pilosulae	3.6%	*Dangshen*
Rhizoma Cyperi	14.2%	*Xiangfu*
Radix Angelicae Sinensis	7.1%	*Danggui*
Fructus Foeniculi	3.6%	*Xiaohuixiang*
Radix Paeoniae Alba	3.6%	*Baishao*
Rhizoma Corydalis	3.6%	*Yanhusuo*
Rhizoma Chuanxiong	7.1%	*Chuanxiong*
Cortex Eucommiae	3.6%	*Duzhong*
Radix Aucklandiae	3.6%	*Muxiang*
Fructus Psoraleae	3.6%	*Buguzhi*

Fructus Amomi	3.6%	*Sharen*
Cortex Ailanthi	14.2%	*Chunpi*
Radix Dipsaci	3.6%	*Xuduan*
Concha Ostreae	3.6%	*Muli*
Indigo Naturalis	3.6%	*Qingdai*
Flos Celosiae Cristatae	14.2%	*Jiguanhua*

Actions: Restoring *Qi* to treat leukorrhagia, adjusting the flow of *Qi* and blood to normalize menstruation.

Indications: Leukorrhea with reddish discharge, irregular menstruation, soreness of the waist and abdominal pain.

Administration and Dosage: Taken orally, 6—9 g each time, 2—3 times daily.

Preparation Form: Water—paste pill.

Package: 18 g in each bag.

Notes: With strengthening and tonifying effects, this drug can induce diuresis and regulating the womb. It is indicated for leukorrhea and irregular menstruation.

Baidai Wan

Ingredients:

Cortex Phellodendri	21.4%	*Huangba*
Cortex Ailanthi	42.9%	*Chunpi*
Rhizoma Cyperi	7.1%	*Xiangfu*
Radix Paeoniae Alba	14.3%	*Baishao*
Radix Angelicae Sinensis	14.3%	*Danggui*

Actions: Clearing away damp—heat and treating leukorrhea with reddish discharge.

Indications: Larger quantity of yellowish—green foul white like pus with reddish discharge and even blood which is as turbid as rice water, pruritus vulvae and scanty dark urine, all due to downward flow fo damp—heat.

Administration and Dosage: Taken orally, 6 g each time, twice daily.

Preparation Form: Water—paste pill.

Package: 18 g in each bag.

Notes: The drug is indicated for leukorrhea.

13.3   Drugs for Treating Diseases in Pregnancy

Baotai Wan

Ingredients:

Radix Astragali	9.3%	*Huangqi*
Poria	9.3%	*Fuling*
Rhizoma Atractylodis Macrocephalae	9.3%	*Baizhu*
Radix Angelicae Sinensis	9.3%	*Danggui*
Folium Artemisiae Argyi	9.3%	*Aiye*
Radix Paeoniae Alba	9.3%	*Baishao*
Radix Rehmanniae Praeparata	9.3%	*Shudihuang*
Rhizoma Chuanxiong	4.7%	*Chuanxiong*
Semen Cuscutae	9.3%	*Tusizi*
Bulbus Fritillariae Cirrhosae	2.3%	*Chuanbeimu*
Fructus Aurantii	4.7%	*Zhiqiao*
Radix Codonopsis Pilosulae	2.3%	*Dangshen*
Cortex Magnoliae Officinalis	2.3%	*Houpu*
Rhizoma seu Radix Notopterygii	1.2%	*Qianghuo*
Ramulus Taxilli	4.7%	*Sangjisheng*
Sbica Schizonepetae	2.3%	*Jingjiesui*
Radix Glycyrrhizae	1.1%	*Gancao*

Actions: Invigorating *Qi* and nourishing blood to prevent miscarriage.

Indications: Syndrome in women due to deficiency of both *Qi* and blood marked by liability to be abortion, threatened abortion, soreness of the waist, abdominal pain, and vaginal bleeding during pregnancy.

Administration and Dosage: Taken Orally, 1 bolus each time, 3 times daily.

Preparation Form: Honeyed bolus.

Package: 6 g in each bolus.

Notes: This drug is clinically indicated for threatened abortion and habitual abortion.

Antai Wan

Ingredients:

Radix Angelicae Sinensis	12%	*Danggui*
Rhizoma Chuanxiong	12%	*Chuanxiong*
Radix Paeoniae Alba	12%	*Baishao*
Radix Scutellariae	12%	*Huangqin*
Rhizoma Atractylodis Macrocephalae	6%	*Baizhu*
Radix Dipsaci	12%	*Xuduan*
Folium Artemisiae Argyi	12%	*Aiye*
Ramulus Taxilli	6%	*Sangjisheng*
Semen Cuscutae	12%	*Tusizi*
Colla Corii Asini	4%	*Ejiao*

Actions: Nourishing blood and preventing miscarriage.

Indications: Threatened and habitual abortion.

Administration and Dosage: Taken Orally, 1 bolus each time, twice daily, in the morning and evening.

Preparation Form: Honeyed bolus.

Package: 6 g in each bolus.

Notes: This drug is clinically indicated for threatened abortion and habitual abortion.

Lutai Gao

Main Ingredients:

Poria	*Fuling*
Colla Cornus Cervi	*Lujiaojiao*
Rhizoma Atractylodis Macrocephalae	*Baizhu*
Radix Rehmanniae Praeparata	*Shudihuang*
Radix Angelicae Sinensis	*Danggui*
Radix Ginseng	*Renshen*
Radix Paeoniae Alba	*Baishao*
Rhizoma Chuanxiong	*Chuanxiong*
Radix Glycyrrhizae	*Gancao*
Colla Corii Asini	*Ejiao*

Actions: Nourishing blood, invigorating *Qi*, warming the kidney and regulating menstruation.

Indications: Syndrome in women due to deficiency of the kidney and deficiency of both *Qi* and blood, marked by irregular menstruation and dysmenorrhea.

Administration and Dosage: Taken orally after dissolved in water, 3 g each time, 2 times daily.

Preparation Form: Medicinal extract.

Package: 50 g in each bottle.

Notes: This drug can be used to treat irregular menstruation, dysmenerrhea and infertility. It is also efficacious for neurosism, sexual neurosism, diabetes and chronic nephritis.

It is contraindicted for syndrome due to heat of excess type and excessive fire.

13.4 Drugs for Treating Puerperal Diseases

Shenghuatang Wan

Ingredients:

Radix Angelicae Sinensis	25.8%	Danggui
Rhizoma Chuanxiong	12.9%	Changxiong
Flos Carthami	1.6%	Honghua
Semen Persicae	3.2%	Taoren
Rhizoma Zingiberis	1.6%	Ganjiang
Radix Glycyrrhizae	3.2%	Gancao
Herba Leonuri	51.7%	Yimucao

Actions: Removing blood stasis, promoting blood circulation, warming the channels and stopping pain.

Indications: Postpartum abdominal pain due to blood stasis and lochiorrhea.

Administrating and Dosage: Taken orally, 1—2 boluses each time, twice daily.

Preparation Form: Honeyed bolus.

Package: 9 g in each bolus.

Notes: This drug has the function of dilating blood vessels, arresting pain, removing blood stasis and regulating the womb. It can be used to treat postpartum pain in the lower abdomen, too much lochia, residue of placental debris and postpartum hematorrhea.

Raw and cold food should be avoided in the course of treatment with this drug.

Bazheng Yimu Wan

Ingredients:

Herba Leonuri	29.7%	*Yimucao*
Radix Codonopsis Pilosulae	7.4%	*Dangshen*
Radix Rehmanniae Praparata	14.8%	*Shudihuang*
Radix Angelicae Sinensis	14.8%	*Danggui*
Rhizoma Atractylodis Macrocephalae	7.4%	*Baizhu*
Poria	7.4%	*Fuling*
Radix Paeoniae Alba	7.4%	*Baishao*
Rhizoma Chuanxiong	7.4%	*Chuanxiong*
Radix Glycyrrhizae	3.7%	*Gancao*

Actions: Invigorating *Qi*, nourishing blood and restoring menstrual flow.

Indications: Chief syndrome in women due to deficiency of both *Qi* and blood marked by general weakness, irregular menstruation, dysmenorrhea, smaller quantity and pale colour of menstruation, and inappetence.

Administration and Dosage: Taken orally, 1 bolus each time, twice daily.

Preparation Form: Hoenyed bolus.

Package: 9 g in each bolus.

Notes: The prescription originates from the book *Jing Yue Quan Shu* compiled by Zhang Jiebin in the Ming Dynasty. The drug has the actions of regulating the womb and arresting pain. It is indicated for irregular menstruation, dysmenorrhea, puerperal fever and other postpartum febrile diseases. It is also efficacious for anemia.

Shixiao San

Ingredients:

Pollen Typhae	50%	*Puhuang*
Faeces Trogopterori	50%	*Wulingzhi*

Actions: Promoting blood circulation to remove blood stasis and alleviating pain.

Indications: Syndrome due to blood stasis marked by chest and epigastric pain, or postpartum lochiostasis, or irregular menstruation and acute pain in the lower abdomen.

Administration and Dosage: Taken orally, 6—9 g each time, 1—2 times daily.

Preparation Form: Powder.

Package: 18 g in each bag.

Notes: The recipe originates from the book *Tai Ping Hui Min He Ji Ju Fang* compiled by Chen Shiwen in the Song Dynasty.

This medicine is clinically indicated for irregular menstruation, dysmenorrhea, amenorrhea, ectopic pregnancy. lochiostasis after childbirth, angina pectoris due to coronary heart disease, acute and chronic gastritis, gastric and duodenal ulcer, virus heapatitis, hematuria, etc.

It is contraindicated for pregnant women.

Xiaru Yongquan San

Main Ingredients:

Radix Angelicae Sinensis	*Danggui*
Radix Paeoniae Alba	*Baishao*
Rhizoma Chuanxiong	*Chuanxiong*

Radix Platycodi	Jiegeng
Radix Rehmanniae	Dihuang
Radix Angelicae Dahuricae	Baizhi
Radix Trichosanthis	Tianhuafen
Radix Glycyrrhizae	Gancao
Radix Bupleuri	Chaihu
Medulla Tetrapanacis	Tongcao
Radix Rhapontici	Loulu
Semen Vaccariae	Wangbuliuxing
Hordei Germinatus	Maiya

Actions: Nourishing blood to stimulate milk secretion.

Indications: Inadequate milk produced in puerperium.

Administration and Dosage: 1 bag of this drug is decocted in water for the decoction and this is done once more. The decoction is mixed and divided into two parts, one of which is drunk each time.

Preparation Form: Powder.

Package: 30 g in each bag.

Notes: Pungent food should be avoided.

Chanhou Shentong Pian

Ingredient:

Zhaoshanbai	100%

Actions: Expelling wind, dispelling cold, and promoting blood circulation to remove obstruction in the channels.

Indications: Syndrome in women marked by lumbago, numbness and pain in the joints of the limbs, irregular menstruation, dysmenorrhea and amenia due to wind—cold affected after giving birth.

Administration and Dosage: Taken orally, 2 tablets each time, 2 times daily.

Preparation Form: Tablet.

Package: 0.25 g in each tablet.

Notes: This drug can be used to treat such disorders in the women occurring after giving birth as lumbago, arthralgia, irregular menstruation, dysmenorrhea and amenorrhea. It is contraindicated for pregnant women, and in the course of treatment with it, raw and cold food should be avoided.

13.5   Drugs for Treating Miscellaneous Diseases

Dahuang Zhechong Wan

Ingredients:

Eupolyphaga seu Steleophaga	2.3%	Tubiechong
Radix et Rhizoma Rhei	22.7%	Dahuang
Hirudo	4.5%	Shuizhi
Semen Persicae	9.1%	Taoren
Tabanus	3.4%	Mangchong
Radix Scutellariae	4.5%	Huangqin
grub	3.4%	Qicao
Radix Rehmanniae	22.7%	Dihuang
Resina Toxicodendri	2.3%	Ganqi
Radix Paeoniae Alba	9.1%	Baishao
Semen Armeniacae Amarum	9.1%	Kuxingren
Radix Glycyrrhizae	6.9%	Gancao

Actions: Promoting blood circulation and removing blood stasis, restoring menstrual flow and disintegrating masses.

Indications: Syndrome due to blood stasis marked by mass

in the abdomen, squamous and dry skin, dull black orbit, tidal fever, emaciation amenorrhea, and lump in the abdomen causing distension and pain.

Administration and Dosage: Taken orally, 1—2 boluses each time, 1—2 times daily.

Preparation Form: Honeyed bolus.

Package: 3 g in each bolus.

Notes: The prescription originates from the book *Jin Gui Yao Lue* compiled by Zhang Zhonjing in the Han Dynasty.

The drug has the effects of dilating blood vessels, removing blood stasis, promoting the absorption of lumps and regulating the womb. It is clinically indicated for lump in the abdomen, trumefaction of liver and spleen, and amenorrhea.

It is contraindicated for pregnant women. If dermal sensitivity appears, this drug should not be used again.

Shaofu Zhuyu Wan

Ingredients:

Fructus Foeniculi	6.6%	*Huixiang*
Radix Angelicae Sinensis	19.7%	*Danggui*
Rhizoma Zingiberis	1.4%	*Gangjiang*
Rhizoma Chuanxiong	6.6%	*Chuangxiong*
Rhizoma Corydalis	6.6%	*Yanhusuo*
Cortex Cinnamomi	6.6%	*Guangui*
Myrrha	6.6%	*Moyao*
Radix Paeoniae Rubra	13.1%	*Chishao*
Faeces Trogopterorum	13.1%	*Wulingzhi*
Pollen Typhae	19.7%	*Puhuang*

Actions: Promoting blood circulation to remove blood stasis, dispelling cold and alleviating pain.

Indications: Syndrome due to accumulation of cold and stagnation of blood marked by mass and pain in the lower abdomen, postpartum lochiostasis with severe pain and blocks of blood stasis, or soreness of the waist and distension of the abdomen during menstruation and irregular menstruation with black—purple colour or lumps of blood stasis.

Administration and Dosage: Taken orally, 1 bolus each time, 1—2 times daily.

Preparation Form: Honeyed bolus.

Package: 6 g in each bolus.

Notes: The recipe originates from the book *Yi Lin Gai Cuo* compiled by Wang Qingren in the Qing Dynasty.

The drug has the actions of dilating blood vessels, removing blood stasis, promoting absorption of lumps, regulating the womb and relieving menalgia. It is clinically indicated for abdominal lumps, postpartum lochiostasis dysmenorrhea and irregular menstruation.

It is contraindicated for pregnant women.

Huazheng Huisheng Wan

Ingredients:

Herba Leonuri	*Yimucao*
Flos Carthami	*Honghua*
Pericarpium Zanthoxyli	*Huajiao*
Radix Angelicae Sinensis	*Danggui*
Hirudo	*Shuizhi*
Lignum Sappan	*Sumu*
Rhizoma Sparganii	*Sanleng*

Rhizoma Chuanxiong	*Chuanxiong*
Rhizoma Anemone	*Zhujiexiangfu*
Lignum Dalbergiae Odoriferae	*Jiangxiang*
Rhizoma Cyperi	*Xiangfu*
Radix Ginseng	*Renshen*
Myrrha	*Moyao*
Rhizoma Galangae	*Gaoliangjiang*
Semen Armeniacae Amarum	*Kuxinren*
Rhizoma Curcumae Longae	*Jianghuang*
Fructus Foeniculi	*Xiaohuixiang*
Radix et Rhizoma Rhei	*Dahuang*
Faeces Trogopterorum	*Wulingzhi*
Rhizoma Corydalis	*Yanhusuo*
Semen Persicae	*Taoren*
Pollen Typhea	*Puhuang*
Tabanus	*Mangchong*
Resina Olibani	*Ruxiang*
Glue of Carapax Trionycis	*Biejiajiao*
Resina Toxicodendri	*Ganqi*
Flos Caryophylli	*Dingxiang*
Fructs Evodiae	*Wuzhuyu*
Radix Paeoniae Alba	*Baishao*
Folium Artemisiae Argyi	*Aiyie*
Resina Ferulae	*Awei*
Radix Rehmanniae	*Dihuang*
Cortex Cinnamomi	*Rougui*
Fructus Perillae	*Suzi*

Actions: Disintegrating lumps and removing blood stasis.

Indications: Syndrome due to lumps and blood-stagnation

marked by lumps, arthralgia, emaciation due to blood disorder in women, postpartum blood—stasis and pain in the lower abdomen worsened by pressure.

Administration and Dosage: Taken orally, 1 bolus each time, 1—2 times daily.

Preparation Form: Honeyed bolus.

Package: 9 g each bolus.

Notes: With the effects of dilating blood vessels, removing blood stasis and promoting absorption of lumps, this drug is clinically indicated for abdominal lumps, postpartum blood stasis, tumefaction of the liver and spleen, hysteromyoma and trauma.

Pregnant women are not allowed to take it.

Tiaojing Zhibao Wan

Ingredients:

Radix et Rhizoma Rhei	72.0%	Dahuang
Radix Aucklandiae	4.0%	Muxiang
Semen Pharbitidis	2.0%	Qianniuzi
Pericarpium Citri Reticulatae	2.0%	Chenpi
Fructus Aurantii Immaturus	2.0%	Zhishi
Radix Scutellariae	2.0%	Huangqin
Rhizoma Atractylodis	2.0%	Cangzhu
Fructus Crataegi	3.2%	Shanzha
Faeces Trogopterorum	2.0%	Wulingzhi
Radix Angelicae Sinensis	1.0%	Danggui
Rhizoma Cyperi	2.8%	Xiangfu
Semen Arecae	2.0%	Binlang
Rhizoma Sparganii	1.0%	Sanleng

| Rhizoma Curcumae | 1.0% | *Ezhu* |
| Carapax Trionycis | 1.0% | *Biejia* |

Actions: Removing blood stasis and restoring menstrual flow.

Indications: Syndrome in women due to blood stasis marked by abdominal mass, amenorrhea and dysmenorrhea.

Administration and Dosage: Taken orally, 6 g each time, 2 times daily.

Preparation.Form: Water—paste pill.

Package: 1 g in every 20 pills.

Notes: This drug has the effects of dilating blood vessels, improving blood circulation, removing blood stasis, relieving menalgia and regulating the womb.

Pregnant women and those debilitated are not allowed to take it.

Jinji Chongji

Ingredients:

Radix Rosa Laevigatae	18.0%	*Jinyinggen*
Caulis Mahoniae	18.0%	*Gonglaomu*
Caulis Spatholobi	33.7%	*Jixeteng*
Radix Zanthoxyli	6.7%	*Liangmianzhen*
Radix Moghania Philippinensis	18.0%	*Qiangjiba*
Herba Andrographitis	5.6%	*Chuanxinlian*

Actions: Clearing away heat, removing toxic materials, promoting blood circulation and restoring menstrual flow.

Indications: Frequent urination, foul leukorrhea with larger quantity, irregular menstruation and dysmenorrhea.

Administration and Dosage: Taken orally, 1 bag each time,

twice daily. 10 days are involved in one course of treatment. 2–3 courses are needed if necessary.

Preparation Form: Granule or powder dissolvable in water.

Package: 6 g in each bag.

Notes: This drug can be used to treat adnexitis, endomatrial inflammation, pelvic inflammation, irregular menstruation, dysmenorrhea, leucorrhea and eczema testicle. It may be also used to prevent infection due to artificial abortion or contraceptive ring.

It is contraindicted for pregnant women.

Fuke Fenqing Wan

Ingredients:

Radix Angelicae Sinensis	16.3%	Danggui
Radix Paeoniae Alba	8.2%	Baishao
Rhizoma Chuanxiong	12.2%	Chuanxiong
Radix Rehmanniae	16.3%	Dihuang
Fructus Gardeniae	8.2%	Zhizi
Rhizoma Coptidis	4.1%	Huanglian
Folium Pyrrosiae	4.1%	Shiwei
Spora Lygodii	2.0%	Haijinsha
Radix Glycyrrhizae	8.2%	Gancao
Caulis Aristolochiae Manshuriensis	8.2%	Guangmutong
Talcum	12.2%	Huashi

Actions: Clearing away heat, promoting diuresis, promoting blood circulation and stopping pain.

Indications: Syndrome due to downward flow of damp–heat into the bladder marked by frequent micturition with urethral twinge and scanty dark and turbid urine.

Administration and Dosage: Taken orally, 9 g each time, twice daily.

Preparation Form: Water—paste pill.

Package: 3 g in every 50 pills.

Notes: The drug is used for cystitis, urethritis, acute prostatitis stone in the urinary system and acute pyelonephritis.

It is cautiously used for pregnant women.

14 Drugs used in the Department of Paediatrics

Xiaoer Zhibao Wan

Main Ingredients:

Herba Pogostemonis	Guanghuoxiang
Folium Perillae	Zisuye
Herba Menthae	Bohe
Rhizoma seu Radix Notopterygii	Qianghuo
Rhizoma Typhonii	Baifuzi
Pericarpium Citri Reticulatae	Chenpi
Semen Sinapis Albae	Baijiezi
Arisaema cun Bile	Dannanxing
Fructus Crataegi	Shanzha
Bulbus Fritillriae Cirrhosae	Chuanbeimu
Massae Medicata Fermentata	Liushenqu
Semen Arecae	Binglang
Fructus Hordei Germinatus	Maiya
Poria	Fuling
Succinum	Hupo
Borneolum Syntheticum	Bingpian
Rhizoma Gastrodiae	Tianma
Ramulus Uncariae cum Uncis	Gouteng
Bombyx Batryticatus	Jiangcan
Pariastracum Cicadae	Chantui
Scorpio	Quanxie

Calculus Bovis man—made	Rengongniuhuang
Realgar	Xionghuang
Talcum	Huashi

Actions: Dispelling wind, relieving convulsion, resolving phlegm and removing stagnancy.

Indications: Syndrome in infants due to wind—cold marked by fever, stuffy nose, cough with profuse sputum, loss of appetite, vomiting, diarrhea and convulsion.

Administration and Dosage: Taken orally. 1 bolus each time, 2—3 times daily.

Preparation Form: Honeyed bolus.

Package: 1.5g in each bolus

Notes: This drug is clinically used for common cold of gastrointestinal type and convulsion caused by acute infectious diseases.

Miaoling Dan

Main Ingredients:

Herba Menthae	Bohe
Radix Puerariae	Gegen
Rhizoma seu Radix Notopterygii	Qianghuo
Bulbus Fritillariae Cirrhosae	Chuanbeimu
Exocarpium Citri Grandis	Huajuhong
Radix Peucedani	Qianhu
Radix Platycodi	Jiegeng
Rhizoma Pinellinae Praeparata	Banxia
Rhizoma Arisaematis	Tiannanxing
Radix Paeoniae Rubra	Chishao
Ramulus Uncarriae cum Uncis	Gouteng

Cinnabaris	*Zhusha*
Borneolum Syntheticum	*Bingpian*
Caulis Aristolochiae Manshuriensis	*Mutong*
Radix Scrophulariae	*Xuanshen*
Radix Rehmanniae	*Dihuang*
Rhizoma Gastrodiae	*Tianma*
Cornus Bubali	*Shuiniujiao*

Actions: Reducing fever and promoting the dispersing fuction of the lung, resolving phlegm and relieving convulsion.

Indications: Common cold in infants marked by fever, headache, vertigo, cough due to interior heat, vomiting with phlegm, dry nasal and oral cavities, sorethroat, difficulty in micturition, crying with fear and disturbed sleep.

Administration and Dosage: Taken orally, 1 bolus each time for those over one year old, 1 / 2 bolus each time for those below one year old, twice daily.

Preparation Form: Honeyed bolus

Package: 1.5g in each bolus

Notes: This drug is clinically indicated for upper respiratory tract infection.

Jieji Ningsou Wan

Ingredients:

Folium Perillae	4.8%	*Zisuye*
Radix Peucedani	8.0%	*Qianhu*
Radix Puerariae	8.0%	*Gegen*
Semen Armeniacae Amarum	8.0%	*Kuxingren*
Radix Platycodi	8.0%	*Jiegeng*
Pericarpium Citri Reticulatae	8.0%	*Chenpi*

Rhizoma Pinelliae	8.0%	Banxia
Radix Trichosanthis	8.0%	Tianhuafen
Bulbus Fritillariae Cirrhosae	8.0%	Chuanbeimu
Fructus Aurantii	8.0%	Zhiqiao
Poria	6.4%	Fuling
Radix Aucklandiae	2.4%	Muxiang
Radix Scrophulariae	8.0%	Xuanshen
Radix Glycyrrhizae	6.4%	Gancao

Actions: Relieving exterior syndrome, promoting the dispersing function of the lung, relieving cough and resolving phlegm

Indications: Common cold in infants marked by fever, headache, cough with profuse sputum, thirst, dry throat, running nose with watery discharge and vomiting with phlegm.

Administration and Dosage: Taken orally, twice daily. 1 / 2 bolus is given to an infant of 1 year old each time; 1 bolus to an infant of 2—3 years old each time.

Preparation Form: Honeyed bolus.

Package: 3g in each bolus.

Notes: The drug can reduce fever, relieve cough and remove phlegm. It is clinically indicated for upper respiratory tract infection and acute bronchitis.

Xiaoer Jindan Pian

Main Ingredients:

Cacumen Tamaricis	Xiheliu
Spica Schizonepetae	Jingjiesui
Radix Peucadani	Qianhu
Herba Menthae	Bohe

Fructus Arctii	*Niubangzi*
Radix Ledebouriellae	*Fangfeng*
Rhizoma seu Radix Notopterygii	*Qianghuo*
Folium Isatidis	*Daqingye*
Cinnabaris	*Zhusha*
Rhizoma Gastrodiae	*Tianma*
Cornu Bubali	*Shuiniujiao*
Bulbus Fritillariae Cirrhosae	*Chuanbeimu*
Rhizoma Pinelliae	*Banxia*
Exocarpium Citri Rubrum	*Juhong*
Fructus Aurantii	*Zhiqiao*
Arisaema cum Bile	*Dannanxing*
Radix Platycodi	*Jiegeng*
Radix Scrophulariae	*Xuanshen*
Caulis Aristolochiae Manshuriensis	*Guanmutong*
Caulis Clematidis Armandii	*Chuanmutong*
Radix Paeoniae Rubra	*Chishao*
Radix Glycyrrhizae	*Gancao*
Borneolum Syntheticum	*Bingpian*
Radix Puerariae	*Gegeng*
Radix Rehmanniae	*Dihuang*

Actions: Expelling wind, clearing away heat, relieving convulsion and resolving phlegm.

Indications: Common cold in infants marked by fever, headache, running nose with watery discharge, cough, shortness of breath, soreness and swelling of the throat, convulsion due to high fever and slow eruption of rash.

Administration and Dosage: Taken orally, three tablets each time, twice daily. The dosage for children within one year old should be reduced accordingly.

Preparation Form: Tablet.

Package: 0.2g in each tablet.

Notes: This drug is clinically indicated for upper respiratory tract infection, infantile convulsion due to acute infection, and early morbillous infectious diseases.

Xiaoer Zhisou Wan

Ingredients:

Radix Scrophulariae	8.7%	Xuanshen
Radix Ophiopogonis	8.7%	Maidong
Semen Armeniacae Amarum	8.7%	Kuxingren
Arisaema cum Bile	8.7%	Dannanxing
Fructus Perillae	4.4%	Zisuzi
Semen Acrecae	6.5%	Binglang
Radix Trichosanthis	6.5%	Tianhuafen
Folium Perillae	4.4%	Zisuye
Bulbus Fritillariae Cirrhosae	6.5%	Chuanbeimu
Rhizoma Anemarrhenae	4.4%	Zhimu
Semen Trichosanthis	6.5%	Gualouzi
Radix Glycyrrhizae	6.5%	Gancao
Radix Platycodi	6.5%	Jiegen
Caulis Bambusae in Taeniam	6.5%	Zhuru
Cortex Mori Radicis	6.5%	Sangbaipi

Actions: Clearing away heat, resolving phlegm, moistening the lung and relieving cough.

Indications: Syndrome in infants marked by fever due to interior heat, dryness of oral cavity, abdominal distention, constipation and protracted cough with profuse yellow sputum.

Administration and Dosage: Taken orally, 1 bolus each time, twice daily, For infants below one year old, the dosage should be reduced accordingly.

Preparation Form: Honeyed bolus.

Package: 3g in each bolus.

Notes: This drug can reduce fever, remove phlegm and relieve cough. It can be used to treat infants with upper respiratory tract infection, fever, cough and constipation.

Xiaoer Zhike Tangjiang

Ingrdients:

Liquid extract of Radix Platycodi	14.3%	Jiegengliujin gao
Liquid extract of Radix Glycyrrhizae	71.4%	Gancaoliujin gao
Orange peel tincture	9.5%	Chengpiding
Ammonium chloride	4.8%	Lühuaan

Actions: Reducing sputum and relieving cough.

Indications: Cough due to common cold in infants.

Administration and Dosage: Taken orally, 3 times daily. Each time, 5 ml is given to infants of 2—5 years old, 5—10 ml to infants over 5, and an accordingly—reduced dossage to infants below 2.

Perparation Form: Syrup.

Package: 100ml in each bottle.

Notes: This drug has the actions of removing phlegm and preventing cough. It is clinically indicated for infants with cough due to upper respiratory tract infection and acute or chronic bronchitis.

Xiaoer Niuhuang Qingxin San

Ingredients:

Rhizoma Gastrodiae	8.5%	Tianma
Arisaema cum Bile	6.8%	Dannanxing
Rhizoma Coptidis	12.8%	Huanglian
Radix Paeoniae Rubra	6.8%	Chishao
Radix et Rhizoma Rhei	12.8%	Dahuang
Scorpio	6.8%	Quanxie
Cornus Bubali	8.5%	Shuiniujiao
Calculus Bovis	0.85%	Niuhuang
Bombyx Batryticatus	8.5%	Jiangcan
Succinum	2.1%	Hupo
Realgar	6.4%	Xionghuang
Borneolum Syntheticum	2.1%	Bingpian
Lapis Micae Aureus	8.5%	Jinmengshi
Cinnabaris	8.5%	Zhusha

Actions: Clearing away heat, resolving phlegm, and relieving convulsion and muscle spasm. .

Indication: Syndrome in infants due to internal heat marked by acute convulsion, dyspnea with phlegm, spasm of the limbs and acute unconsciousness.

Administration and Dosage: Taken orally, 1—2 times daily. Each time, 1 / 2 bag of the drug is given to infants within 1 year old, 1 bag to infants of 1—3 years old, and an accordingly—increased dosage to infants over 3.

Preparation Form: Powder

Package: 0.6g in each bag.

Notes: This drug is clinically indicated for infants with high fever and convulsion due to acute infection.

It is contraindicated for common cold due to wind—cold, interior heat—fever due to measles or varicella.

Baoying Zhenjing Wan

Ingredients:

Radix et Rhizoma Rhei	53.6%	Dahuang
Cinnabaris	10.7%	Zhusha
Radix Glycyrrhizae	35.7%	Gancao

Actions: Purging heat, removing stagnancy and relieving convulsion.

Indications: Syndrome in infants marked by constipation due to excess heat, abdominal distention, vomiting, convulsion, conjunctival congestion and aphthae.

Administration and Dosage: Taken orally, once daily. 1 bolus is given to infants between 1—6 years old, 1 / 2 bolus to infants within 1 year old.

Preparation Form: Honeyed bolus.

Package: 1.5g in each bolus

Notes: This drug can be used to treat infants with constipation, convulsion and tic of limbs.

Xiaoer Jingfeng Wan

Main Ingredients:

Herba Ephaedrae	Mahuang
Rhizoma Atractylodis	Cangzhu
Flos Caryophylli	Dingxiang
Herba Asari	Xixin
Fructus Gardeniae	Zhizi

Rhizoma Gastrodiae	*Tianma*
Radix Glycyrrhizae	*Gancan*
Bombyx Batryticatus	*Jiangcan*
Fructus Glenitsine Abnormalis	*Zhuyazao*
Scorpio	*Quanxie*
Scolopendra	*Wugong*
Arisaema cum Bile	*Dannanxing*
Ramulus Uncariae cum Uncis	*Gouteng*
Borneolum Syntheticum	*Bingpian*
Cinnabaris	*Zhusha*

Actions: Expelling wind, clearing away cold, inducing resuscitation and relieving convulsion.

Indications: Syndromes in infants marked by acute convulsion, common cold in the four seasons, and alternate attacks of chills and fever.

Administration and Dosage: Taken orally, 3 times daily. Each time, 5 pills is given to newborns, 10 pills to babies of 6 months to 1 year old, 15 pills to infants of 1—2 years old, and 20 pills to infants above 2 years old.

Preparation Form: Water—paste pill.

Package: 0.6g in every 100 pills.

Notes: This drug is clinically indicated for babies or infants with convulsion due to acute infection, and upper respiratory tract infection.

Yingeran Pian

Ingredients:

Endothelium Corneum Gigeriae Galli	15%	*Jineijin*
Rhizoma Pinelliae	10%	*Banxia*

Bulbus Fritillariae Cirrhosae	10%	*Chuangbeimu*
Concretio Silicae Bambusae	10%	*Tianzhuhuang*
Pericarpium Citri Reticulatae	10%	*Chenpi*
Ramulus Uncariae cum Uncis	10%	*Gouteng*
Rhizoma Gastrodiae	10%	*Tianma*
Cinnabaris	10%	*Zhusha*
Succinum	15%	*Hupo*

Actions: Dispelling wind, relieving convulsion, promoting digestion, resolving phlegm and reducting fever.

Indications: Syndrome in infants marked by fever, cough, retention of food and convulsion due to accumulation of phlegm and heat.

Administration and Dosage: Taken orally, once in the evening. 1／2 tablet is given to infants below 1 year old, 1 to those between 1—3 years old, 2 to young children between 4—7 years old, and 3 to children between 8—12 years old.

Preparation Form: Tablet.

Package: 0.32g in each tablet.

Notes: This drug can be used to treat children with fever, cough, dyspepsia, convulsion and tic of limps. Cold or greasy food is avoided.

Xiaoer Jianpi Wan

Ingredients:

Radix Ginseng	4.6%	*Renshen*
Rhizoma Atractylodis Macrocephalae	1.3%	*Baizhu*
Radix Glycyrrhizae	4.6%	*Gancao*
Poria	1.3%	*Fuling*
Rhizoma Pinellinae Praeparata	4.6%	*Zhibanxia*

Pericarpium Citri Reticulatae	9.3%	*Chenpi*
Semen Dolichoris Album	9.3%	*Baibiandou*
Rhizoma Dioscoreae	9.3%	*Shanyao*
Semen Nelumbinis	9.3%	*Lianzi*
Fructus Amomi	4.6%	*Sharen*
Massa Fermentata Medicinalis	9.3%	*Shenqu*
Radix Platycodi	4.6%	*Jiegeng*
Fructus Hordei Germinatus	9.3%	*Maiya*
Rhizoma Polygonati Odorati	9.3%	*Yuzhu*
Fructus Crataegi	9.3%	*Shanzha*

Actions: Strengthening the spleen, regulating the stomach and removing stagnancy.

Indications: Syndrome in infants due to weakness of the spleen and stomach marked by anorexia, loose stools, general weakness and acratia.

Administration and Dosage: Taken orally, 2 boluses each time, 3 times daily.

Preparation Form: Honeyed bolus.

Package: 2g in each bolus.

Notes: The drug has the actions of strengthening the stomach and promoting digestion. It can be used to treat children with dyspepsia, anorexia and malnutrition.

Xiaoer Xiaoshi Pian

Ingredients:

Fructus Crataegi	Shanzha
Endothelium Corneum Gigeriae Galli	Jineijin
Massa Fermentata Medicinalis	Shenqu
Semen Arecae	Binglang

| Fructus Hordei Germinatus | Maiya |
| Pericarpium Citri Reticulatae | Chenpi |

Actions: Promoting digestion to eliminate indigested food, strengthening the spleen, to regulate the stomach.

Indications: Syndrome due to incoordination between the spleen and stomach, marked by and dyspepsia, anorexia, abdominal distension, constipation, retention of food and malnutrition.

Administration and Dosage: Taken orally, 3 times daily. Each time, 2—4 tablets is given to infants of 1—3 years old, and 4—6 to young children of 3—7.

Preparation Form: Tablet.

Package: 0.3g in each tablet.

Notes: This drug has the actions of strengthening the stomach to promote digestion, It can be used to treat infants with dyspepsia, anorexia, constipation and malnutrition.

Xiaoer xiaoji Wan

Ingredients:

Fructus Aurantii	4.1%	Zhiqiao
Radix Scutellaria	2.5%	Huangqin
Rhizoma Sparganii	4.1%	Sanleng
Semen Arecae	16.4%	Binglang
Rhizoma Zedoariae	4.1%	Ezhu
Pericarp ium Citri Reticulatae	4.1%	Chenpi
Cortex Magnoliae Officinalis	4.1%	Houpo
Radix et Rhizoma Rhei	8.2%	Dahuang
Pericarpium Citri Reticulatae Viride	4.1%	Qingpi
Radix Aucklandiae	4.1%	Muxiang
Semen Pharbitidis	4.1%	Qiannuzi

Pulvis Crotonis Tiglium	8.2%	*Badoushuang*
Rhizoma Cyper	16.4%	*Xiangfu*
Cinnabaris	3.2%	*Zhusha*

Actions: Promoting digestion to remove indigested food, activating the flow of Qi to regalate the stomach.

Indications: Syndrome in infants marked by retention of milk and food, abdominal distention and pain.

Administration and Dosage: Taken orally, twice daily. Each time, 5 pills is given to babies of 1—3 months old, 10 to those of 4—6 months old, 30 to infants of 1—2 years old, and 80 to children of 7—12 years old.

Preparation Form: Water—paste pill.

Package: 1g in every 320 pills.

Notes: This drug can be used to treat dyspepsia and constipation. It is contraindicated for those with diarrhea and general weakness.

Xiangsu Zhengwei Wan

Ingredients:

Herba Pogostemonis	11.8%	*Guanghuoxiang*
Folium Perillae	23.6%	*Zisuye*
Cortex Magnoliae Officinalis	11.8%	*Houpo*
Herba Elsholtziae	11.8%	*Xiangru*
Fructus Aurantii	2.9%	*Zhiqiao*
Pericarpium Citri Reticulatae	5.9%	*Chenpi*
Semen Dolichoris Album	5.9%	*Baibiandou*
Fructus Amomi	2.9%	*Sharen*
Fructus Crataegi	2.9%	*Shanzha*

Poria	2.9%	*Fuling*
Massa Fermentata Medicinalis	2.9%	*Shenqu*
Radix Glycyrrhizae	1.6%	*Gancao*
Fructus Horei Germinatus	2.9%	*Maiya*
Talcum	9.7%	*Huashi*
Cinnabaris	0.5%	*Zhusha*

Actions: Relieving exterior syndrome, regulating the middle—*Jiao*, promoting digestion and eliminating indigested food.

Indications: Common cold in infants due to summer—dampness marked by loss of appetite, headache and fever, vomiting and diarrhea, distention and fullness in the abdomen and dribbling urination.

Administration and Dosage: Taken orally, 1 bolus each time, 1—2 times daily. For infants within one year old, the dosage should be reduced accordingly.

Preparation Form: Honeyed bolus.

Package: 3g in each bolus.

Notes: This drug can be clinically used to treat common cold of gastrointestinal type and acute gastroenteritis.

Xiangju Wan

Ingredients:

Poria	7.8%	*Fuling*
Rhizoma Atractylodis Macrocephalae	7.8%	*Baizhu*
Rhizoma Atractylodis	7.8%	*Cangzhu*
Pericarpium Citri Reticulatae	7.8%	*Chenpi*
Rhizoma Cyperi	7.8%	*Xiangfu*
Rhizoma Dioscoreae	5.2%	*Shanyao*

Semen Dolichoris Album	5.2%	*Baibiandou*
Rhizoma Pinellinae Praeparata	5.2%	*Fabanxia*
Semen Coicis	5.2%	*Yiyiren*
Semen Nelumbinis	5.2%	*Lianzi*
Fructus Crataegi	5.2%	*Shangzha*
Rhizoma Alismatis	2.6%	*Zexie*
Fructus Aurantii Immaturus	5.2%	*Zhishi*
Radix Aucklandiae	1.2%	*Muxiang*
Fructus Amomi	2.6%	*Sharen*
Fructus Hordei Germinatus	5.2%	*Maiya*
Cortex Magnoliae Officinalis	5.2%	*Houpo*
Radix Glycyrrhizae	2.6%	*Gancao*
Massa Fermentata Medicinalis	5.2%	*Shenqu*

Actions: Strengthening the spleen, promoting appetite, eliminating dampness and arresting diarrhea.

Indications: Syndrome in infants due to weakness of the spleen and stomach marked by abdominal distension, vomiting, diarrhea and anorexia.

Administration and Dosage: Taken orally. 1 bolus each time, 3 times daily. For infants within three years old, the dosage should be reduced accordingly.

Preparation Form: Honeyed bolus.

Package: 3g in each bolus

Notes: The drug has the actions of strengthening the stomach to promote digestion, It can be used to treat infants with chronic consumptive diseases such as parastosis and pure infantile dyspepsia.

Yingér San

Ingredients:

Semen Dolichoris Album	4.5%	*Baibiandou*
Bulbus Fritilariae Cirrhosae	0.97%	*Chuanbeimu*
Endothelium Cormeum Gigeriae Galli	13.5%	*Jineijin*
Radix Aucklandiae	13.5%	*Muxiang*
Rhizoma Dioscoreae	13.5%	*Shanyao*
Calculus Bovis	0.03%	*Niuhuang*
Rhizoma Atractylodis Macrocephalae	13.5%	*Baizhu*

Actions: Reinforcing the spleen, promoting digestion and arresting diarrhea.

Indications: Dyspepsia, loss of appetite, abdominal pain and diarrhea.

Administration and Dosage: Taken orally, twice daily. Each time, 0.25g is given to infants within 1 year old, and 0.5—1g to those between 1—3 years old.

Preparation Form: Powder.

Package: 2.5g in each bag.

Notes: The drug has the actions of strengthening the stomach, promoting digestion and arresting diarrhea. It can be clinically used to treat children with dyspepsia, anorexia and diarrhea.

Xiaoer Zhixie Pian

Main Ingredients:

Rhizoma Dioscoreae	*Shanyao*
Rhizoma Atractylodis Macrocephalae	*Baizhu*
Alumen	*Baifan*

| Semen Plantanginis | Cheqianzi |
| Cortex Ziziphi Jujubae | Zaoshupi |

Actions: Strenthening the spleen, reducing diuresis, normalizing the function of the intestines and relieving diarrhea.

Indications: Syndrome in infants due to weakness of the spleen and stomach marked by diarrhea, abdominal pain, dyspepsia, anorexia, and emaciation with sallow complexion.

Administration and Dosage: Taken orally. 3 times daily. Each time, 2 tablet, is given to infants within 1 year old, 3 to those between 1—2 years old, and to those between 3—4. 4 tables each time.

Preparation Form: Tablet.

Package: 0.25g in each tablet

Notes: This drug can be used to treat infants with diarrhea.

Niuhuang Baolong Pian

Main Ingredients:

Calculus Bovis	Niuhuang
Cinnabaris	Zhusha
Succinum	Hupo
Arisaema cum Bile	Dannanxing
Scorpio	Quanxie
Poria	Fuling
Concretio Silicea Bambusae	Tianzhuhuang
Bombyx Batryticatus	Jiangcan

Actions: Clearing away heat. dissolving phlegm, dispelling wind and relieving convulsion.

Indications: Syndrome in infants due to sudden convulsion marked by fever, sopor, trismus, clonic spasm of hands and feet, dyspnea with phlegm and upward looking eyes.

Administration and Dosage: Taken orally, two tablets each time, 1—2 times daily. For infants within one year old, the dosage should be reduced accordingly.

Preparation Form: Tablet.

Package: 4 tablets in one bag

Notes: This drug can be used to treat infants with fever cough, and convulsion caused by acute infection as well.

Qizhen Wan

Main Ingredients:

Bombyx Batryticatus (fried)	*Jiangcan*
Scorpio	*Quanxie*
Cinnabaris	*Zhusha*
Realgar	*Xionghuang*
Arisaema cum Bile	*Dannanxing*
Concretio Silicea Bambusae	*Tianzhuhuang*
Pulvis Crotonis Tiglium	*Badoushuang*

Actions: Arresting convulsion, eliminating phelgm, promoting digestion and relaxing the bowels.

Indications: Syndrome in infants due to sudden convulsion marked by fever, sopor, dyspnea, dysphoria, lots of phlegm, loss of appetite and constipation.

Administration and Dosage: Taken orally, 1—2 times daily. Each time, 3 pills is given to babies of 3—4 months old, 4—5 to those of 5—7 months old, and 6—7 to those of 1 year old. The dosage for infants over one year old or with general insufficiency of *Qi* should be increased accordingly.

Preparation Form: Water—paste pill

Package: 3g in every 200 pills.

Notes: This drug can be used to treat convulsion caused by acute infection, fever, anorexia and constipation.

The drug contains Pulvis Crotonis Tiglium, so the dosage should be controlled and it can not be used for a long time.

Niuhuang Zhenjing Wan

Ingredients:

Ariseama cum Bile	*Dannanxing*
Calculus Bovis	*Niuhuang*
Bulbus Fritillariae Cirrhosae	*Chuanbeimu*
Concretio Silicea Bambusae	*Tianzhuhuang*
Realgar	*Xionghuang*
Radix et Rhizoma Rhei	*Dahuang*
Ramulus Uncariae cum Uncis	*Gouteng*
Scorpio	*Quanxie*
Rhizoma Typhonii	*Baifuzi*
Lumbricus	*Dilong*
Borneolum Syntheticum	*Bingpian*
Radix Curcumae	*Yujin*
Rhizoma Acori Graminei	*Shichangpu*
Lignum Aquilariae Resinatum	*Chenxiang*
Rhizoma seu Radix Notopterygii	*Qianghuo*
Herba Menthae	*Bohe*
Radix Aconoti	*Chuangwu*
Rhizoma Chuanxiong	*Chuangxiong*
Poria	*Fuling*
Margarita	*Zhenzhu*
Succinum	*Hupo*

Cinnbaris   *Zhusha*

Actions: Clearing away heat, relieving convulsion, expelling wind and resolving phlegm.

Indications: Infantile sudden convulsion marked by fever, dyspnea, lots of phlegm, spasm, trismus, and unconsciousness.

Administration and Dosage: Taken orally, 1 bolus each time, 2 times daily, For children within one year old, the dosage should be reduced accordingly.

Preparation Form: Honeyed bolus.

Package: 1.5g in each bolus.

Notes: This drug can be used to treat infantile epilepsy and convulsion caused by acute infection.

Daochi Wan

Ingredients:

Fructus Forsythiae	12.5%	*Lianqiao*
Rhizoma Coptidis	6.3%	*Huanglian*
Fructus Gardeniae	12.5%	*Zhizi*
Caulis Aristlochiae Manshuriensis	6.2%	*Mutong*
Radix Scrophulariae	12.5%	*Xuanshen*
Radix Peaoniae Rubra	6.2%	*Chishao*
Radix Trichosanthis	12.5%	*Tianhuafen*
Radix et Rhizoma Rhei	6.3%	*Dahuang*
Radix Scutellariae	12.5%	*Huangqin*
Talcum	12.5%	*Huashi*

Actions: abating fever, purging fire, reducing diuresis and relaxing the bowels.

Indications: Sore oral cavity and throat, dysphoria with smothery sensation in the chest, scanty dark urine and constipation.

Administration and Dosage: Taken orally, 1 bolus each time, twice daily. For children within one year old, the dosage should be reduced accordingly.

Preparation Form: Honeyed bolus.

Package: 3g in each bolus.

Notes: The drug can be used to treat oral ulcer, acute pharyngitis, laryngitis, tonsillitis, acute cystitis, acute urethritis and acute pyelonephritis

It is contraindicated for those with diarrhea or weakened body.

Baochi San

Ingredients:

Massa Fermentata Medicinalis	23.8%	Shenqu
Pulvis Crotonis Tiglium	14.3%	Badou shuang
Rhizoma Arisaematis	38.1%	Tiannanxing
Cinnabaris	23.8%	Zhusha

Actions: Promiting digestion, eliminating indigested food, resolving phlegm and tranquilizing the mind.

Indications: Syndrome in infants marked by retention of food due to cold, loss of appetite, constipation, distention and fullness in the abdomen, abundant phlegm, and palpitation due to fright.

Administration and Dosage: Taken orally, 1−2 times daily. Each time, 0.09g is given to infants of 6 months to 1 year old, and 0.18g to those of 2−4 years old. For babies within 6 month, the dosage should be reduced accordingly.

Preparation Form: Powder.

Package: 0.09g in each bottle.

Notes: The drug can be used to treat infants with anorexia, dyspepsia, constipation, abdominal distention and psychological syndrome due to convulsion.

The drug contains Pulvis Crotonis Tiglium, therefore overdose must be avoided. Besides, it is contraindicated for those with diarrhea.

Xiaoer Shengxueling Chongi

Main Ingredients:

Fructus Ziziphi Jujubae	*Dazao*
KAL(SO4)2,12H2O	*Zaofan*
Frucuts Crataegi	*Shanzha*

Actions: Invigorating *Qi*, enriching blood, removing stagnated food and regulating the spleen.

Indications: Deficiency of blood and consumptive diseases. in infants.

Administration and Dosage: Taken after being infused in boiling water, 3 times daily. Each time, 5g is given to infants within 1 year old, 10g to those of 1—3 years old, and 15g to young children of 3—7.

Preparation Form: Granule or powder dissolvable in water.

Package: 10g in each bag.

Notes: The drug has the actions of increasing the quantity of red blood cells and promoting the function of hemoglobin. It can be used to treat children with iron—deficiency anemia.

According to clinical reports, 300 children having iron—deficiency anemia were treated with the drug. After 10 days' treatment, 67% of the children were cured, after 20 days' treatment, 79% and after 30 days, 91.7%.

This drug can't be taken with tea.

Zhierling Chongji

Main Ingredients:

Radix Salviae Miltiorrhizae	Dangshen
Radix Pseudostellariae	Haiershen
Radix Adenophorae	Nanshashen
Radix Rehmanniae	Dihuang
Radix Polygoni Multiflori	Shouwu
Radix Angelicae Sinensis	Danggui
Rhizoma Atractylodis Macrocephalae	Baizhu
Semen Sojae Nigrum	Heidadou
Radix Paeoniae Alba	Baishao
Radix Aucklandiae	Muxiang
Semen Dolichoris Album	Baibiandou
Rhizoma Dioscoreae	Shanyao
Herba Agrimoniae	Xianhecao
Poria	Fuling
Fructus Schisandrae	Wuweizi
Rhizoma Acori Gramine	Shichangpu
Fructus Tritici Levis	Fuxiaomai
Radix Glycyrrhizae	Gancao
Concha Ostreae	Muli
Pericarpium Citri Reticulatae	Chenpi
Radix Polygala	Yuanzhi
Fructus Ziziphi Jujubae	Dazao

Actions: Invigorating *Qi*, strengthening the spleen, tonifying the brain and building up the body.

Indications: Symptoms in infants such as anorexia, loose stools, emaciation with sallow complexion, disturbed sleep, night sweat, etc.

Administration and Dosage: Taken after being infused in boiling water. 9—15g each time, twice daily.

Preparation Form: Granule or powder dissolvable in water.

Package: 400g in a bottle.

Notes: This drug can be used to treat infants with anorexia, dystrophy, dyspesia, and developmental retardation.

Wuli Huichun Dan

Main Ingredients:

Cacumen Tamaricis	Xiheliu
Flos Lonicerae	Jinyinhua
Fructus Arctii	Niubangzi
Periostracum Cicadae	Chantui
Fructus Forsythiae	Lianqiao
Herba Menthae	Bohe
Folium Mori	Sangye
Radix Ledebouriellae	Fangfeng
Herba Ephedrae	Mahuang
Rhizoma seu Radix Notopterygii	Qianghuo
Bombyx Batryticatus	Jiangcan
Citri Reticulatae	Juhong
Arisaema cum Bile	Dannanxing
Bulbus Fritillariae Cirrhosae	Chuanbeimu
Semen Armeniacae Amarum	Kuxingren
Poria	Fuling

Radix Paeoniae Rubra	Chisho
Herba Lophatheri	Danzhuye
Radix Glycyrrhizae	Gancao
Cornu Saigae Tataricae	Lingyangjiao
Borneolum Syntheticum	Bingpian
Calculus Bovis man—made	Rengongniu huang

Actions: Ventilating the lung, expelling exogenous pathogenic factors, clearing away heat and removing toxic materials.

Indications: Syndrome in infants due to virulent pathogens mark by headache, high fever, running nose, delacrimation cough with dyspnea, dysphoria, thirst, and early measles without adequate eruption.

Administration and Dosage: Paste—pill.

Package: 3g in every 100 pills.

Notes: The drug can be used to treat infants with acute in fection, erysipelas in face, scarlet fever, diphtheria, epidemic parotitis and early meales.

Cold, raw or greasy food should be avoided.

Qingzhen San

Ingredients:

Gypsum Fibrosum	Shigao
Cornu Bubali	Shuiniujiao
Rhizoma Anemarrhenae	Zhimu
Periostracum Cicadae	Chantui
Rhizoma Paridis	Chonglou
Herba Menthae	Bohe

Flos Lonicerae	Jinyinhua
Fructus Forsythiae	Lianqiao
Bombyx Batryticatus	Jiangcan
Rhizoma Phargmitis	Lugen

Actions: Clearing away heat, removing toxic materials, relieving exterior syndrome and promoting eruption.

Indications: Measles without adequate eruption, congestion of throat, hoarseness, rapid breathing, abdominal pain, loose stools, coma, delirium, and clonic convulsion.

Administration and Dosage: Taken orally. 1 / 2 bag is for infants above 1 year old, 1 bag for those above 3, and 1.5 bag for those above 5.

Preparation Form: Powder.

Package: 0.652g in each bag.

Notes: The drug has the actions of reducing fever and resisting bacteria. It can be used to treat infants with such acute eruptive diseases as measles, rubella, scarlet fever, diphtheria, etc.

Niuhuang Zhibao Wan

Main Ingredients:

Radix Ginseng Silvestris	Yerenshen
Cinnabaris	Zhusha
Calculus Bovis man—made	Rengongniuhua
Rhizoma Arisaematis	Tiannanxing
Borneolum Syntheticum	Bingpian
Concretio Silicae Bambusae	Tianzhuhuang
Succinum	Hupo
Cornus Bubali	Shuiniujiao
Garapax Eretomochelydis	Daimao

Actions: Clearing away heat, removing toxic materials, relieving convulsion and inducing resuscitation.

Indications: Syndrome in infants due to sanking of pathogenic warmth into the interior and invasion of pathogenic heat into the pericardium, marked by coma, delirium, faint skin eruption and sudden convulsion.

Administration and Dosage: Taken orally, after dissolved in boiling water, 1 bolus each time.

Preparation Form: Honeyed bolus.

Package: 3g in each bolus.

Notes: This drug can be used to treat epidemic encephalitis B, epidemic cerebrospinal meningitis, hematosepsis, toxic pneumonitis, coma due to toxic bacillary dysentery, and infantile convulsion due to acute infective diseases.

It should be cautiously given to pregnant women.

Xiaoer Tuire Chongji

Main Ingredients:

Flos Longicerae	9.0%	Jinyinhua
Fructus Forsythiae	9.0%	Lianqiao
Folium Isatidis	14.9%	Daqingye
Radix Isatidis	9.0%	Banlangen
Radix Scutellariae	9.0%	Huangqin
Fructus Gardeniae	9.0%	Zhizi
Cortex Moutan Radicis	9.0%	Mudanpi
Herba Lophatheri	5.9%	Danzhuye
Lumbricus	5.9%	Dilong
Rhizoma Paridis	4.4%	Chonglou
Radix Bupleuri	9.0%	Chaihu

Radix Ampelopsis   5.9%   *Bailian*

Actions: Clearing away heat and relieving exterior syndrome.

Indications: Fever in infants due to common cold or influenza.

Administration and Dosage: Taken orally, 3 times daily. Each time, 5g is given to young children below 5 years old, 15g to those of 5—10.

Preparation Form: Powder.

Package: 6g in each bag.

Notes: The drug can be used to treat children with upper respiratory tract infection, epidemic influenza and fever.

Xiaoer Qiying Wan

Main Ingredients:

Lignum Aguilariae Resinatum	*Chenxiang*
Realgar	*Xionghuang*
Pulvis Cornus Bubali Concentratus	*Shuiniujiao Nongsuofen*
Rhizoma Pinellinae	*Banxia*
Cinnabaris	*Zhusha*
Radix Salviae Miltiorrhizae	*Dangshen*
Radix Platycodi	*Jiegeng*
Rhizoma Typhonii	*Baifuzi*
Quinine Hydrochloride	*Yansuan Kuining*
Camphora	*Zhangnao*
Calculus Bovis man—made	*Rengongniuhuang*
Borneolum Synthencum	*Bingpian*
Extractum Fel Bovis	*Niudanzhiqingao*

Actions: Clearing away heat, relieving convulsion and calming the mind.

Indications: Syndrome in infants marked by sudden or slow convulsion, high fever, cough due to common cold, measles without adequate eruption and malnutrition.

Administration and Dosage: Taken orally, twice daily usually, 3 times daily when the case is serious. Each time, 6—8 pills is given to infants within 1 year old, 12 to those of 1 to 3 years old, 15 to young children of 4—6, and 20 to those of 7—10.

Preparation Form: Water—paste pill.

Package: 0.05g in every 10 pills.

Notes: This drug can be used to treat infantile convulsion due to acute infection, or tic of limps due to chronic diseases. high fever and early measles.

Xiaoer Jiere Shuan

Ingredients:

Flos Lonicerae	22.3%	Jinyinhua
Rhizoma seu Radix Notopterygii	11.1%	Sanqi
Folium Isatidis	44.4%	Daqingye
Radix Scrophulariae	111.1%	Xuanxhen
Radix et Rhzima Rhei	11.1%	Dahuang

Actions: Clearing away heat, removing toxic materials, expelling wind, relieving exterior syndrome, resolving blood stasis and promoting the subsidence of swelling.

Indications: Common cold, mumps and high fever.

Administration and Dosage: Put into the point of the rectum which is 2 cm from the anus after the area around the anus is washed. 1 suppository each time, 2—3 times daily.

Preparation Form: Suppository.

Package: 1g in each suppository.

Notes: This drug can be used to treat infants with high fever, upper respiratory tract infection, epidemic influenza or mumps.

Ganji San

Ingredients:

Fossil of Cyrtiospirifer	18.2%	*Shiyan*
Poria	18.2%	*Fuling*
Concha Haliotidis	18.2%	*Shijueming*
Flos Eriocauli	9.0%	*Gujingcao*
Fructus Quisqualis	18.2%	*Shijunzi*
Radix Clematidis	9.1%	*Weilingxian*
Endothelium Corneum Gigeriae Galli	9.1%	*Jineijin*

Actions: Removing retention of food to treat infantile malnutrition,

Indications: Emaciation, sallow complexion, abdominal distention due to infantile malnutrition, conjunctivitis and night blindness.

Administration and Dosage: Taken after mixed with hot rice soup plus sugar, 9g each time, twice daily. For infants within 3 years old, the dosage should be reduced accordingly.

Preparation Form: Powder.

Pacage: 3g in each bottle.

Notes: The drug has the actions of promoting digestion and killing parasites. It can be used to treat infantile malnutrition and dyspepsia, and magersucht due to parasitosis, tuberculosis and other chronic consumptive diseases.

Feier Wan

Ingredients:

Semen Myristicae	10.6%	*Roudoukou*
Radix Aucklandiae	4.3%	*Muxiang*
Fructus Hordei Germinatus	10.6%	*Maiya*
Rhizoma Picrorhizae	21.3%	*Huhuanglian*
Massa Fermentata Medicinalis	21.3%	*Shenqu*
Semen Arecae	10.6%	*Binglang*
Fructus Quisqualis	21.3%	*Shijunzi*

Actions: Strengthening the stomach, removing indigested food and killing parasites.

Indications: Symproms in infants such as dyspepsia, abdominal pain due to enterositosis, emaciation with sallow complexion, inappetence, distension of the abdomen and diarrhea.

Administration and Dosage: Taken oraly, 1—2 boluses each time, 1—2 times daily. For children within 3 years old, the dosage should be reduced accordingly.

Preparation Form: Hoeyed bolus.

Package: 3g in each bolus.

Notes: This prescription originates from the book Tai Ping Hui Min He Ji Ju Fang compiled by Chen Shiwen in the Song dynasty.

The drug has the actions of strengthening the stomach, promoting digestion and expelling intestinal parasites. It can be used to treat infantile ascariasis, dyspepsia and malnutrition.

Generally, the course of treatment involves no more than 3 days. Usualy, it is stopped after defecation with foul stools or round worm occurs

Xiaòer Ganyan Chongji

Main Ingredients:

Herba Artemisiae Scopariae	24.2%	*Yinchen*
Radix Scutellariae	12.1%	*Huangqin*
Fructus Gardeniae	6.1%	*Zhizi*
Cortex Phellodendri	12.1%	*Huangbai*
Fructus Crataegi	18.2%	*Shanzha*
Radix Curcumae	3.0%	*Yujin*
Medulla Tetrapanacis	6.1%	*Tongcao*

Actions: Clearing away heat, promoting diuresis and treating jaundice.

Indications: Syndrome in infants due to damp—heat marked by jaundice with yellow eyes and skin, abdominal distention, nausea, fever and lassitude, inappetence and hepatalgia.

Administration and Dosage: Taken orally, 3 times daily. Each time, 0.5—1 piece is given to infants of 1—3 years old, 2 to those of 3—7, and more to those above 7 accordingly.

Preparation Form: Granule.

Package: 7.5g in each piece.

Notes: The drug can be used to treat infantile acute interohepatitis.

Wanying Ding

Main Ingredients:

Rhizoma Picrorhizae	*Huhuanlian*
Rhizoma Coptidis	*Huanglian*
Catechu	*Ercha*
Borneolum Syntheticum	*Bingpian*

Actions: Clearing away heat, relieving convulsion, removing toxic material, eliminating summer—heat, cooling blood and reducing swelling.

Indications: Syndromes in infants such as high fever, convulsion, sunstroke, aphthae, toothache, swelling and pain of gum and throat, and skin disorders.

Administration and Dosgae: Taken orally, 2—4 pills each time, 1—2 times daily. For infants within 3 years old, the dosage should be reduced acordingly.

Preparation Form: Water—paste pill.

Package: 1.5g in every 10 pills.

Notes: The prescription originates from the book Qing Nei Ting Fà Zhi Wan San Gao Dan Ge Yao Pei Ben.

This drug can be used to treat infants with convulsion, nail—like boil, furuncle, carbuncle, acute pharyngitis, acute tonsiutis aphthous stomatitis and acute achilles abscess, all of which are due to high fever, infection, poisoning, dystrophy and metabolic disturbance, epylepsy and sunstroke.

Wufu Huadu Wan

Ingredients:

Pulvis Cornus Bubali Concentratus	4.7%	Shuiniujiao Nongshufen
Fructus Forsythiae	14.8%	Lianqiao
Indigo Naturalis	4.7%	Qingdai
Rhizoma Coptidis	1.2%	Huanglian
Fructus Arctii	11.6%	Niubangzi
Radix Scrophulariae	14.0%	Xuanshen
Radix Rehmanniae	11.5%	Dihuang

Radix Platycodi	11.5%	*Jiegeng*
Natrii Sulphas	1.2%	*Mangxiao*
Radix Paeoniae Rubra	11.6%	*Chishao*
Radix Glycyrrhizae	14.0%	*Gancao*

Actions: Clearing away heat, removing toxic materials, cooling blood and reducing swelling.

Indications: Syndromes in infants due to noxious heat and excessive fire marked by skin and external diseases, swelling and pain of the throat, aphthae, gingival bleeding and mumps.

Administration and Dosage: Taken orally, 1 bolus each time, 2—3 times daily.

Preparation Form: Bolus.

Package: 3g in each bolus.

Notes: The prescription originates from the book Shou Shi Bao Yuan compiled by GongYanxian in the Ming Dynasty.

The drug can be used to treat disorders of infants such as nail—like boil, furuncle, carbuncle, acute pharyngitis and tonsillitis, aphthous stomatitis, parotitis and late infection diseases with rash.

Bairike Pian

Ingredients:(omitted)

Actions: Stopping cough, dissolving sputum and relieving asthma.

Indications: Infantile chin cough.

Adminisreation and Dosage: Taken orally, three times daily. Each time, 1 tablet is given to an infant of 1 year old and 1 more tablets to an infant of 1 more year old.

Preparation Form: Tablet.

Package: 150mg in each tablet.

Notes: The drug is a kind of thick medicinal extract made from domestic fowl's bile. It can be used to treat infantile chin cough.

15 Drugs used in the Department of Eye, Ear, Nose and Throat

15.1 Drugs used in the Department of Ophthalmology

Qiju Dihuang Wan

Ingredients:

Fructus Lycii	6.9%	Gouqizi
Flos Chrysanthemi	6.9%	Shanjuhua
Fructus Corni	13.8%	Shanzhuyu
Rhizoma Dioscoreae	13.8%	Shanyao
Cortex Moutan Radicis	10.3%	Mudanpi
Rhizoma Alismatis	10.3%	Zexie
Radix Rehmanniae Praeparata	27.7%	Shudihuang
Poria	10.3%	Fuling

Actions: Nourishing both the kidney and liver.

Indications: Vertigo, tinnitus, photophobia, irritated epiphora and blurred vision due to deficiency of Yin of the liver and kidney.

Administration and Dosage: Taken orally, 1 bolus each time, twice daily.

Preparation Form: Honeyed bolus.

Package: 9g in per bolus.

Notes: The recipe is recorded in the book Yi Ji. This drug can nourish and protect the liver and diminish inflammation. It is efficacious for dacryorrhea, glaucoma, photophobia, senile cataract, vitreous opacity, acute optic neuritis, central retinis, retinal detachment, optic atrophy, herpes simplex retinitis, trachomatous retinitis, viral retinitis, tinnitus and aural vertigo.

Shihu Yeguang Wan

Ingredients:

Radix Ginseng	*Renshen*
Poria	*Fuling*
Radix Asparagi	*Tianmendong*
Rhizoma Dioscroreae	*Shanyao*
Radix Ophiopogonis	*Maimendong*
Radix Rehmanniae Praeparata	*Shudihuang*
Radix Rehmanniae	*Dihuang*
Fructus Lycii	*Gouqizi*
Semen Cassiae	*Juemingzi*
Radix Acyranthis Bidentatae	*Niuxi*
Semen Cuscutae	*Tusizi*
Flos Chrysanthemi	*Juhua*
Semen Armeniacae Amarum	*Kuxingren*
Herba Dendrobii	*Shihu*
Herba Cistanchis	*Roucongrong*
Radix Glycyrrhizae	*Gancao*
Fructus Schisandrae	*Wuweizi*
Radix Ledebouriellae	*Fangfeng*
Fructus Tribuli	*Baijili*
Rhizoma Coptidis	*Huanglian*
Fructus Aurantii	*Zhiqiao*
Rhizoma Chuanxiong	*Chuanxiong*

Semen Celosiae   *Qingxiangzi*
Pulvis Cornu Bubali Concetratus   *Shuiniujiaonongsuofen*

Actions: Nourishing *Yin* to reduce pathogenic fire and improving visual acuity.

Indications: Internal oculopathy, blurred vision, mydriasis or colour change of the pupil and photophobia due to deficiency of liver—*Yin* and kidney—*Yin*, and hyperactivity of fire caused by *Yin* deficiency.

Administration and Dosage: Taken orally, 1 bolus each time, twice daily.

Preparation From: Honeyed bolus.

Package: 9g in per bolus.

Notes: The recipe is recorded in the book *Shen Shi Yao Han* written by Fu Renyu in the Ming Dynasty.

The drug can nourish and protect the liver, diminish inflammation and induce purgation. It is clinically active against cataract, glaucoma, retinitis, choroiditis, optic neuritis, nervous headache, vitreous opacity and photophobia.

Mingmu Dihuang Wan

Ingredients:

Radix Rehmanniae Praeparata	18.6%	*Shudihuang*
Rhizoma Dioscoreae	9.2%	*Shanyao*
Fructus Corni	9.2%	*Shanzhuyu*
Poria	7.0%	*Fuling*
Cortex Moutan Radicis	7.0%	*Mudanpi*
Rhizoma Alismatis	7.0%	*Zexie*
Fructus Lycii	7.0%	*Gouqizi*
Flos Chrysanthemi	7.0%	*Juhua*

Fructus Tribuli	7.0%	*Baijili*
Radix Angelicae Sinensis	7.0%	*Danggui*
Concha Haliotidis	7.0%	*Shijueming*
Radix Paeoniae Alba	7.0%	*Baishao*

Actions: Nourishing the liver and kidney and improving visual acuity.

Indications: Xenophthalmia, photophobia, irritated epiphora, epiphora induced by wind, and night blindness due to deficiency of liver—*Yin* and kidney—*Yin* and flaring—up of fire of *Yin* deficiency.

Administration and Dosage: Taken orally, 1 bolus each time, twice daily.

Praparation From: Honeyed bolus.

Package: 9g in per bolus.

Notes: This bolus can nourish and protect the liver and diminish inflammation. It is clinically efficacious for central retinitis, retinal detachment, optic neuritis, optic atrophy, vitreous opacity, dacryorrhea, photophobia and night blindness.

Huanglian Yanggan Wan

Ingredients:

Rhizoma Coptidis	3.2%	*Huanglian*
Flos Buddlejae	5.6%	*Mimenghua*
Semen Cassiae	5.6%	*Juemingzi*
Radix Gentianae	3.2%	*Longdan*
Concha Haliotidis	5.6%	*Shijueming*
Crotex Phellodendri	3.2%	*Huangbai*
Fructus Leonuri	5.6%	*Chongweizi*
Radix Scutellariae	5.6%	*Huangqin*

Faeces Vespertilionis	5.6%	*Yemingsha*
Radix Bupleuri	5.6%	*Chaihu*
Rhizoma Picrorhizae	5.6%	*Huhuanglian*
Herba Equiseti Hiemalis	5.6%	*Muzei*
Pericarpium Citri Reticulatae Viride	5.6%	*Qingpi*
fresh sheep liver	25.6%	*Xianyanggan*

Actions: Purging intense heat and improving visual acuity.

Indications: Blurred vision, photophobia and pterygium due to hyperactivity of liver—fire.

Administration and Dosage: Taken orally, 1 bolus each time, once or twice daily.

Preparation From: Honeyed bolus.

Package: 9g in per bolus.

Notes: This drug can reduce fever. It is not only an antibiotic but an antiphogistic and is good for pterygium, photophobia, night blindness, glaucoma and cataract.

Mingmu Yanggan Wan

Ingredients:

fresh sheep liver	20.8%	*Xianyanggan*
Herba Equiseti Hiematis	6.9%	*Muzei*
Fructus Lycii	3.6%	*Gouqizi*
Radix Rehmanniae	6.9%	*Dihuang*
Semen Cassiae	6.9%	*Juemingzi*
Radix Angelicae Sinensis	6.9%	*Danggui*
Faeces Vespertilionis	6.9%	*Yemingsha*
Periostracum Cicadae	6.9%	*Chantui*
Semen Astragali Complanati	6.9%	*Shayuanzi*
Rhizoma Coptidis	6.9%	*Huanglian*

Fructus Tribuli	6.9%	*Jili*
Flos Chyranthemi	6.9%	*Juhua*
Spica Schizonepetae	1.0%	*Jingjiesui*
Radix Ledebouriellae	3.6%	*Fangfeng*
Rhizoma seu Radix Notopterygii	1.0%	*Qianghuo*
Rhizome Chuanxiong	1.0%	*Chuanxiong*

Actions: Nourishing the liver and kidney, expelling wind and improving visual acuity.

Indications: Night blindness, irritated epiphobia and blurred vision.

Administration and Dosage: Taken orally, 1 bolus each time, twice daily.

Preparation Form: Honeyed bolus.

Package: 9g in per bolus.

Notes: This drug can nourish and protect the liver and diminish inflammation. It is used for night blindness, dacryorrhea and vitreous opacity.

Zhangyanming Pian

Ingredients:

Fructus Corni	8%	*Shanyurou*
Nux Prinsepiae	10%	*Ruirenrou*
Fructus Lycii	12%	*Gouqizi*
Herba Cistanchis	12%	*Roucongrong*
Radix Codonopsis Pilosulae	12%	*Fangdangshen*
Radix Astragali	15%	*Mianhuangqi*
Flos Buddlejae	8%	*Mimenghua*
Rhizoma Cimicifugae	2%	*Shengma*
Fructus Viticis	6%	*Manjingzi*

Rhizoma Chuanxiong	3%	*Chuanxiong*
Rhizoma Acori Graminei	2%	*Shichangpu*
Flos Chrysanthemi	10%	*Juhua*

Actions: Tonifying the liver and kidney, invigorating the spleen, regulating the middle—*Jiao*, and removing nebula to improve visual acuity.

Indications: Cataract, blurred vision, vitreous opacity, asthenopia, listlessness, dizziness, soreness of lower back, and poor memory.

Administration and Dosage: Taken orally, 4 tablets each time, 3 times daily. 1 treatment course involves 3—6 months.

Preparation Form: Tablet.

Package: 100 tablets in each bottle.

Notes: This drug is used to promote the metabolism of the eyes and the regeneration of the corneal epithelium. It is clinically efficacious for senile cataract at early and intermediate stages, blockage of the central retinal vessels, retinal periphlebitis, retinal detachment, acute optic neuritis, central choroido—retinitis, vitreous opacity, pigmentary degeneration of the retina, optic atrophy and asthenopia.

Guangming Yangao

Ingredients:

Calamina	72.5%	*Luganshi*
Borneolum Syntheticum	20.3%	*Bingpian*
Borax	3.4%	*Pengsha*
Copper Sulfate	2.4%	*Liusuantong*
Berberine Bisulfate	1.4%	*Zhongliusuan huangliansu*

Actions: Clearing away heat, removing toxic materials, eliminating dampness and alleviating pain.

Indications: Acute conjunctivitis and trachoma.

Administration and Dosage: Apply the drug to the inner side of the eyelid and then take a short rest, and do this 3—4 times daily.

Preparation From: Ointment.

Package: 2g in each tube.

Notes: This drug can diminish inflammation and act as an astringent. It is clinically indicated for conjunctivitis, conjunctival ulcer, pterygium and trachoma.

15.2 Drugs used in Ear—Nose—Throat Department

Erlong Zuoci Wan

Ingredients:

Magnetitum	3.7%	Cishi
Radix Rehmanniae Praeparata	29.6%	Shudihuang
Fructus Corni	14.7%	Shanzhuyu
Rhizoma Dioscoreae	14.7%	Shanyao
Cortex Moutan Radicis	11.2%	Mudanpi
Poria	11.2%	Fuling
Radix Bupleuri	3.7%	Chaihu
Rhizoma Alismatis	11.2%	Zexie

Actions: Nourishing the kidney and subduing the hyperactivity of the liver.

Indications: Tinnitus, deafness and dizziness due to deficiency of liver—Yin and kidney—Yin.

Administration and Dosage: Taken orally, 1 bolus each time, twice daily.

Preparation Form: Honeyed bolus.

Package: 9g in each bolus.

Notes: This drug can nourish and protect the liver. It is clinically efficacious for tinnitus, deafness, acute and chronic non—suppurative otitis media and Meniere's disease.

Huodan Wan

Ingredients:

Herba Pogostemonis	90%	*Guanghuoxiang*
extract of pig bile	10%	*Zhudangao*

Actions: Removing wind—heat, and clearing the nasal passage.

Indications: Stuffy and running nose due to disturbance of up—flowing wind—heat.

Administration and Dosage: Taken orally, 3—6g each time, twice daily.

Preparation Form: Water—paste pill.

Package: 36g in per bottle.

Notes: The recipe is recorded in the book *Yi Zong Jin Jian* written by Wu Qian in the Qing Dynasty.

This drug can diminish inflammation, relieve swelling and reduce fever. It is clinically suitable for chronic rhinitis, chronic accessary nasosinusitis, and nasosinusitis.

Biyan Pian

Ingredients:

Fructus Xanthii   *Cangerzi*

Flos Magnoliae	*Xinyi*
Radix Angelicae Dahuricae	*Baizhi*
Radix Ledebourieliae	*Fangfeng*
Herba Schizonepetae	*Jingjie*
Fructus Forsythiae	*Lianqiao*
Cortex Phellodendri	*Huangbai*
Rhizoma Anemarrhenae	*Zhimu*
Flos Crysanthemi Indici	*Yejuhua*
Herba Ephedrae	*Mahuang*
Herba Asari	*Xixin*
Radix Platycodi	*Jiegeng*
Fructus Schisandrae	*Wuweizi*
Radix Glycyrrhizae	*Gancao*

Actions: Reducing fever, dispelling wind, relieving swelling and clearing the nasal passage.

Indications: Stuffy nose due to affection of wind.

Administration and Dosage: Taken orally, 3 or 4 tablets each time, 3 times daily. Appropriate reduction of the dosage is done for children.

Preparation Form: Tablet.

Package: 0.3g in per tablet

Notes: This drug has antiseptic effects and can relieve inflammation. It is clinically efficacious for acute and chronic rhinitis and accessary nasosinusitis.

Biyan Tangjiang

Ingredients:

Radix Scutellariae	16.8%	*Huangqin*
Radix Angelicae Dahuricae	16.8%	*Baizhi*

Fructus Xanthii	16.8%	*Cangerzi*
Flos Magnoliae	16.8%	*Xinyi*
Herba Centipedae	16.8%	*Ebushicao*
Herba Ephedrae	7.9%	*Mahuang*
Herba Menthae	8.1%	*Bohe*

Actions: Reducing fever, removing toxic materials, relieving swelling and clearing the nasal passage.

Indications: Stuffy nose due to invasion of wind.

Administration and Dosage: Taken orally, 20ml each time, 3 times daily.

Preparation Form: Syrup.

Package: 200ml in per bottle.

Notes: This drug can reduce fever and relieve swelling and has antiseptic effects. It is clinically used for acute and chronic rhinitis.

Biyuan Wan

Main Ingredients:

Flos Lonicerae	*Jinyinhua*
Flos Chrysanthemi Indici	*Yejuhua*
Flos Magnoliae	*Xinyi*
Fructus Xanthii	*Cangerzi*

Actions: Clearing away heat, removing toxic materials and clearing the nasal passage.

Indications: Stuffy nose and rhinorrhea with turbid discharge.

Administration and Dosage: Taken orally, 5 pills each time, 3 times daily.

Preparation Form: Concentrated pills.

Package: 1g in per pill.

Notes: This drug has antiseptic effects and can diminish inflammation. It is indicated for acute and chronic rhinitis and nasosinusitis.

Liushen Wan

Ingredients: (omitted)

Actions: Clearing away heat, removing toxic materials, relieving swelling and alleviating pain.

Indications: Diphtheria, swelling and pain of the throat, unilateral or bilateral tonsillitis, acute throat trouble, scarlet fever, etc.

Administration and Dosage: Sucked, 1—2 times daily. 1 pill is taken each time by an infant of 1 year old, 5—6 pills by a young child of 4—8 years old, 8 pills by a child of 9—15, and 10 pills by an adult. Or, 10 pills are mixed with a little boiled water or rice vinegar into a paste and applied to the affected part, and this is done several times a day.

Preparation Form: Pill.

Package: 1g in per 330 pills.

Notes: With antivirotic and cordiac effects, this drug can diminish inflammation and alleviate pain. It is efficacious for diphtheria, acute pharyngitis and laryngitis, lonsillitis, stomatitis, pericoronitis, acute periapical abscess, parotitis, scarlet fever and ordinary sores.

Reportedly, this drug can be used as a cardiac stimulant and is efficacious for pulmonary heart disease associated with heart failure, and hepatalgia of chronic hepatitis. It is contraindicated for pregnant women and those with ulcerated sore.

Houzheng Wan

Ingredients:

Radix Isatidis	41.3%	*Banlangen*
Borneolum Syntheticum	1.4%	*Bingpian*
Calculus Bovis Factitius	2.9%	*Rengongniu huang*
Indigo Naturatis	1.2%	*Qingdai*
pig bile	39.2%	*Zhudanzhi*
Realgar	4.5%	*Xionghuang*
Natrii Sulfas Exsiccatus	2.0%	*Xuanmingfen*
Borax	2.0%	*Pengsha*
Venenum Bufonis	3.9%	*Chansu*
Fuligo Plantae	1.5%	*Baicaoshuang*

Actions: Clearing away heat, removing toxic materials, relieving swelling and alleviating pain.

Indications: Swelling and pain of the throat, unilateral and bilateral tonsillitis, and ordinary sores.

Administration and Dosage: Sucked, twice daily, with 3—5 pills each time for those of 3—10 years old and 5—10 pills for adults. Or, Several pills are mixed with cool boiled water and applied to the area with swelling and pain due to early sore or boil.

Preparation Form: Pill.

Package: 1g in per 224 pills.

Notes: This drug is used clinically for pharyngitis, laryngitis, tonsillitis and ordinary sores.

It is contraindicated for pregnant women and those with ulcerated sore.

Qingyin Wan

Ingredients:

Radix Platycodi	15.5%	*Jiegeng*
Calcitum	15.2%	*Hanshuishi*
Herba Menthae	15.1%	*Bohe*
Fructus Chebulae	15.2%	*Hezi*
Radix Glycyrrhizae	15.1%	*Gancao*
Fructus Mume	15.2%	*Wumei*
Borax	3.0%	*Pengsha*
Indigo Naturalis	3.0%	*Qingdai*
Borneolum Syntheticum	3.0%	*Bingpian*

Actions: Removing intense heat from the throat and chest.

Indications: Acute laryngeal infection caused by the retention of pathogenic heat in the lung and stomach marked by dry mouth and tongue, low sound intensity and hoarseness.

Administration and Dosage: Taken orally or sucked in the mouth, 1 pill each time, twice daily.

Preparation from: Honeyed bolus.

Pacage: 6g in per bolus.

Notes: This drug has antiseptic effect and can diminish inflammation. It is clinically efficacious for acute laryngitis.

Yandeping Jiaonang

Ingredient:

Herba Andrographitis	100%	*Chuanxinlian*

Actions: Clearing away heat, removing toxic materials, cooling blood and relieving swelling.

Indications: Cough caused by lung—heat, swelling and pain

of the throat, sore in the oral cavity, diarrhea, and dysentery.

Administration and Dosage: Taken orally, 2 capsules each time, 3 times daily.

Preparation Form: Capsule.

Package: 0.3g in per capsule.

Notes: This drug has an antiseptic effect and can diminish inflammation. It is clinically efficacious for acute tonsillitis, laryngopharyngitis, epidemic mumps, bronchitis, pneumonia, bacillary dysentery, acute gastroenteritis, and infection from trauma.

15.3   Drugs used in the Department of Stomatology

Bingpeng San

Ingredients:

Borax	45.0%	*Pengsha*
Borneolum Syntheticum	4.5%	*Bingpian*
Cinnabaris	5.5%	*Zhusha*
Natrii Sulfas Exsiccatus	45.0%	*Xuanmingfen*

Actions: Clearing away heat, removing toxic materials, relieving swelling and alleviating pain.

Indications: Swelling and pain of the throat and gum, and sore in oral cavity.

Administration and Dosage: A little is applied to the affected part or blown into the throat.

Preparation From: Powder.

Package: 3g in per bottle.

Notes: The recipe is recorded in the book *Wai Ke Zheng*

Zong written by Chen Shigong in the Ming Dynasty.

This powder has antiseptic and tranquilizing effects. It is clinically efficacious for acute pharyngitis, acute laryngitis, acute laryngemphraxia, neurosis of pharynx, acute tonsillitis, stomatitis, glossitis, ulcer of tongue, periodentitis, acute periapical abscess, otitis media suppuratira, rhinitis, acute conjunctivitis, and *Candida albicans* infection of vagina.

Xilei San

Ingredients:

Indigo Naturalis	41.6%	*Qingdai*
Calculus Bovis man—made	3.8%	*Rengongniu huang*
Uroctea compactilis	7.0%	*Biqian*
Borneolum Syntheticum	2.1%	*Bingpian*
elephant—tusk scraps	21.0%	*Xiangyaxia*
Margarita	21.0%	*Zhenzhu*
human nail	3.5%	*Renzhijia*

Actions: Clearing away heat, removing toxic materials and eliminating putridity.

Indications: Redness, swelling and erosion of the throat, and swelling and pain of the lips and tongue.

Administration and Dosage: A little is blown onto the affected part, or a proper amount determined by a physician is taken orally.

Preparation Form: Powder.

Package: 0.3g in per bottle.

Notes: The recipe is found in the book *Jin Kui Yi* written by *You Zaijing* in the Qing Dynasty.

This drug can reduce fever, diminish inflammation and alleviate pain. It is efficacious for ulcer of oral mucosa, stomatitis, thrush, acute pharyngitis, acute laryngitis, tonsillitis, abscess of retropharynx and acute epiglottiditis, all of which are treated externally, and chronic bacillary dysentery, chronic colitis, and gastric and duodenal ulcer, all of which are treated internally.

Shuangliao Houfeng San

Main Ingredients:

Margarita	*Zhenzhu*
Calculus Bovis man-made	*Rengongniuhuang*
Indigo Naturalis	*Qingdai*
Borneolum Syntheticum	*Bingpian*
Rhizoma Coptidis	*Huanglian*
Radix Glycyrrhizae	*Gancao*

Actions: Clearing away heat, removing toxic materials, relieving swelling, and alleviating pain.

Indications: Swelling and pain of the throat, erosion of mouth cavity, pain of the gum, rhinorrhea with turbid discharge and cervical carcinoma with cachexia.

Administration and Dosage: A little is blown onto the affected part, or applied under the instruction of a physician.

Preparation Form: Powder.

Package: 1.25g in per bottle.

Notes: This drug has antiseptic, anti-inflammatory and sedative effects. It is clinically efficacious for pharyngitis, laryngitis, tonsillitis, stomatitis, pericoronitis, abscess of nasal sinuses, inflammation of nasopharyngeal carcinoma, otitis media suppurativa, and skin ulcer.

Niuhuang Yijin Pian

Main Ingredients:

Cortex Phellodendri	*Huangbai*
Calculus Bovis man—made	*Rengongniuhuang*

Actions: Clearing away heat to relieve swelling and pain of the throat.

Indications: Swelling and pain of the throat, sore in the oral cavity, globus hystericus and constipation.

Administration and Dosage: Sucked, 1—2 tablets each time, 3 times daily; or swallowed, 4—6 tablets each time, 3 times daily; or taken according to the order of a physician.

Preparation Form: Tablet.

Package: About 0.5g in per tablet.

Notes: This drug can reduce fever and has sedative and anti—inflammatory effects. It is clinically efficacious for acute and chronic pharyngitis, neurosis of the pharynx, stomatocace, and constipation.

Yatong Yili Wan

Ingredients:

Venenum Bufonis	41.0%	*Chansu*
Cinnabaris	8.0%	*Zhusha*
Realgar	10.0%	*Xionghuang*
Radix Glycyrrhizae	41.0%	*Gancao*

Actions: Alleviating pain and swelling.

Indications: Toothache and swelling and pain of the gum due to pathogenic wind—fire.

Administration and Dosage: The hole of a decayed tooth or

the interproximal space between decayed teeth is filled with 1 or 2 pills, and covered with a piece of sterillized cotton to prevent the pills from escaping. The salvia due to the above treatment is to be spitted out but not swallowed.

Preparation Form: Pill.

Package: 0.3g in per 125 pills.

Notes: This drug has anti—inflammatory and tranquilizing effects. It is clinically efficacious for toothache, caries, and periodentitis.

16 Drugs used in the Department of Dermatology

Fuman Ling Ruangao

Main Ingredients:

Semen Chaulmoograe	*Dafengziren*
Semen Armeniacae Amarum	*Kuxingren*

Actions: Destroying parasites, and relieving itching and pain.

Indication: Rosacea.

Administration and Dosage: Applied to the affected part in the evening after the face is washed with lukewarm water and medicated soap.

Preparation Form: Ointment.

Package: 5 g in each box.

Notes: This drug powerfully kills vermiform mites and is efficacious for the rosacea of vermiform mite. It is not suitable for patients with photosensitive or allergic dermatitis or with eczema in the face, and not for pregnant women. If redness, allergic reaction, swelling, itching, or desquanmation is caused by the drug, the medication should be stopped until the above symptoms vanish. In addition, cosmetics are kept away in the course of treatment.

Yangrong Quban Yaogao

Main Ingredients:

Stearic acid		*Yingzhisuan*
Lanolin		*Yangmaozhi*
Extractum Folium Kaki		*Shiyetiquye*
Margarita (powder)		*Zhenzhufen*

Actions: Removing ecchymoses and nourishing the skin.

Indications: Facial chloasma and mild freckle.

Administration and Dosage: Applied to the affected part after the face is washed and wiped, and this is done once or twice daily.

Preparation Form: Cream.

Package: 30g in each tube.

Notes: This drug can improve microcirculation and metabolism of the epidermal chromocytes to protect the skin. It is used as an adjuvant in treating facial chloasma, freckle and allergic itching.

It is not to be taken orally.

Baidianfeng Wan

Ingredients:

Fructus Psoraleae	3.7%	*Buguzhi*
Radix Astragali	3.7%	*Huangqi*
Flos Carthami	3.7%	*Honghua*
Rhizome Chuanxiong	3.7%	*Chuanxiong*
Radix Angelicae Sinensis	3.7%	*Danggui*
Rhizoma Cyperi	3.7%	*Xiangfu*
Semen Persicae	3.7%	*Taoren*
Radix Salviae Miltiorrhizae	3.7%	*Danshen*
Zaocys	3.7%	*Wushaoshe*
Radix Arnebiae	3.7%	*Zicao*

Cortex Dictamni	3.7%	*Baixianpi*
Rhizoma Dioscoreae	3.7%	*Shanyao*
Fructus Tribuli	48.1%	*Baijili*
Rhizoma Zingiberis	3.7%	*Ganjiang*
Cuperic Sulfate	0.1%	*Liusuantong*
Radix Gentianae	3.7%	*Longdan*

Actions: Stimulating blood circulation to getrid of obstruction in the channels, removing toxic materials, dispelling dampness, expelling wind, relieving itching, invigorating *Qi* and eliminating ecchymoses.

Indication: Vitiligo.

Administration and Dosage: Taken orally, 1 honeyed bolus or 6 concentrated pills each time, twice daily.

Preparation Forms: Honeyed bolus and concentrated pill.

Package: 6 g in each bolus; 2 g in every 10 pills.

Notes: This drug can improve microcirculation and promote the production of melamin of skin. It is good for vitiligo.

Zigui Zhilie Gao

Ingredients:

Radix Arnebiae	11.1%	*Zicao*
Radix Angelicae Sinensis	11.1%	*Danggui*
Radix Ampelopsis	5.6%	*Baiwei*
Radix Glycyrrhizae	5.6%	*Gancao*
Lanolin	3.9%	*Yangmaozhi*
Borneolum Syntheticum	2.2%	*Bingpian*
Zinc chloride	21.1%	*Lühuaxin*
Rosin	16.7%	*Songxiang*
liquid paraffin	1.7%	*Yezhuangshila*

Rubber	17.8%	*Xiangjiao*
dimethyl sulfocide	1.1%	*Erjiajiyafeng*
vaseline	2.1%	*Fanshilin*

Actions: Promoting blood circulation, stimulating tissue regeneration, and alleviating pain.

Indication: Rhagades of hands and feet.

Administration and Dosage: Applied to the affected part after it is washed and steeped in warm water for a moment and wiped, with dressing change done every 2—3 days.

Preparation Form: Salve.

Package: 5 × 7 cm per piece.

Notes: This salve can dilate blood vessels, alleviate pain and promote wound healing. It is efficacious for rhagades of hands and feet.

Dongchuang Shui

Ingredients:

| Fructus Capsici | *Lajiao* |
| Camphora | *Zhangnao* |

Actions: Warming the channels, promoting blood circulation, and relieving swelling.

Indication: Chilblain without ulceration.

Administration and Dosage: Applied to the affected part, 3—5 times daily.

Preparation From: Tincture.

Package: 10 ml in each bottle.

Notes: This drug can improve microcirculation and promote the regeneration of epidermic cells, being clinically good for chilblain without ulceration.

Ezhangfeng Yaoshui

Ingredients:

Cortex Pseudolaricis	20%	*Tujingpi*
Fructus Cnidii	10%	*Shechuangzi*
Semen Chaulmoograe	10%	*Dafengziren*
Radix Stemonae	10%	*Baibu*
Radix Ledebouriellae	4%	*Fangfeng*
Radix Angelicae Sinensis	8%	*Danggui*
Caulis Impatientis	10%	*Fengxiantou gucao*
Cacumen Biotae	8%	*Cebaiye*
Fructus Evodiae	3.9%	*Wuzhuyu*
Pericarpium Zanthoxyli	10%	*Huajiao*
Periostracum Cicadae	6%	*Chantui*
Mylabris	0.2%	*Banmao*

Actions: Expelling wind, dispelling dampness, relieving itching, and destroying parasites.

Indications: Tinea unguium, onychomycosis, exudative dermatitis, and tinea pedis.

Administration and Dosage: Externally used. Applied to the affected part after it is washed, 3—4 times daily. When onychomycosis is treated, the disjointed part of the nail is cut off to facilitate the penetration of the drug.

Preparation From: Tincture.

Package: 20 ml in each bottle.

Notes: This tincture can destroy parasites, relieve itching and fight against mycetes. It is efficacious for parasitic and mycotic exudative dermatitis, tinea pedis and tinea manus.

17　Drugs with Nourishing and Strengthening Effects

17.1　Drugs for Regulating the Functions of the Organism and Preventing Decrepitude

Qingchunbao

Main Ingredidents:

Radix Ginseng	*Renshen*
Radix Asparagi	*Tianmendong*
Radix Rehmanniae	*Dihuang*

Actions: Invigorating *Qi*, enriching blood, nourishing *Yin* and promoting the production of body fluid.

Indications: Premature senility, breakdown of the normal physiological coordination between the heart and kidney, amnesia, insomnia, lassitude in the loins and knees, and inappetence owing to deficiency of both *Qi* and blood.

Administration and Dosage: Taken orally, 3–5 tablets each time, twice daily.

Preparation Form: Tablet.

Notes: Without toxic and side effects, this drug can invigorate the brain to relieve mental stress, prevent fatigue and raise the body's immunity. It is clinically efficacious for premature senility, premature grey hair, anemia, neurasthenia and cardiopathy. It can also promote recovery from various diseases.

Experiments have shown that the tablet of this kind can extend the life span of old rats, enhance phagocytic function of macrophages, promote immunological function of the body and reduce radiation damage to organs.

Raw radish is avoided during the medication of this drug.

Buzhong Yiqi Wan

Ingredients:

Radix Astragali	30.3%	Huangqi
Radix Codonopsis Pilosulae	9.1%	Dangshen
Radix Glycyrrhizae	15.1%	Gancao
Rhizoma Atractylodis Macrocephalae	9.1%	Baizhu
Radix Angelicae Sinensis	9.1%	Danggui
Rhizoma Cimicifugae	9.1%	Shengma
Radix Bupleuri	9.1%	Chaihu
Pericarpium Citri Reticulatae	9.1%	Chenpi

Actions: Reinforcing the spleen to replenish and elevata *Qi*

Indications: Fatigue, poor appetite, abdominal distension, protracted diarrhea, proctoptosis and hysteroptosis due to weakness of the spleen and stomach and sinking of *Qi* of the middle—*Jiao*.

Administration and Dosage: Taken orally, 1 bolus each time, 2 or 3 times daily.

Preparation Form: Honeyed bolus.

Package: 9 g in each bolus.

Notes: The recipe was first recorded in the book *Pi Wei Lun* written by Li Gao in the Jin Dynasty.

This bolus can reinforce the body's resistance and regulate

the function of the intestines and stomach. It is clinically efficacious for various dystrophic anemia, neurasthenia, simple orthostatic hypotension, hysteroptosis, gastroptosis, chronic enterogastritis, chronic hepatitis, and hemorrhage caused by various factors.

Shiquan Dabu Wan

Ingredients:

Radix Codonopsis Pilosulae	10.8%	Dangshen
Rhizoma Atractylodis		
Macrocephalae	10.8%	Baizhu
Poria	10.8%	Fuling
Radix Glycyrrhizae	5.4%	Gancao
Radix Angilicae Sinensis	16.2%	Danggui
Rhizoma Chuanxiong	5.4%	Chuanxiong
Radix Paeoniae Alba	10.8%	Baishao
Cortex Cinnamomi	2.3%	Rougui
Radix Rehmanniae Praeparata	16.2%	Shudihuang
Radix Astragali	10.8%	Huangqi

Actions: Warming and tonifying *Qi* and blood.

Indications: Pale complexion, dyspnea, palpitation, dizziness, spontaneous perspiration, fatigue and clammy limbs due to deficiency of both *Qi* and blood.

Administration and Dosage: Taken orally, 1 bolus each time, 2 or 3 times daily.

Preparation Form: Honeyed bolus.

Package: 9 g in each bolus.

Notes: The recipe is quoted from the book *Tai Ping Hui Mi He Ji Ju Fang* compiled by Chen Shiwen in the Song Dynasty.

This drug can regulate the function of the stomach and the intestines, reinforce adrenocortical function, improve microcirculation, fight against gastric ulcer and anemia, and raise the body's immunity. As an adjuvent, it is effective in the treatment of gynecopathy and chronic diseases such as anemia, gastroptosis, diabetes, cirrhosis and pulmonary emphysema.

Renshen Jing

Ingredient:
Radix Ginseng   100%   *Renshen*

Actions: Invigorating *Qi*, promoting the production of body fluid, quenching thirst, tranquilizing the mind and relieving mental stress.

Indications: Palpitation owing to deficiency of *Qi*, thirst caused by deficiency of body fluid, and spontaneous perspiration, prostration syndrome, amnesia, an insomnia resulting from kindey deficiency.

Administration and Dosage: Taken orally, 2—3 ml each time, 3 times daily.

Perpartion Form: Oral liquid.

Pockage: 10 ml in each bottle.

Notes: This drug can regulate the body function and has an antiaging effect. It is clinically efficacious for neurasthenia, psychosis, angiocardiopathy, anemia, sexual hypofunction, diabetes, and hemorrhagic shock.

Shuangbaosu

Ingredients:
Radix Ginseng   *Renshen*

Lac Regis Apis   *Fengwangjiang*

Actions: Nourishing the body, invigorating *Qi* and strenthening the spleen.

Indications: Weakness after illness, fatigue, inappetence, amnesia and insomnia.

Administration and Dosage: Taken orally, 1 capsule or 2 each time, 3 times daily; or 10 ml of oral liquid each time, twice a day.

Preparation Form: Capsule and oral liquid.

Package: 30 capsules in each per bottle; 10 ml of oral liquid in each bottle.

Notes: This drug can promote metabolism, improve the function of the brain and reinforce body immunity. It is clinically efficacious for cardiopathy, hepatitis, gastric ulcer, anemia, premature senility, rheumatic arthritis, and neurasthenia.

Wangjiang Pian

Ingredient:

Lac Regis Apis   *Wangjiang*

Actions: Nourishing and strengthening the body.

Indications: Inappetence, dizziness, tinnitus, amnesia, insomnia and palpitation owing to *Qi* deficiency of the spleen and stomach.

Administration and Dosgae: Taken orally, 2 or 3 tablets each time, 2 or 3 times daily.

Preparation Form: Tablet.

Package: 0.25 g in each tablet.

Notes: This drug is efficacious for neurosis, neuritis, malnutrition, rheumatic arthritis, rheumatic fever and neuritis. It can be used as an adjuvant in the treatment of hypertension, duodenal ulcer, angiocadiopathy, tuberculosis and diabetes.

Wujiashen Chongji

Ingredient:

Radix Acanthopanacis Senticosi   *Ciwujia*

Actions: Invigorating the brain, relieving mental stress, tonifying the kidney, reinforcing the spleen, and strengthening muscles and bones.

Indications: General weakness, fatigue, inappetence, amnesia, insomnia, palpitation and dyspnea.

Administration and Dosgae: Taken orally, 1 cube each time, 2 or 3 times daily.

Preparation Form: Medicinal cube.

Package: 12.25 g in each cube.

Notes: This drug can reinforce body function, fight against allergy, fatigue and radiation, regulate blood pressure and help increase the coronary blood flow. It is clinically efficacious for chronic tracheitis, neurosis, primary hypertension, sexual dysfunction, rheumatic arthritis, and all types of anemia.

Liuwei Dihuang Wan

Ingredients:

Radix Rehmanniae Praeparata	32.0%	*Shudihuang*
Fructus Corni	16.0%	*Shanzhuyu*
Cortex Moutan Radicis	12.0%	*Danpi*
Rhizoma Dioscoreae	16.0%	*Shanyao*
Poria	12.0%	*Fuling*
Rhizoma Alismatis	12.8%	*Zexie*

Actions: Nourishing *Yin* and reinforcing the kidney.

Indications: Dizziness, tinnitus, lassitude in the knees, hectic fever, night sweating, emission and diabetes due to deficiency of kidney−*Yin*.

Administration and Dosage: Taken orally. 1 pill each time, twice daily.

Preparation Form: Honeyed bolus.

Package: 9 g in each bolus.

Notes: The recipe is quoted from the book *Xiao Er Yao Zheng Zhi Jue* written by Qian Yi in the Song Dynasty.

This drug can improve the function of the kidney, lower blood pressure, induce diuresis, and fight against inflammation and cancers. It is clinically efficacious for congenital hypoevolutism in infants, chronic nephritis, hypertension, diabetes, rheumatoid arthritis, vertebral hyperostosis, pulmonary tuberculosis, hyperthyroidism, optic neuritis, glaucoma, and periodontal abscess.

Lingzhi Pian

Ingredient:

Gaboderma Lucidum   *Lingzhi*

Actions: Strengthening the body and relieving mental stress.

Indications: Amnesia, insomnia, dreaminess, and inappetence.

Administration and Dosage: Take orally, 3 tablets each time, 3 times daily.

Preparation Form: Tablet.

Package: 1 g in each tablet.

Notes: This drug can reinforce body immunity, strengthen

the heart, lower blood fat, regulate blood pressure, normalize the function of the central nervous system, relieve cough, and remove the phlegm. It is efficacious for asthmatic trachitis, bronchial asthma, infectious hepatitis, chronic enteritis, bacillary dysentery, thrombocytopenic purpura, rheumatic arthritis, coronary heart disease, gastric ulcer, and duodenal ulcer.

Bazhen Wan

Ingredients:

Radix Codonopsis Pilosulae	12.1%	]Dangshen
Rhizoma Astractylodis Macrocephalae	12.1%	Baizhu
Poria	12.1%	Fuling
Radix Angilicae Sinensis	18.2%	Danggui
Radix Glycyrrhizae	6.1%	Gancao
Radix Paeoniae Alba	12.1%	Baishao
Rhizoma Chuanxiong	9.1%	Chuangxiong
Radix Rehmanniae Praeparata	18.2%	Shudihuang

Actions: Invigorating *Qi* and replenishing blood.

Indications: Sallow complexion, inappetence, myasthenia of limbs and irregular menstruation due to deficiency of both *Qi* and blood.

Administration and Dosage: Taken orally, 1 bolus each time, 2 times daily.

Preparation Form: Bolus.

Package: 9 g in each bolus.

Notes: The recipe is recorded in the book *Rui Zhu Tang Jing Yan Fang*.

This drug can regulate the function of the stomach and intestine and promote the regeneration of erythrocytes. It is efficacious for all types of anemia, chronic gastritis, gastric ulcer, duodenal ulcer, optic atrophy, and irregular menstruation.

Dabuyin Wan

Ingredients:

Radix Rehmanniae Praeparata	21.4%	*Shudihuang*
Rhizoma Anemarrhenae	14.4%	*Zhimu*
Cortex Phellodendri	14.4%	*Huangbai*
Plastrum Testudinis	21.4%	*Guiban*
pig marrow	28.4%	*Zhugusui*

Action: Nourishing *Yin* to reduce fire.

Indications: Hectic fever, night sweat, hemoptysis, tinnitus and emission caused by hyperactivity of fire due to *Yin*—deficiency.

Administration and Dosage: Taken orally, 6 g each time, 2 or 3 times daily.

Preparation Form: Honeyed bolus.

Package: 3 g in each bolus.

Notes: The recipe is recorded in the book *Dan Xi Xin Fa* written by Zhu Zhenheng in the Yuan Dynasty.

This drug can improve the function of the kidney, lower blood pressure, induce diuresis and diminish inflammation. It is efficacious for hyperthyroidism, renal tuberculosis, bone tuberculosis, and diabetes.

Shenling Baizhu Wan

Ingredients:

Radix Ginseng	13.8%	*Renshen*

Poria	13.8%	*Fuling*
Rhizoma Atractylodis		
Macrocephalae	13.8%	*Baizhu*
Rhizoma Dioscoreae	13.8%	*Shanyao*
Semen Dolichoris Album	10.3%	*Baibiandou*
Fructus Amomi	6.9%	*Sharen*
Semen Coicis	6.9%	*Yiyiren*
Radix Platycodi	6.9%	*Jiegeng*
Radix Glycyrrhizae	13.8%	*Gancao*

Actions: Tonifying the spleen and stomach, and benefiting lung—*Qi*.

Indications: Inappetence, loose stools, dyspnea, cough and myasthenia of limbs due to weakness of the spleen and stomach.

Administration and Dosage: Taken orally, 6—9 g each time, 2 or 3 times daily.

Preparation Form: Water—paste pill.

Package: 1 g in every 20 pills.

Notes: The recipe is quoted from the book *Tai Ping Hui Min He Ji Ju Fang* compiled by Chen Shiwen in the Song Dynasty.

This drug can regulate the function of the stomach and intestines, diminish inflammation, aid digestion, and reinforce body immunity. It is efficacious for chronic gastroenteritis, anemia, pulmonary tuberculosis, chronic nephritis and dyspepsia.

Kangbao Koufuye

Main Ingredients:

Lac Regis Apis	*Fengwangjiang*
Radix Acanthopanacis Senticosi	*Ciwujia*
Rhizoma Polygonati	*Huangjing*

Radix Codonopsis Pilosulae	*Dangshen*
Fructus Mori	*Sangshen*
Fructus Amomi	*Sharen*
Radix Astragali	*Huangqi*
Fructus Crataegi	*Shanzha*
Fructus Lycii	*Gouqizi*
Herba Epimedii	*Yinyanghuo*

Actions: Replenishing *Qi*, tonifying the kidney, strengthening the spleen, regulating the stomach, nourishing the heart, and tranquilizing the mind.

Indications: Amnesia, insomnia, dizziness, tinnitus, poor vision and hearing, inappetence, lassitude in the loins and knees, palpitation, dyspnea, and sequel from apoplexy.

Administration and Dosage: Taken orally, 10—20 ml each time, twice daily.

Preparation Form: Oral liquid.

Package: 10 ml in each bottle.

Notes: This drug can improve the function of the brain and promote metabolism. It is efficacious for neurasthenia, coronary heart disease, baldness, chronic nephritis, cerebral embolism and menopausal syndrome.

Renshen Fengwang Jiang

Ingredients:

Radix Ginseng	*Renshen*
Lac Regis Apis	*Wangjiang*
Mel	*Fengmi*

Actions: Nourishing the body and replenishing *Qi* to strengthen the spleen.

Indications: Inappetence, weakness after illness, and fatigue.

Administration and Dosage: Taken orally on an empty stomach in the morning or evening, 10 ml each time, once daily.

Preparation Form: Oral liquid.

Package: 10 ml in each bottle.

Notes: This liquid can improve the function of the brain, promote metabolism, and nourish and strengthen the body. It is efficacious for all types of anemia, neurasthenia, neurosis, chronic hepatitis, pulmonary heart disease, chronic trachitis, rheumatic arthritis, chronic nephritis, and pulmonary tuberculosis.

Shenqi Chongji

Ingredients:

Radix Condonopsis Pilosulae   *Dangshen*

Fructus Lycii   *Gouqizi*

Actions: Invigorating *Qi*, enriching blood, strengthening the spleen and stomach, and nourishing the liver and kidney.

Indications: Dizziness, dim eyesight and fatigue due to weakness of the spleen and stomach.

Administration and Dosage: Taken orally, 1 sack each time, twice daily.

Preparation Form: Granule.

Package: 10 g in each sack.

Notes: This drug can improve the function of the body and reduce blood fat. It is efficacious for chronic hepatitis, arteriosclerosis, hyperlipemia, anemia, and neurosis.

Taishan Lingzhi Jing

Ingredients:

Gaboderma Lucidum	38.2%	Lingzhi
Radix Ginseng	0.5%	Renshen
Radix Salviae Miltiorrhizae	1.5%	Danshen
Cortex Eucommiae	1.5%	Duzhong
Fructus Lycii	1.5%	Gouqizi
Radix Polygoni Multiflori	1.5%	Heshouwu
Semen Ziziphi Spinosae	1.5%	Suanzaoren
Fructus Schisandiae	1.5%	Wuweizi
Radix Rehmanniae Praeparata	1.5%	Shudihuang
Radix Angelicae Sinensis	1.2%	Danggui
Mel	49.6%	Fengmi

Actions: Invigorating *Qi*, enriching blood, nourishing the heart, and relieving mental stress.

Indications: Severe palpitation due to fright, amnesia, insomnia, lassitude in the loins and knees and inappetence owing to deficiency of both *Qi* and blood and incoordination between the heart and the kidney.

Administration and Dosage: Taken orally, 10 ml each time, twice daily, respectively before breakfast and bedtime in the evening.

Preparation Form: Oral liquid.

Package: 10 ml in each bottle.

Notes: This drug can regulate the function of the body, promote blood circulation and remove phlegm. It is clinically efficacious for neurasthenia, coronary heart disease, chronic hepatitis, duodenal and gastric ulcer, neurosis, alopecia and anemia.

Danggui Buxue Jing

Ingredients:

Radix Angelicae Sinensis	76.2%	*Danggui*
Radix Rehmanniae Preparata	4.8%	*Shudihuang*
Radix Paeoniae Alba	4.8%	*Baishao*
Rhizoma Chuanxiong	2.3%	*Chuanxiong*
Radix Condonopsis Pilosulae	4.8%	*Dangshen*
Radix Astragali	4.8%	*Huangqi*
Radix Glycyrrhizae	2.3%	*Gancao*

Actions: Invigorating *Qi* and enriching blood.

Indications: Anemia, dizziness, palpitation, amnesia, irregular menstruation, and postpartum weakness owing to defciency of blood.

Administration and Dosage: Taken orally. 5 ml each time, twice daily.

Preparation Form: Syrup.

Package: 150 ml in each bottle.

Notes: This drug has nourishing and tranquilizing effects and can reinforce body immunity. It is clinically efficacious for all types of anemia, functional uterine bleeding, irregular menstruation, neurasthenia, and allergic purpura.

Shouwu Wan

Ingredients:

Radix Polygoni Multiflori	42.7%	*Heshouwu*
Radix Rehmanniae	2.4%	*Dihuang*
Radix Achyranthis Bidentatae	4.7%	*Niuxi*
Extractum Fructus Mori	8.3%	*Sangshengao*
Fructus Ligustri Lucidi	4.7%	*Nüzhenzi*
Folium Mori	4.7%	*Sangye*
Semen Sesami Nigrum	1.9%	*Heizhima*

Extractum Herba Ecliptae	5.7%	*Mohanliangao*
Fructus Psoraleae	4.7%	*Buguzhi*
Herba Siegesbeckiae	9.5%	*Xixiancao*
Flos Lonicerae	2.4%	*Jinyinhua*
Extractum Fructus Rosae		
Laevigatae	8.3%	*Jinyingzigao*

Actions: Invigorating the liver and kidney, strengthening muscles and bones, and blackening hair.

Indications: Dizziness, tinnitus, lassitude in the loins and knees, and premature greying of hair owing to deficiency of both the liver and kidney.

Administration and Dosage: Taken orally, 6 g each time, twice daily.

Preparation Form: Water—paste pill.

Package: 1 g in every 20 pills.

Notes: This drug can dimnish inflammation and lower blood fat and cholestol. It is clinically efficacious for rheumatic arthritis, premature greying of hair, arteriosclerosis, coronary heart disease, urticaria, neurasthenia and mental disorders.

Yupingfeng Wan

Ingredients:

Radix Astragali	50.0%	*Huangqi*
Radix Ledebouriellae	16.7%	*Fangfeng*
Rhizoma Astractylodis	33.3%	*Baizhu*
Macrocephalae		

Actions: Invigorating *Qi*, dispelling pathogenic factors from the exterior of the body and suppressing sweating.

Indications: Spontaneous perspiration owing to deficiency of

Qi and symptoms of wind—cold type owing to exterior weakness.

Administration and Dosage: Taken orally, 6 g each time, twice a day.

Preparation Form: Water—paste pill.

Package: 125 g in each bottle.

Notes: The recipe was recorded in the book *Jing Yue Quan Shu* written by Zhang Jiebin in the Ming Dynasty.

This drug can reinforce the immunity of the body. It is clinically efficacious for chronic tracheitis, common cold owing to weakness, chronic rhintis and urticaria. It can also be used for the prevention of common cold.

Qing'e Wan

Ingredients:

Cortex Eucommiae	48.5%	*Duzhong*
Fructus Psoraleae	24.2%	*Buguzhi*
Semen Juglandis	15.2%	*Hetaoren*
Bulbus Allii	12.1%	*Dasuan*

Actions: Tonifying the kidney to strengthen the waist.

Indications: Lumbago, limited movement, weakness of the knees and acratia due to deficiency of the kidney.

Administration and Dosage: Taken orally, 1 bolus each time, 2 or 3 times daily.

Preparation Form: Honeyed bolus.

Package: 9 g in each bolus.

Notes: The recipe is quoted from the book *Tai Ping Hui Min He Ji Ju Fang* compiled by Chen Shiwen in the Song Dynasty.

This drug can improve the function of the kidney, lower blood pressure and induce diuresis. It is clinically efficacious for chronic nephritis, renal tuberculosis, lumbar—vertebrae tuberculosis and bone tuberculosis.

Rehshen Yangrong Wan

Ingredients:

Radix Codonopsis Pilosulae	8.3%	*Dangshen*
Radix Astragali	8.3%	*Huangqi*
Pericarpium Citri Reticulatae	8.3%	*Chenpi*
Radix Glycyrrhizae	8.3%	*Gancao*
Radix Paeoniae Alba	12.4%	*Baishao*
Poria	5.8%	*Fuling*
Rhizoma Zingiberis Recens	4.1%	*Shengjiang*
Cortex Cinnamoni	8.3%	*Rougui*
Radix Rehmanniae Preparata	5.7%	*Shudihuang*
Radix Angelicae Sinensis	8.3%	*Danggui*
Radix Polygalae	4.1%	*Yuanzhi*
Rhizoma Astractylosis		
Macrocephalae	8.3%	*Baizhu*
Fructus Schisandrae	5.7%	*Waweizi*
Fructus Jujubae	4.1%	*Dazao*

Actions: Invigorating *Qi*, enriching blood, strengthening the spleen, and relieving mental stress.

Indications: Inappetence, palpitation, night sweat and amnesia owing to insufficiency of Qi and blood due to hypofunction of the spleen and lung.

Administration and Dosage: Taken orally. 9 g each time, twice a day.

Preparation Form: Water—paste pill.

Package: 1 g in each pill.

Notes: This pill can regulate gastrointestinal function and has tranquilizing effect. It is clinically efficacious for thromboangiitis, all kinds of tumors, and chronic gastroenteritis. In addition, it is used as an adjuvant in the convalescence of operation and advanced stages of infectious diseases.

Shengfa Wan

Ingredients:

Radix Angelicae Sinensis	12.3%	Danggui
Cacumen Biotae	12.3%	Cebaiye
Radix Rehmanniae	12.3%	Dihuang
Fructus Ligustri Lucidi	12.3%	Nüzhenzi
Semen Biotae	12.4%	Baiziren
Fructus Lycii	3.7%	Gouqizi
Fructus Mori	12.4%	Sangshenzi
Cortex Phellodendri	3.7%	Huangbai
Semen Cuscutae	12.4%	Tusizi
Cortex Dictamni Radicis	6.2%	Baixianpi

Actions: Nourishing the liver, kidney and blood, and promoting hair—growth.

Indications: Baldness and Jonston's arc.

Administration and Dosage: Taken orally, 1 bolus each time, twice daily. A larger dose may be given to severe cases.

Preparation Form: Big honeyed bolus.

Package: 9 g in each bolus.

Notes: This drug aids hair—growth. It is clinically efficacious for seborrheic dermatitis, neurasthenia and baldness owing to dysbolism.

Nervousness and diet with animal fat should be avoided during this midicaiton.

Wufa Wan

Ingredients:

Radix Rehmanniae	25.0%	Dihuang
Herba Ecliptae	12.5%	Hanliancao
Radix Polygoni Multiflori	25.0%	Heshouwu
Semen Sojae Nigrum	12.5%	Heidou
Fructus Ligustri Lucidi	12.5%	Nuzhenzi
Semen Sesami Nigrum	12.5%	Heizhima

Actions: Nourishing the kidney, tonifying the brain, enriching blood and blackening the hair.

Indication: Poliosis in teen—agers.

Administration and Dosage: Taken orally, 1 bolus each time, 2 or 3 times daily.

Preparation Form: Honeyed bolus.

Package: 9 g in each bolus.

Notes: This drug can reinforce body immunity. It is clinically efficacious for poliosis caused by various factors.

Nervousness and pungent food should be avoided during this medication.

Qibao Meiran Wan

Ingredients:

Radix Polygoni Multiflori	42.2%	Heshouwu
Semen Cuscutae	10.5%	Tusizi
Radix Achyranthis Bidentatae	10.5%	Niuxi
Fructus Psoraleae	5.3%	Buguzhi
Radix Angelicae Sinensis	10.5%	Danggui

Fructus Lycii	10.5%	*Gouqizi*
Poria	10.5%	*Fuling*

Actions: Nourishing the liver and kidney, replenishing essence and enriching blood.

Indications: Poliosis due to deficiency of essence and blood.

Administration and Dosage: Taken orally, 1 bolus each time, twice daily.

Preparation Form: Honeyed bolus.

Package: 9 g in each bolus.

Notes: The recipe was recorded in the book *Jing Yan Fang* written by Shao Yuanjie in the Tang Dynasty.

This drug can regulate the function of the body and promote metabolism. It is clinically efficacious for premature senility and poliosis.

17.2 Drugs for Treating Sexual Neurasthenia

Zhibao Sanbian Wan

Ingredients:

Mel	*Fengmi*
Radix Astragali	*Huangqi*
Radix Ginseng	*Renshen*
Radix Angelicae Sinensis	*Danggui*
Cornu Cervi Pantotrichum	*Lurong*
Male deer externalia	*Meihualubian*
Gecko	*Gejie*
Semen Cuscutae	*Tusizi*
Radix Rehmanniae	*Dihuang*
Fructus Lycii	*Gouqizi*

Lac Regis Apis	*Fengru*
Fructus Foeniculi	*Xiaohuixiang*
Pericarpium Zanthoxyli	*Chuanjiao*
Rhizoma Nardostachydis	*Gansong*
Lignum Aquilariae Resinatum	*Chenxiang*
Testis et Penis Callorhini	*Haigoubian*
Testix et Penis Canitis	*Guanggoubian*
Hippocampus	*Dahaima*
Actinolitum	*Feiyangqishi*
Os Draconis	*Wuhualonggu*
Fructus Corni	*Jingyurou*
Fructus Psoraleae	*Buguzhi*
Radix Achyranthis Bidentatae	*Niuxi*
Herba Epimedii	*Yinyanghuo*
Poria	*Yunling*
Öitheca Mantidis	*Sangpiaoxiao*
Rhizoma Dioscoreae	*Shanyao*
Radix Morindae Officinalis	*Bajitian*
Cortex Eucommiae	*Duzhong*
Cortex Cinnamomi	*Rougui*
Fructus Rubi	*Fupenzi*
Radix Polygoni Multiflori	*Heshouwu*
Cortex Moutan Radicis	*Fendanpi*
Cortex Phellodendri	*Chuanhuangbai*
Radix Paeoniae Alba	*Hangbaishao*
Rhizoma Atractylodis	
Macrocephalae	*Baizhu*
Herba Cistanchis	*Roucongrong*
Rhizoma Alismatis	*Zexie*

Acorus Calamus	Jiechangpu
Radix Polygalae	Yuanzhi

Actions: Enriching blood, promoting the generation of vital essence, strengthening the brain and tonifying the kidney.

Indications: General asthenia, soreness and pain in the back and loins; emission, amnesia and insomnia owing to deficiency of the kidney; inappetence, anemia and dizziness owing to deficiency of *Qi;* blood insufficiency of women and dyspnea of the aged.

Administration and Dosage: Taken orally, 8 concentrated pills or 1 honeyed bolus each time, once daily.

Preparation Forms: Concentrated pill and honeyed bolus.

Package: 6.25 g in each honyed bolus; 0.2 g in each concentrated pill.

Notes: This drug can improve the function of the brain and the sexual gland. It is clinically efficacious for all types of hypofunction of the body, sexual neurasthenia, all types of anemia, chronic gastroenteritis, gastric and duodenal ulcer and neurasthenia.

Guiling Ji

Ingredients:

Radix Ginseng	Renshen
Cornu Cervi Pantotrichum	Lurong
Hippocampus	Haima
Semen Nelumbinis	Lianzi
Poria	Fuling
Radix Asparagi	Tiandong
Radix Ophiopogonis	Maidong
Squama Manitis	Chuanshanjia

Herba Cistanchis	*Roucongrong*
Herba Cynomorii	*Suoyang*
Fructus Psoraleae	*Buguzhi*
Herba Epimedii	*Yinyanghuo*
Semen Trigonellae	*Huluba*
Semen Cuscutae	*Tusizi*
Semen Astragali Complanati	*Shayuanzi*
Cortex Eucommiae	*Duzhong*
Radix Aconiti Lateralis Preparata	*Fuzi*
Spongilla Fraqilla Fraqilis	*Zishaohua*
Radix Achyranthis Bidentatae	*Huainiuxi*
Herba Asari	*Xixin*
Radix Rehmanniae	*Dihuang*
Herba Dendrobii	*Shihu*
Radix Angelicae Sinensis	*Danggui*
Fructus Amoni	*Sharen*
Fructus Flos Caryophylli	*Mudingxiang*
Flos Chrysanthemi	*Juhua*
Semen Plantaginis	*Cheqianzi*
Semen Raphani	*Laifuzi*
Fossilia Spiriferis	*Shiyan*
Salt	*Shiyan*
Rhizoma Dryopteris Crassirhizomae	*Guanzhong*
Colla Corii Asini	*Ejiao*
Cinnabaris	*Zhusha*
Radix Glycyrrhizae	*Gancao*

Action: Nourishing kidney—*Yang*.

Indications: Deficiency of kidney—*Yang*, marked by impotence, emission and cough owing to deficiency of *Qi*, cold pain in the loins and knees, cramping sensation in the lower abdomen, dizziness, tinnitus, hypomnesis, metrorrhagia, metrostaxis, leukorrhea with reddish discharge and diarrhea before dawn.

Administration and Dosage: Taken orally, 1.5 g each time, once or twice a day.

Preparation Form: Powder.

Package: 0.3 g in each bottle.

Notes: This drug can regulate the function of the adrenal cortex, promote growth and development and reinforce body resistance. It is clinically efficacious for weakness, sexual neurasthenia, chronic nephritis, abnormal menstruation, menopausal syndrome and infertility.

It is contraindicated for pregnant women. Raw and cold foods must be avoided during this medicaiton.

Hailong Gejie Jing

Main Ingredients:

Syngnathus	*Hailong*
Gecko	*Gejie*
Radix Ginseng	*Renshen*
Penis Caprae seu Ovis	*Yangbian*
Cornu Cervi Pantotrichum	*Lurong*
Radix Rehmanniae	*Dihuang*
Herba Cistanchis	*Roucongrong*
Pericarpium Citri Reticulatae	*Chenpi*
Lignum Aquilariae Resinatum	*Chenxiang*
Fructus Lycii	*Gouqizi*
Radix Astragali	*Huangqi*

Cortex Cinnamomi	*Rougui*
Radix Angelicae Sinensis	*Danggui*
Rhizoma Chuanxiong	*Chuanxiong*
Fructus Amoni Rotundus	*Baikou*
Radix Glycyrrhizae	*Gancao*

Actions: Nourishing the liver and kidney, replenishing vital essence and enriching blood.

Indications: Amnesia, insomnia, dizziness, tinnitus, lassitude of the loins and knees, impotence, emission and metrorrhagia owing to deficiency of both Qi and blood.

Administration and Dosage: Taken orally, 10 ml each time, twice daily.

Preparation Form: Oral liquid.

Package: 10 ml in each bottle.

Notes: This drug can improve the function fo the brain, promote energy metabolism and enhance the function of the sexual gland. It is clinically efficacious for neurasthenia, neurosis, sexual neurasthenia, all type of anemia, pulmonary emphysema, chronic gastroenteritis, bronchial asthma, male infertility, prostatitis and menopausal syndrome.

Huanshao Dan

Main Ingredients:

Radix Morindae Officinalis	*Bajitian*
Fructus Foeniculi	*Xiaohuixiang*
Herba Cistanchis	*Roucongrong*
Radix Ginseng	*Renshen*
Rhizoma Dioscoreae	*Shanyao*
Fructus Lycii	*Gouqi*

Fructus Corni	*Shanzhuyu*
Radix Achyranthis Bidentatae	*Niuxi*
Cortex Eucommiae	*Duzhong*
Fructus Schisandrae	*Wuweizi*
Poria	*Fuling*
Radix Rehmanniae	*Dihuang*
Radix Angelicae Sinensis	*Danggui*
Cortex Cinnamomi	*Rougui*
Radix Astragali	*Huangqi*
Colla Corii Asini	*Ejiao*

Actions: Nourishing and strengthening the body, and calming the mind.

Indications: Deficiency of kidney—*Qi* marked by cold lower limbs and nocturnal emission, dizziness and dim eyesight owing to deficiency of both *Qi* and blood; lassitude of the loins and knees and leukorrhea with reddish discharge owing to deficiency of the spleen and stomach.

Administration and Dosage: Taken orally, 1 bolus each time, twice daily.

Preparation Form: Honeyed bolus.

Package: 10 g in each bolus.

Notes: The recipe was recorded in the book *Dan Xi Xin Fa* written by Zhu Zhenheng in the Yuan Dynasty.

This drug can strengthen the body, stimulate the adrenal cortex, and reinforce the immunologic function of the body. It is clinically efficacious for weakness of the aged, sexual hypofunction and various hematopoietic disorders.

It is contraindicated for pregnant women and those with hypertension.

Quanlu Wan

Ingredients:

fresh deer meat	39.2%	*Xianlurou*
Colla Cornu Cervi	0.9%	*Lujiaojiao*
Cornu Cervi Pantotrichum	0.5%	*Lurong*
Penis et Testis Cervi	0.4%	*Lushen*
Cauda Cervi	0.2%	*Luwei*
Radix Ginseng	2.0%	*Renshen*
Radix Astragali	2.0%	*Huangqi*
Rhizoma Atractylodis		
Macrocephalae	2.0%	*Baizhu*
Poria	2.0%	*Fuling*
Radix Glycyrrhizae	1.9%	*Gancao*
Rhizoma Dioscoreae	1.9%	*Shanyao*
Radix Rehmanniae Preparata	1.9%	*Shudihuang*
Radix Rehmanniae	1.9%	*Shengdihuang*
Radix Angelicae Sinensis	1.9%	*Danggui*
Rhizoma Chuanxiong	1.9%	*Chuanxiong*
Fructus Lycii	1.9%	*Gouqizi*
Semen Cuscutae	1.9%	*Tusizi*
Fructus Broussonetiae	2.0%	*Gouzi*
Fructus Rubi	2.0%	*Fupenzi*
Semen Trigonellae	2.0%	*Huluba*
Cortex Eucommiae	2.0%	*Duzhong*
Radix Dipsaci	2.0%	*Xuduan*
Radix Achyranthis Bidentatae	2.0%	*Niuxi*
Fructus Psoraleae	2.0%	*Buguzhi*
Radix Morindae Officinalis	2.9%	*Bajitian*

Herba Cistanchis	2.0%	*Roucongrong*
Herba Cynomorii	2.0%	*Suoyang*
Halitum	0.9%	*Daqingyan*
Autumn stone	2.0%	*Qiushi*
Radix Asparagi	2.0%	*Tianmendong*
Radix Ophiopogonis	2.0%	*Maimendong*
Fructus Foeniculi	0.9%	*Huixiang*
Pericarpium Zanthoxyli	0.9%	*Huajiao*
Lignum Aquilariae Resinatum	0.9%	*Chenxiang*
Pericarpium Citri Reticulatae	2.0%	*Chenpi*
Semen Euryales	2.0%	*Qianshi*
Fructus Schisandrae	2.0%	*Wuweizi*

Actions: Invigorating *Yang*, enriching essence, replenishing *Qi* and nourishing blood.

Indications: Weakness, dizziness, tinnitus, nocturnal emission, lassitude of the loins and knees, inappetence, acratia, spontaneous perspiration, night sweat, metrorrhagia, metrostaxis and leukorrhea, all of which are due to deficiency of both *Yin* and *Yang*.

Administration and Dosage: Taken orally, 1 bolus each time, twice daily.

Preparation Form: Honeyed bolus.

Package: 9 g in each bolus.

Notes: The recipe was recorded in the book *Jing Yue Quan Shu* written by Zhang Jiebin in the Ming Dynasty.

This drug is clinically efficacious for sexual neurasthenia, neurosis, diabetes, prostatitis, chronic nephritis, chronic enterogastritis, pulmonary tuberculosis and neurasthenia.

Nanbao

Ingredients:

Testis et Penis Equi	Lüshen
Testis et Penis Cantis	Goushen
Radix Ginseng	Renshen
Radix Angelicae Sinensis	Danggui
Cortex Eucommiae	Duzhong
Cornu Cervi Pantotrichum	Lurong
Hippocampus	Haima
Colla Coril Asini	Ejiao
Cortex Moutan Radicis	Danpi
Radix Astragali	Huangqi
Radix Rehmanniae Preparata	Shudihuang
Poria	Fuling
Rhizoma Atractylodis Macrocephalae	Baizhu
Fructus Corni	Shanzhuyu
Herba Epimedii	Yinyanghuo
Fructus Psoraleae	Buguzhi
Fructus Lycii	Gouqizi
Semen Cuscutae	Tusizi
Radix Aconiti Lateralis Preparata	Fuzi
Radix Morindae Officinalis	Bajitian
Herba Cistanchis	Roucongrong
Fructus Rubi	Fupenzi
Semen Trigonellae	Huluba
Radix Ophiopogonis	Maimendong
Herba Cynomorii	Suoyang

Rhizoma Curculiginis	*Xianmao*
Radix Dipsaci	*Xuduan*
Radix Achysanthis Bidentatae	*Niuxi*
Radix Scrophulariae	*Xuanshen*
Radix Glycyrrhizae	*Gancao*

Actions: Reinforcing the kidney to strengthen *Yang*.

Indications: Impotence, emission, pain of the loins and legs, dampness and cold of the scrotum, listlessness and inappetence owing to deficiency of kidney—*Yang*.

Administration and Dosage: Taken orally, 2 or 3 capsules each time, twice daily, in the morning and evening respectively.

Preparation Form: Capsule.

Package: 0.3 g in each capsule.

Notes: This drug can strengthen the body, regulate the function of the adrenal cortex and promote the function of the sexual gland. It is clinically efficacious for sexual hypofunction, chronic nephritis, prostatitis, neurasthenia, gastrointestinal neurosis and hematopoietic disorders.

Sanshen Wan

Ingredients:

Testis et Penis Cervi	*Lushen*
Testis et Penis Canitis	*Goushen*
Testis et Penis Equi	*Lüshen*
Radix Astragali	*Huangqi*
Plastrum Testudinis	*Guiban*
Radix Ginseng	*Renshen*
Fructus Corni	*Shanzhuyu*
Radix Angelicae Sinensis	*Danggui*

Radix Aconiti Lateralis Preparata	*Fuzi*
Radix Rehmannine Preparata	*Shudihuang*
Herba Epimedii	*Yinyanghuo*
Poria	*Fuling*
Fructus Psoraleae	*Buguzhi*
Fructus Lycii	*Gouqizi*
Fructus Tribuli	*Shajili*
Rhizoma Atractylodis Macrocephalae	*Baizhu*
Fish bladder	*Yubiao*
Colla Corni Asini	*Ejiao*
Cortex Eucommiae	*Duzhong*
Semen Cuscutae	*Tusizi*
Cornu Cervi Pantotrichum	*Lurong*
Cortex Cinnamomi	*Rougui*

Actions: Nourishing *Yin,* invigorating *Qi* and reinforcing the kidney to strengthen *Yang.*

Indications: Impotence, pain of the loins and knees, listlessness and inappetence.

Administration and Dosage: Taken orally, 1 bolus each time, once or twice a day.

Preparation Form: Honeyed bolus.

Package: 6 g in each bolus.

Notes: This drug can sttrengthen the body, relieve mental stress and enhance sexual function and body immunity. It is clinically efficacious for sexual hypofunction, neurasthenia, various anemia, chronic nephritis, prostatitis and infertility.

Wuzi Yanzong Wan

Ingredients:

Fructus Lycii	34.8%	*Gouqizi*
Semen Cuscutae	34.8%	*Tusizi*
Fructus Rubi	17.4%	*Fupenzi*
Fructus Schisandrae	4.3%	*Wuweizi*
Semen Plantaginis	8.7%	*Cheqianzi*

Actions: Nourishing the kidney and replenishing vital essence.

Indications: Lumbago, dripping urination, emission, prospermia, and impotence with sterility due to deficiency of the kidney.

Administration and Dosage: Taken orally, 1 bolus each time, twice daily.

Preparation Form: Honeyed bolus.

Package: 9 g in each bolus.

Notes: The recipe is quoted from the book *Dan Xi Xin Fa* written by Zhu Zhenheng in the Yuan Dynasty.

With a sedative effect, this drug can promote the function of the sexual gland, induce diuresis and strengthen the body. It is clinically efficacious for sexual neurasthenia, aspermatogenesis, chronic cystitis, chronic nephritis and chronic prostatitis.

Haima Bushen Wan

Ingredients:

Hippocampus	*Dahaima*
Radix Gingseng	*Renshen*
Cornu Cervi Pantotrichum	*Lurong*

Ligamentum Cervi	Lujin
dog bone	Gougu
Os Draconis	Longgu
Fructus Lycii	Gouqizi
Radix Angelicae Sinensis	Danggui
Radix Rehmanniae Preparata	Shudihuang
Gecko	Gejie
Radix Astragali	Huangqi
Poria	Fuling
fresh prawn	Xianduixia
Fructus Corni	Shanyurou
Fructus Caryophylli	Mudingxiang
Semen Juglandis	Hetaoren

Actions: Nourishing *Yin* and the kidney, strengthening the loins and building up the brain.

Indications: Dizziness, tinnitus, soreness and pain in the waist and knees, weakness, palpitation, dyspnea and nocturnal emission owing to deficiency of *Qi*, blood and kidney.

Administration and Dosage: Taken orally, 10 pills each time, twice daily.

Preparation Form: Concentrated pill.

Package: 120 pills in each bottle.

Notes: This drug can promote metabolism and reinforce body resistance. It is clinically efficacious for neurasthenia, rheumatic arthritis, chronic nephritis, chronic bronchitis and sexual neurasthenia.

Chufeng Jing

Main Ingredients:

chicken embryo	*Jipei*
Testis et Penis Canitis	*Goubian*
Male sheep externalia	*Yangbian*
sheep testicle	*Yangwaishen*
Radix Ginseng	*Rensen*
Cornu Cervi Pantotrichum	*Lurong*
Rhizoma Dioscoreae	*Shanyao*
Cortex Eucommiae	*Duzhong*
Fructus Lycii	*Gouqizi*
Radix Rehmanniae Preparata	*Shudihuang*
Fructus Amomi	*Sharen*
Cortex Cinnamomi	*Rougui*
Lignum Aquilariae Resinatum	*Chenxiang*
Fructus Psoraleae	*Buguzhi*
Fructus Rubi	*Fupenzi*
Radix Angelicae Sinensis	*Danggui*

Actions: Warming the kidney, strengthening *Yang*, invigorating *Qi* and nourishing blood.

Indications: Soreness of the waist and pain in the back, dizziness, tinnitus, amnesia, insomnia and palpitation owing to deficiency of both *Qi* and blood; emission, cold of the uterus and abnormal menstruation owing to deficiency of the kidney.

Administration and Dosage: Taken orally, 10 ml each time, twice daily.

Preparation Form: Oral liquid.

Package: 10 ml in each bottle.

Notes: This drug can strengthen the body, promote blood circulation and activate metabolism. It is clinically efficacious for all types of anemia, abnormal menstruation, functional uterine bleeding, infertitlity, neurasthenia, chronic nephritis, chronic gastroenteritis, sexual neurasthenia, neurosis and menopausal syndrome.

Bushenning Pian

Ingredients:

Testis Ovis seu Caprae   *Yangwaishen*

Radix Ginseng   *Renshen*

Actions: Warming the kidney to strengthen *Yang*, in vigorating *Qi* to increase body resistance.

Indications: Impotence, emission, lassitude of the loins and knees, and amnesia; cold of uterus, leukorrhea and metrorrhagia in women; all of which are owing to deficiency of kidncy−*Yang*.

Administration and Dosage: Taken orally, 3−5 tablets each time, 3 times daily.

Preparation Form: Tablet.

Package: 0.2 g in each tablet.

Notes: This drug can regulate the function of the adrenal cortex and promote the function of the sexual gland. It is clinically efficacious for sexual neurasthenia, prostatitis, chronic nephritis, and menopausal syndrome.

Erxian Gao

Main Ingredients:

Radix Ginseng   *Rehshen*

Colla Cornus Cervi   *Lujiaojiao*

Cornu Cervi Pantotrichum   *Lurong*

Actions: Noruishing *Yin*, strengthening *Yang*, reinforcing *Qi* and enriching blood.

Indications: Listlessness, weakness, impotence, emission, palpitation, dyspnea and lassitude of the loins and knees owing to deficiency of both *Qi* and blood.

Administration and Dosage: Taken orally, 20 g each time, twice daily.

Preparation Form: Soft extract.

Package: 250 g in each bottle.

Notes: This drug can improve the function of the brain, promote the function of the sexual gland and reinforce body resistance. It is clinically efficacious for sexual neurasthenia, chronic nephritis, prostatitis, all types of anemia and puerperal asthenia.

Suoyang Gujing Wan

Ingredients:

Herba Cynmorii	3.8%	*Suoyang*
Herba Cistanchis	4.7%	*Roucongrong*
Radix Morindae Officinalis	5.7%	*Bajitian*
Fructus Psoraleae	4.7%	*Buguzhi*
Semen Cuscutae	3.8%	*Tusizi*
Cortex Eucommiae	4.7%	*Duzhong*
Fructus Anisi Stellati	4.7%	*Dahuixiang*
Semen Allii Tuberosi	3.8%	*Jiucaizi*
Semen Euryales	3.8%	*Qianshi*
Semen Nelumbinis	3.8%	*Lianzi*
Stamen Nelumbinis	4.7%	*Lianxu*
Concha Ostreae	3.8%	*Muli*
Os Draconis	3.8%	*Longgu*
Cornu Cervi Degelatinatum	3.8%	*Lujiaoshuang*

Radix Rehmanniae Preparata	10.6%	*Shudihuang*
Fructus Corni	3.2%	*Shanzhuyu*
Cortex Moutan	2.1%	*Mudanpi*
Rhizoma Dioscoreae	10.6%	*Shanyao*
Poria	2.1%	*Fuling*
Rhizoma Alismatis	2.1%	*Zexie*
Rhizoma Anemarrhenae	0.7%	*Zhimu*
Cortex Phellodendri	0.7%	*Huangbai*
Radix Achyranthis Bidentatae	3.8%	*Niuxi*
Halitum	4.5%	*Daqingyan*

Actions: Warming the kidney to control nocturnal emission.

Indications: Spermatorrhea, lassitude of the loins and knees, vertigo, tinnitus and myasthenia of limbs owing to deficiency of the kidney.

Administration and Dosage: Taken orally, 1 bolus each time, twice daily.

Preparation Form: Honeyed bolus.

Package: 9 g in each bolus.

Notes: This drug can regulate the function of the adrenal cortex and promote metabolism. It is clinically efficacious for sexual neurasthenia, chronic nephritis, neurosis, and chronic gastroenteristis.

Bushen Qiangshen Pian

Ingredients:

Herba Epimedii	29.4%	*Yinyanhuo*
Semen Cuscutae	17.6%	*Tusizi*
Fructus Rosae Laevigatae	17.6%	*Jinyingzi*
Rhizoma Cibotii	17.7%	*Gouji*

Fructus Ligustri Lucidi   17.7%   *Nüzhenzi*

Actions: Noruishing the kidney to strengthen the body.

Indications: Soreness of the waist, weakness of the feet, dizziness, tinnitus, dim eyesight, palpitation, impotence and emission.

Administration and Dosage: Taken orally. 3 tablets each time, 3 times daily.

Preparation Form: Tablet.

Package: About 0.25 in each tablet.

Notes: This drug can promote the function of the sexual gland and produce a tranquilizing effect. It is clinically efficacious for neurasthenia, chronic nephritis, sexual hypofunction, chronic bronchitis and neurosis.

Lujiaojiao

Ingredient:

Cornu Cervi   100%   *Lujiao*

Actions: Warming the kidney, strengthening *Yang*, and supplementing vital essence and enriching marrow.

Indications: Impotence, coldness of the uterus, metrorrhagia, metrostaxis and leukorrhea owing to deficiency of the kidney.

Administration and Dosage: Taken orally, 3—6 g each time, once or twice daily.

Preparation Form: Gelatin.

Package: About 4.5 g in each cube.

Notes: This drug can promote growth and development, and improve hematopoiesis. It is clinically efficacious for sexaul neurasthenia, dysplasia of children, all types of anemia, rheumatic heart disease and functional uterine bleeding.

Hailongjiao

Ingredients:

Syngnathus	53.3%	Hailong
Gelatin	40.0%	Huangmingjiao
Radix Angelicae Sinensis	0.8%	Danggui
Rhizoma Chuanxiong	0.5%	Chuanxiong
Herba Cistanchis	0.5%	Roucongrong
Radix Astragali	0.5%	Huangqi
Radix Paeoniae Alba	0.3%	Baishao
Cortex Cinnamomi	0.8%	Rougui
Fructus Lycii	0.3%	Gouqizi
Pericarpium Citri Reticulatae	0.3%	Chenpi
Radix Glycyrrhizae	2.7%	Gancao

Actions: Warming the kidney, nourishing blood, supplementing vital essence and enriching marrow.

Indications: Impotence, dysmenorrhea due to deficiency of blood, lassitude of the loins and knees, dizziness and tinnitus.

Administration and Dosage: 6—9 g is mected in hot water and taken orally, once or twice daily.

Preparation Form: Gelatin.

Package: 15 g in each cube.

Notes: This drug can strengthen the body. It is clinically efficacious for sexual neurasthenia, irregular menstruation, menopausal syndrome and all types of anemia.

18 Other Drugs

Huoxiang Zhengqi Shui

Ingredients:

Rhizoma Atractylodis	11.6%	Cangzhu
Pericarpium Cirti Reticulatae	11.6%	Chenpi
Cortex Magnoliae Officinalis	11.6%	Houpo
Radix Angelicae Dahuricae	17.4%	Baizhi
Poria	17.4%	Fuling
Pericarpium Pinelliae	17.4%	Dafupi
Rhizoma Pinelliae	11.6%	Shengbanxia
Extractum Glycyrrhizea	1.2%	Gancaojingao
Oleum Pogostemonis	0.1%	Guanghuoxiangyou
Oleum Perillae Folium	0.1%	Zisuyeyou

Actions: Dispelling pathogenic factors from the exterior of the body, resolving dampness, activating the flow of Qi and regulating the middle—Jiao.

Indications: Headache, dizziness, distending pain in the epigastric region, vomiting and diarrhea due to affection of exogenous wind—cold and accumulation of endogenous dampness.

Administration and Dosage: Shaked evenly and taken orally. 5—10 ml each time, twice a day.

Preparation Form: Tincture

Package: 10 ml in each bottle.

Notes: The prescription was recorded in the book *Tai Ping Hui Min He Ji Ju Fang* compiled by Chen Shiwen in the Song Dynasty.

This drug can clear away heat, strengthen the stomach and arrest vomiting. It is clinically efficacious for dizziness, vomiting, abdominal pain and diarrhea owing to summer—heat, influenza of gastrointestinal type, and acute gastroenteritis.

Qushu Wan

Ingredients:

Herba Agastachis	18.8%	*Huoxiang*
Folium Perillae	18.8%	*Zisuye*
Herba Elasholtziae	7.5%	*Xiangru*
Fructus Chaenomelis	5.8%	*Mugua*
Poria	29.3%	*Fuling*
Lignum Santali Albi	2.8%	*Tanxiang*
Flos Caryophylli	2.8%	*Dingxiang*
Radix Glycyrrhizae	14.2%	*Gancao*

Actions: Eliminating summer—heat, removing dampness, regulating the stomach and arresting diarrhea.

Indications: Affection of summer—heat marked by chills, fever, headache, fatigue, abdominal distention, vomiting and diarrhea.

Administration and Dosage: Taken orally. 1 bolus each time, once or twice daily.

Preparation Form: Honeyed bolus.

Package: 9 g in each bolus.

Notes: The prescription is quoted from the book *Tai Ping Hui Min He Ji Ju Fang* compiled by Chen Shiwen in the Song

Dynasty.

This drug can reduce fever, strengthen the stomach, tranquilize the mind, and arrest diarrhea. It is clinically efficacious for common cold owing to summer—heat, and acute gastroenteritis.

Qingshu Yiqi Wan

Ingredients:

Radix Astragali	9.6%	Huangqi
Rhizoma Atractylodis	9.6%	Cangzhu
Cortex Phellodendri	2.9%	Huangbai
Pericarpium Citri Reticulatae Viride	3.8%	Qingpi
Radix Angelicae Sinensis	5.8%	Danggui
Radix Codonopsis Pilosulae	9.6%	Dangshen
Radix Ophiopogonis	5.8%	Maimendong
Rhizoma Atrachylodis Macrocephalae	11.5%	Baizhu
Massa Fermentata Medicinalis	9.6%	Liushenqu
Pericarpium Crtri Reticulatae	9.6%	Jupi
Radix Puerariae	3.9%	Gegen
Rhizoma Alismatis	9.6%	Zexie
Fructus Schisandrae	2.9%	Wuweizi
Radix Glycyrrhizae	3.9%	Gancao
Rhizoma Cimicifugae	1.9%	Shengma

Actions: Eliminating summer—heat, removing dampness, supplementing *Qi* and promoting the production of body fluid.

Indications: Headache, fever, lassitude of limbs, thirst, vexation, spontaneous perspiration, and deep—colored urine owing to general weakness and affection of summer—evils.

Administration and Dosage: Taken orally, 1 bolus or 2 each time, twice daily.

Preparation Form: Honeyed bolus.

Package: 9 g in each bolus.

Notes: The prescription was recorded in the book *Pi Wei Lun* written by Li Gao in the Jin Dynasty.

This drug can reinforce the body immunity, eliminate heat and relieve pain. It is clinically suitable for weak cases with fever, dry throat, headache and difficulty in micturition caused by summer—heat.

Liuyi San

Ingredients:

Pulvis Talci	85.7%	*Huashifen*
Radix Glycyrrhizae	14.3%	*Gancao*

Actions: Clearing away summer—heat and dispelling dampness.

Indications: Fatigue, thirst, diarrhea, and scanty and dark urine caused by summer—heat. This drug is used externally in treating prickly heat with itching.

Administration and Dosage: Mixed with boiled water or wrapped and decocted in water for the decoction which is taken orally, 6—9 g each time, once or twice a day. Or, applied directly to the affected part.

Preparation Form: Powder.

Package: 18 g in each bag.

Notes: The prescription was recorded in the book *Shang Han Biao Ben* wirtten by Liu Hejian in the Jin Dynasty.

This durg can diminish inflammation, induce diuresis and eliminate heat. It is clinically efficacious for influenza of gastro—intestinal type in summer, acute nephritis, and acute cystitis.

Shayao

Main Ingredients:

Flos Caryophylli	*Dingxiang*
Rhizoma Atractylodis	*Cangzhu*
Rhizoma Gastrodiae	*Tianma*
Herba Ephedrae	*Mahuang*
Radix et Rhizoma Rhei	*Dahuang*
Radix Glycyrrhizae	*Gancao*
Borneloum Syntheticum	*Bingpian*
Venenum Sufonis	*Chansu*
Realgar	*Xionghuang*
Cinnabaris	*Zhusha*

Actions: Eliminating summer—heat, removing toxic materials, clearing away pestilence and inducing resuscitation.

Indications: Sudden fidgetiness, abdominal pain, vomiting, diarrhea, trismus and clammy limbs, all owing to excessive intake of cold drinks in summer.

Administration and Dosage: Taken orally, 5—10 pills each time, once daily; or, ground into fine powder for nasal insufflation to induce sneeze.

Preparation Forms: Powder or water—paste pill.

Package: 1 g in every 33 pills.

Notes: The recipe was recorded in the book *Ji Shi Yang Sheng Ji*.

This drug can induce perspiration and exert a tonic effect on the heart. It also has antibiotic and anti—inflammatory effects. It is clinically efficacious for acute gastroenteritis and food poisoning in summer.

It is contraindicated for pregnant women.

Shuzheng Pian

Ingredients:

Fructus Gleditsiae Abnormalis	10.3%	Zhuyazao
Herba Asari	10.3%	Xixin
Herba Menthae	8.8%	Bohe
Herba Pogostemonis	8.9%	Guanghuoxing
Radix Angelicae Dahuricae	2.9%	Baizhi
Radix Ledebouriellae	5.9%	Fangfeng
Pericarpium Citri Reticulatae	5.9%	Chenpi
Radix Platycodi	5.9%	Jiegeng
Alumen	2.9%	Baifan
Radix Aucklandiae	5.9%	Muxiang
Cinnabaris	7.3%	Zhusha
Realgar	7.3%	Xionghuang
Rhizoma Dryopteris Crassirhizomae	5.9%	Guanzhong
Rhizoma Pinelliae	5.9%	Banxia
Radix Glycyrrhizae	5.9%	Gancao

Actions: Clearing away summer—heat, inducing resuscitation, eliminating pestilence, and removing toxic material.

Indications: Faint, trismus, abdominal pain, vomiting, diarrhea, and numbness of the etremities owing to heliosis.

Administration and Dosage: Taken orally. 2 tablets each

time, 2 or 3 times daily.

Preparation Form: Tablet.

Package: 0.8 g in each tablet.

Notes: This drug can eliminate heat, exert a tonic effect on the heart, strengthen the stomach and arrest vomiting. It is clinically efficacious for shock due to summer−heat, and acute gastroenteritis.

Shushi Zhengqi Wan

Main Ingredients:

Herba Pogostemonis	*Guanghuoxiang*
Rhizoma Pinelliae	*Banxia*
Radix Aristolochiae	*Qingmuxiang*
Pericarpium Citri Reticulatae	*Chenpi*
Flos Caryophylli	*Dingxiang*
Cortex Cinnamoni	*Rougui*
Rhizoma Atractylodis	*Cangzhu*
Rhizoma Atractylodis Macrocephalae	*Baizhu*
Poria	*Fuling*
Cinnabaris	*Zhusha*
Nitre	*Xiaoshi*
Borax	*Pengsha*
Realgar	*Xionghuang*
Lapis Micae Aureus	*Jinmengshi*
Borneolum Syntheticum	*Bingpian*

Actions: Eliminating summer−heat, dispelling cold, alleviating pain and arresting diarrhea.

Indications: Abdominal pain, vomiting, diarrhea, headache,

chills, and soreness and heaviness of the limbs owing to affection of cold in summer.

Administration and Dosage: Taken orally, 1.5—3 g each time once or twice daily.

Preparation Form: Water—paste pill.

Package: 3 g in each bottle (200 pills).

Notes: With tranquilizing effect, this drug can eliminate heat, strengthen the stomach, and arrest vomiting. It is clinically efficacious for acute gastroenteritis, food poisoning and dyspepsia.

Yiyuan San

Ingredients:

Talcum	82.2%	Huashi
Radix Glycyrrhizae	13.7%	Gancao
Cinnabaris	4.1%	Zhusha

Actions: Eliminating summer—heat, dispelling dampness, and relieving mental stress.

Indications: Fatigue, vexation, thirst and scanty·dark urine owing to heliosis.

Administration and Dosage: 3—6 g of the drug is wrapped and decocted in water for the decoction, which is taken orally, and this is done once or twice daily.

Preparation Form: Powder.

Package: 30 g in each bag.

Notes: The prescription was recorded in the book *He Jian Liu Shu* written by Liu Hejian in the Jin Dynasty.

This drug can induce diuresis and has antiphlogistic and tranquilizing effects. It is clinically efficacious for urinarry infection, stomatitis, and acute gastroenteritis.

Xingjun San

Main Ingredients:

Margarita	*Zhenzhu*
Calcilus Bovis man—made	*Rengongniuhuang*
Borneloum Syntheticum	*Bingpian*
Nitre	*Xiaoshi*
Borax	*Pengsha*
Pulvis Zingiberis	*Jiangfen*
Realgar	*Xionghuang*

Actions: Eliminating pestilence, removing toxic material, and inducing resuscitation.

Indications: Dizziness, abdominal pain, vomiting, and diarrhea owing to heliosis.

Administration and Dosage: Taken orally, 0.3—0.9 g each time, once or twice a day.

Preparation Form: Powder.

Package: 0.9 g in each bag.

Notes: This drug can eliminate heat and has antibacterial and antiphlogistic effects. It is clinically efficacious for common cold accompanied by gastrointestinal tract symptoms and acute gastroenteritis caused by heliosis.

It is contraindicated for pregnant women.

RenDan

Main Ingredients:

Mentholum	*Bohenao*
Semen Alpininae Katsumadai	*Caodoukou*
Borneolum Syntheticum	*Bingpian*

Rhizoma Zingiberis	Ganjiang
Cortex Cinnamomi	Rougui
Flos Caryophylli	Dingxiang
Radix Aucklandiae	Muxiang
Radix Glycyrrhizae	Gancao

Actions: Expelling wind, invigorating *Qi*, promoting the production of the body fluid, and strengthening the stomach.

Indications: Motion sickness and indigestion caused by megathermal climate.

Administration and Dosage: Taken orally or sucked, 4—8 pills each time.

Preparation Form: Water—paste pill.

Package: 3 g in every 75 pills.

Notes: This drug has the effects of reducing fever, strengthening the stomach, arresting vomiting and promoting digestion. It is clinically efficacious for headache, dizziness and dyspepsia due to heliosis.

This drug is not allowed to be taken along with postassium bromide, sodium bromide or sodium iodide simultaneously.

Qingliang Dan

Ingredients:

Mentholum	Bohenao
Oleum Menthae	Boheyou
Camphora	Zhangnao
Semen Myristicae	Roudoukou
Rhizoma Zingiberis Recens	Shengjiang
Flos Caryophylli	Dingxiang
Catechu	Ercha

Radix Glycyrrhizae	Gancao
Cortex Cinnamoni	Roukou
Fructus Piperis Nigri	Hujiao
Borneolum Syntheticum	Bingpian

Actions: Expelling wind, strengthening the stomach, cooling the throat and quenching thirst.

Indications: Dizziness, dry throat, burning sensation of the tongue, motion sickness and discomfort caused by summer—heat.

Administration and Dosage: To be sucked. 1 small square or 2 each time.

Preparation Form: Piece.

Package: 5 g in each piece which is subdived into 25 smaller ones.

Notes: This drug can eliminate heat, and strengthen the stomach. it is clinically efficacious for dry mouth, dizziness and dyspepsia.

Qingliang You

Ingredients:

Mentholum	Bohenao
Camphora	Zhangnao
Oleum Menthae	Boheyou
Oleum Eucalyptus	Anyeyou
Oleum Camphorae	Zhangnaoyou
Oleum Cortex Cinnamomi	Guipiyou
Oleum Flos Caryophylli	Dingxiangyou

Actions: It is a local stimulant and has a cooling effect.

Indication: Headache, skin pruritus, mosequito and insect bites, and mild burn, etc.

Administration and Dosage: Applied to the point *Taiyan,* or directly to the affected part.

Preparation Form: Ointment.

Package: 3 g in each bottle.

Notes: This drug has antiphlogistic, analgesic and antipruritic effects. It is clinically efficacious for headache caused by common cold, and mosequito and insect bites.

Fengyoujing

Main Ingredients:

Oleum Menthae	*Boheyou*
Oleum Eucalyptus	*Anyeyou*
Camphora	*Zhangnao*
Oleum Flos Caryophylli	*Dingxiangyou*
Essential oil	*Xiangjingyou*
Chlorophyll	*Yelusu*

Actions: It is a local stimulant and has a cooling effect.

Indications: Headache, dizziness and toothache due to common cold, and mosequito and insect bites.

Administration and Dosage: Applied to the affected part, or taken orally 4—6 drops each time.

Preparation Form: Liquid.

Package: 10 ml in each bottle.

Notes: With local antiphlogistic, analgesic and antipruritic effects, this drug can expell pathogenic wind. It is clinically efficacious for headache caused by common cold and dermatosis caused by mosequito and insect bites.

Shidi Shui

Ingredients:

Camphorae Pulvis	*Zhangnaofen*
Cortex Cinnamomi	*Guipi*
Radix et Rhizoma Rhei	*Daihuang*
Rhizoma Zingiberis	*Ganjiang*
Fructus Capsici	*Lajiao*
Fructus Anisi	*Dahuixiang*
Oleum Eucalyptus	*Anyeyou*

Action: Eliminating Summer—heat.

Indications: Dizziness, nausea, abdominal pain and gastrointestinal discomfort owing to heliosis.

Administration and Dosage: Taken orally, 0.5—1.0 ml each time.

Preparation Form: Tincture.

Package: 10 ml in each bottle.

Notes: This drug has the effects of tranquilizing the mind, relieving pain, strengthening the stomach and arrsting vomiting. It is clinically efficacious for dizziness, vomiting, abdominal pain and dyspepsia caused by heliosis.

Bingshuang Meisu Wan

Ingredients:

Herba Menthae	*Bohe*
Folium Perillae	*Zisuye*
Fructus Mume	*Wumei*
Radix Puerariae	*Gegen*
White Sugar	*Baitang*

Actions: Eliminating summer—heat, promoting the production of body fluid, and quenching thirst.

Indications: Thirst, dry throat, fullness in the chest and dizziness due to affection of summer—heat.

Administration and Dosage: Sucked, 1 or 2 pills each time several times daily.

Preparation Form: Water—paste pill.

Package: 30 g in each bag.

Notes: The recipe was recorded in the book *Tang Tou Ge Jue* written by Wang Ang in the Qing Dynasty.

This drug can dispel pathogenic factors from the exterior of the body, invigorate the function of the stomach and arrest vomiting. It is clinically efficacious for thirst and dyspepsia caused by heliosis.

Feizi Fen

Ingredients:

Pulvis Talci	*Huashifen*
Borneolum Syntheticum	*Bingpian*

Actions: Refreshing the body, removing dampness, and relieving itching.

Indications: Prickly heat with itching in summer.

Administration and Dosage: Applied to the affected part, 4—6 times daily.

Preparation Form: Powder.

Package: 100 g in each box.

Notes: This drug produces a local anti—inflammatory effect and is clinically efficacious for hidradenitis in summer.

Appendix 1

Index of Chinese Herbal Formulae by TCM Division

Department of Internal Medicine

Phlegm Syndrome due to Wind

Renshen Zaizao Wan

Dahuoluo Wan

Xiaohuo luo Wan

Wanshi Niuhuang Qingxin Wan

Niuhuang Zhibao Dan

Niuhuang Jiangya Pian

Mugua Wan

Xinkeshu Pian

Tianma Wan

Fengshi Zhitong Gao

Wujiapi Yaojiu

Fengshi Yaojiu

Baijin Wan

Fengliaoxing Yaojiu

Zaizao Wan

Yangxianfeng Wan

Shangshi Baozhen Gao

Shangshi Qutong Gao

Honghua Zhusheye

Shangshi Zhitong Gao

Jiufang Niuhuang Qingxin Wan

Yixian Wan

Subing Diwan

Shenjindan Jiaonang

Duzhong Jiangya Pian

Jixueteng Jingao Pian

Kanlisha

Huanxin Dan

Luobuma Jiangya Pian

Jiangyaping Pian

Jiangzhiling Jiaowan

Jinbuhuan Gaoyao

Goupi Gao

Guogong Jiu

Wuli Bahan San

Guci Wan

Duhuo Jisheng Wan

Huoxin Wan

Guanxin Suhe Wan

Qufeng Shujin Wan

Fufang Danshen Pian

Fufang Luobuma Pian

Mailuotong Pian

Guanxin Tongmailing Pian

Guci Xiaotong Ye

Fufang Danshen Zhusheye

Fufang Danggui Zhusheye

Maian Chonji

Xiaoshuan Zaizao Wan

Naoliqing Wan

Yixin Wan

Suxiao Jiuxin Wan

Xiaoluotong Pian

Xiaoshuan Tongluo Pian

Shuxin Jiangya Pian

Shujin Huoluo Jiu

Yuxin Ningxin Pian

Jiexintong Pian

Xijian Wan

Zhenjiang Gaoyao

Baoxin Wan

Invigoration

Shiquan Dabu Wan

Qibao Meiran Wan

Bazhen Wan

Renshen Guipi Wan

Renshen Yangrong Wan

Renshen Jianpi Wan

Erxian Gao

Renshen Jing

Renshen FengWang Jing

Sanshen Pian

Dabuyin Wan

Shandong Ejiao Gao

Wufa Wan

Liuwei Dihuang Wan

Liujunzi Wan

Shuangbao Su

Wangjiang Pian

Wuweizi Chongji

Wujiashen Chongji

Shengfa Wan

Yuquan Wan

Yuping Feng Wan

Sijunzi Wan

Shengmaiyin Koufuye

Zhibao Saibianwa

Zhusha Anshen Wan

Quanlu Wan

Danggui Buxue Jing

Danggui Yangxue Pian

Huanshao Dan

Buzhong Yiqi Wan

Nanbao

Guilingji

Bushen Qiangli Wan

Lingzhi Pian

E'jiao

Jingui Shengqi Wan

Qing'e Wan

Zhengzhong Dan

Shenling Baizhu Wan

Qingchunbao

Shenqi Chongji

Baizi Yangxin Wan

Guzhi Zengsheng Wan

Shouwu Wan

Guxian Pian

Gu ci Pian

Jiannao Wan

Jiannao Bushen Wan

Xiaoke Wan

Naolingsu Pian

Hailong Jiao

Hailong Gajie Jing

Huangmingjiao

Lujiaojiao

Kangbao Koufuye

Suoyang Gujing Wan

Yaotong Wan

Xin Ejiao

Chufengjiang

Productive Cough Division

Ermu Ningsou Wan

Erchen Wan

Erdong Gao

Chuanbei Zhike Tangjiang

Xiaoqinglong Heji

Xiaobanxia Heji

Zhisou Qingguo Wan

Zhisou Dingchuan Wan

Zhikechuan Reshen Pian

Chuanbei Pipa Zhike Chongji

Banxia Lu

Aiyeyou Qiwuji

Baihe Gujin Wan

Baihua Dingchuan Wan

Suzi Jiangqi Wan

Xingren Zhike Tangjiang

Mujingyou JiaoWan

Yunxiangyou Diwan

Dingchuan Wan

Zhigancao Heji

Luohanguo Chongji

Yangyin Qingfei Gao

Fuling Wan

Fufang Chuanbeijing Pian

Fufang Baibu Zhike
 Tangjiang

Tongxuan Lifei Wan

Xiaokechuan Tangjiang

Taohua San

Runfei Bugao

Laiyangli Zhike Tangjiang

Qingfei Yihuo Wan

Maxing Zhike Tangjiang

Qingqi Huatan Wan

Kongxian Wan

Shedan Chuanbei Me

Shedan Chenpi Me

Gejie Dingchuan Wan

Zhihua Dujuan Pian

Chuanshu Pian

Tanchuan Wan

Tanke Jing

Xianzhuli Koufuye

Juhong Wan

Mengshi Guntan Wan

Stagnation of Qi and Accumulation

Jiuqi Niantong Wan

Yuanhu Zhitong Pian

Kaixiong Shunqi Wan

Muxiang Shunqi Wan

Muxiang Binlang Wan

Pingwei Wan

Dutong Wan

Chenxiang Huaqi Wan

Chenxiang Huazhi Wan

Liangfu Wan

Xiangsha Liujun Wan

Xiangsha Zhizhu Wan

Langji Wan

Fuganning Pian

Xiaoyao Wan

Yiganling Pian

Jiangan Pian

Shugan Wan

Shugan Hewei Wan

Yueju Wan

Epidemic and Pestilence

Jiuwei Qianghuo Wan

Wanshi Niuhuang Qingxin

Chuanxiong Chatiao Wan

Xiaoqinglong Heji
Niuhuang Qingnao Pian
Angong Niuhuang Wan
Fangfeng Tongsheng Wan
Fanggan Pian
Jufang Zhi bao Dan
Fufang Chaihu Zhusheye
Sangju Ganmao Pain
Yingqiao Jiedu Wan
Lingqiao Jiedu Wan

Yinhuang Pian
Qingwen Jiedu Wan
Yingqiao Jiedu Pian
Xiling Ganmao Pian
Xiling Jiedu Pian
Zixue Dan
Saixianyan Pian
Ganmao Chongji
Ganmao Qingre Chongji

Summer—heat and Dampness

Shizao Shui
Shidi Wan
Bazheng Heji
Sanjin Pian
Sanren Heji
Rendan
Fenqing Zhenglin Wan
Wuling San
Liiuyi San
Yushu Dan
Fengyoujing
Shilintong Pian
Zhouche Wan
Bingshuang Meisu Pian
Xingjunsan
Lidan Pian

Lidan Paishi Pian
Shenyan Siwei Wan
Jieyinhua Lu
Qushu Wan
Yenchen Wuling Wan
Xiaoyan Lidan Pian
Yiyuan San
Qingshu Yiqi Wan
Qingliangyou
Qingliang Dan
Paishi Chongji
Shushi Zhengqi Wan
Shayao
Shuzheng Pian
Feizi Fen
Huoxiang Zhengqi Shui

Dryness—heat

Qianliguang Pian

Niuhuang Shangqing Wan

Niuhuang Jiedu Wan

Niuhuang Xiaoyan Wan

Wurenchun Jiaonang

Yunzhi Gantai Chongji

Zuojin Wan

Longdan Xiegan Wan

Wuji Wan

Sijiqing Pian

Liangqiao Baidu Wan

Jigucao Wan

Kangjun Xiaoyan Pian

YandePing Jiaonang

Banlangen Ganfenjiang

Fufang Daqingye Zhusheye

Fuganning Pian

Zhgizi Jinhua Wan

Yiganling Pian

Yinhuang Pian

Huangqinsulu Jiaonang

Qingning Wan

Huanglian Shangqing Wan

Qingnao Wan

Shugan Hewei Wan

Xiling Jiedu Pian

Blood Malarial Disease Divisio

Shihui San

Sanqi Pian

Huazheng Huisheng Wan

Heye Wan

Spleen and Stomach Division

Dashanzha Wan

Xiaojianzhong Heji

Wuren Runchang Wan

Sishen Wan

Sixao Wan

Anwei Pian

Fuzi Lizhong Wan

Zhishi Daozhi Wan

Baohe Wan

Maren Wan

Qingning Wan

Qingwei Baoan Pian

Qianggan Wan

Binglang Sixiao Wan

Purgative Dysentery Division

Xianglian Wan

Xiaoyan Kangjun Wan

Libiling Pian

Department of Surgery

Skin and Exernlal Disease Divisison

Yilizhu

XiaojinDan

Neixiao Luoli Pian

Huazhiling Pian

Niuhuang xiaoyan Pian

Fengshi Zhitong Gao

Yanghe Wan

Ruyi Jinhuang San

Yanghe Jiening Gao

Shenyang Hongyao

Dongchuang Shui

Badu Gao

Zhizi Jinhua Wan

Jingfang Baidu Wan

Gongjing'ai Pian

Zanglian Wan

Haizao Wan

Taohua San

Xiakucao Gao

HeKui Zhusheye

Xioaozhiling Pian

Meihua Dianshe Dian

E'zhang Feng Yaoshui

Zigui Zhilie Gao

Hougujun Pian

Lanwei Xiaoyan Pian

Xihuang Wan

Huaijiao Wan

Xinhuang Pian

Biejiajian Wan

Xingxiao Wan

Chansu Wan

Trauma

Yili Zhitong Dan

Qili San

Sanqi Shanyao Pian

Jufeng San

Wanying San

Pianzi huang

Wuhu San

Yunnan Sheyao

Yunnan Beiya

Zhonghua Dieda Wan

Zhenggu Shui

Jingwanhong Tangshang
 Yaogao

Jidesheng Sheyao Pian

Guzhe Cuoshang San

Shaoshang Qiwuji

Jiegu San

Dieda Yaojing

Zicao Gao

Dieda Huoxue San

Dieda Sunshang Wan

Dieda Wan

Huanyou

Department of Gynecoiogy

Gynecopathy

Bazhen Yimu Wan

Qizhe Xiangfu Wan

Daihuang Zhechong Wan

Niujin Dan

Qianjin Zhidai Wan

Shaofu Zhuyu Wan

Wuji Baifeng Wan

Aifu Nuangong Wan

Baidai Wan

Danggui Buxue Jing

Danggui Yangxue Wan

Dangui Jingao Wan

Xuefu Zhuyu Wan

Euke Shiwei Pian

Fuke Wulin Wan

Fuke Tongjing Wan

Fuke Tiaojing Pian

Kunshun Wan

Gujing Wan

Tinji Chongji

Yimu Wan

Tiaojing Zhibao Wan

Yimucao Gao

Lutai Gao

Tongjing Wan

Wenjing Wan

Prefetal Division

Antai Wan

Baotai Wan

Lutai Gan

Postpartum Division

Xiaru Tongquan San

Shenghuatang Wan

Shixiao San

Chanhou Shentong Pian

Yimucao Gao

Yimu Wan

Department of Pediatrics

Infantile Conrulsion Division

Qizhen Dan

Xiaoer Qiying wan

Xiaoer Jingfeng Wan

Xiaoer Niuhuang Qingxin San

Niuhuang Zhibao Dan

Niuhuang Zhenjing Wan

Niuhuang Baolong Pian

Wuli Huichun Dan

Baoying Zhenjing Wan

Yingeran Pian

Infantile Malnutrition

Xiaoer Jianpi Wan

Xiaoer Xiaoji Wan

Xiaoer Qiying Wan

Xiaoer Xiaoshi Pia

Wumei Wan

Wumei Anwei Wan

Feier Wan

Baochi Wan

Xiangju Wan

Xiangsu Zhengwei Wan

Yinger San

Other Division of Pediatrics

Xiaoer Zhisou Wan

Xiaoer Zhibao Wan

Wanying Ding

Xiaoer Zhike Tangjiang

Xiaoer Ganyan Chongji

Xiaoer Tuire Chongji

Xiaoer Jiere Shuan

Xiaoer Shengxueling

Xiaoer Zhixie Pian

Wuli Huichun Dan

Wufu Huadu Dan

Epidemic Cerebrospinal Meningitis

Angong NiuHuang Wan

Jufang Zhibao Dan

Zixue Dan

Fufang Daqing Ye Zhusheye

Banlan Gen Gantangjiang

Zcterohepatitis

Yunzhi Gantai Chongji

Longdan Xiegan Wan

Jiangan Pian

Lingzhi Tangjiang

Yinchen Yuling Wan

Fugan Ning Pian

Wuling San

Chronic Hepatitis

Yueju Wan

Muxiang Shunqi Wan

Kaixiong Shunqi Wan

Liangfu Wan

Shugan Wan

Xiaoyao Wan

Shugan Hewei Wan

Jigu Cao Wan

Wuren Chun Jiaonang

Jiangan Pian

Yigan Ling Pian

Shixiao San

Xiangsha Yangwei Wan

Jiuqi Niantong Wan

Chenxiang Huazhi Wan

Huangqi Jianzhong Wan

Xiaojian Zhong Heji

Buzhong Yiqi Wan

Shenqi Chongji

Qili San

Naoling Su Pian

Bacillary Dysentery

Libi Ling

Xianglian Wan

Huangqin Sulu Jiaonang

Gegen Qinlian Pian

Muxiang Binlang Wan

Zhishi Daozhi Wan

Zuojin Wan

Wuji Wan

Fuzi Lizhong Wan

Yinhuang Pian

Qianli Guang Pian

Yande Ping Jiaonang

Roundworm Diseases

Wumei Wan

Wumei Anwei Wan

Chuanlian Su Pian

Quchong Pian

Shijunzi Wan

Huachong Wan

Pharyngolaryngitis

Liushen Wan

Houzheng Wan

Shuangliao Houfeng San

Niuhuang Yijin Pian

Meihua Dianshe Dan

Bingpeng San

Niuhuang Xiaoyan Wan

Qingyin Wan

Yande Ping Jiaonang

Baihe Gujin Wan

Niuhuang Jiedu Pian

Zhizi Jinhua Wan

Huanglian Shangqing Wan

Chuanbei Pipa Zhike Chongji

Xingren Zhike Tangjiang

Erdong Gao

Tankejing

Luohan Guo Chongji

Yangyin Qingfei Gao

Tonsillitis

Houzheng Wan

Bingpeng San

Shuangliao Houfeng San

Meihua Dianshe Dan

Niuhuang Jiedu Wan

Siji Qing Pian

Yangyin Qingfei Gao

Appendicitis

Lanwei Xiaoyan Pian

Qianli Guang Pian

Urticaria

Maxing Zhike Tangjiang

Fangfeng Tongsheng Wan

Shouwu Wan

Biliary Calculi

Lidan Pian

Lidan Paishi Pian

Xiaoyan Lidan Pian

Mumps

Xiaku Cao Gao

Zijin Ding

Liushen Wan

Meihua Dianshe Dan

Shaixian Yan Pian

Niuhuang Jiedu Wan

Yinqiao Jiedu Pian

Huanglian Shangqing Wan

Ruyi Jinhuang San

Banlan Gen Gantangjiang

Mastitis

Xingxiao Wan

Jingfang Baidu Wan

Xiaojin Wan

Xihuang Wan

Yili Zhu

Optic Neuritis

Shihu Yeguang Wan

Qiju Dihuang Wan

Mingmu Dihuang Wan

Huanglian Yanggan Wan

Zhangyan Ming Pian

Rhinitis

Huodan Wan

Biyan Pian

Biyan Wan

Biyan Tangjiang

Qingxuan Wan

Liushen Wan
Shuangliao Houfeng San
Xiongju Shangqing Wan

Chuanxiong Chatiao San
Xiaojian Zhong Heji

Nephritis

Yinchen Wuling Wan
Zhouche Wan
Wuling San
Shanren Heji
Bazheng Heji
Ermiao Wan
Fenqing Wulin Wan
Shilin Tong Pian
Sanjin Pian
Jiannao Bushen Wan
Fuke Fenqing Wan

Shenling Baizhu San
Liuwei Dihuang Wan
Wuzi Yanzhong Wan
Haima Bushen Wan
Bushen Ning
Suoyang Gujing Wan
Bushen Qiangshen Pian
Qinge Wan
Quanlu Wan
Liuyi San
Naoling Su

Hyperthyroidism

Haizao Wan
Xiaku Cao Gao
Liuwei Dihuang Wan

DabuYin Wan
Tianwang Buxin Dan

Diabetes

Xiaoke Wan
Xiaoke Ping Pian
Liuwei Dihuang Wan
Yuquan Wan
Suoquan Wan

DabuYin Wan
Quanlu Wan
Lutai Gao
Naoling Su
Renshen Jing

Aplastic Anaemia

Ajiao

Renshen Guipi Wan

Xiaojian Zhong Heji

Anaemia

Ajiao

Xin Ajiao

Huangmingjiao

Fufang Ajiao Jiang

Shengxue Gao

Jiannao Bushen Wan

Danggui Buxue Jing

Jixue Teng Pian

Buzhong Yiqi Wan

Bazhen Wan

Qingchun Bao

Shuangbao Su

Renshen Jing

Shandong Ajiao Gao

Plumonary Tuberculosis

Gajie Dingchuan Wan

Baihe Gujin Wan

Qingfei Yihuo Wan

Zhigan Cao Heji

Shengmai Yin Koufuye

Hypertension

Niuhuang Jiangya Pian

Niuhuang Qingnao Pian

Shuxin Jiangya Pian

Duzhong Jiangya Pian

Fufang Luobu Ma Pian

Luobu Ma Jiangya Pian

Jiangya Ping Pian

Naoli Qing

Qingnao Wan

Qiongju Shangqing Wan

Yufeng Ningxin Pian

Lingzhi Tangjiang

Zaizao Wan

Fangfeng Tongsheng Wan

Liuwei Dihuang Wan

Artery Arteriosclerosis

Maile Tong

Huoxin Wan

Shenqi Chongji

Shouwu Wan

Wanshi Niuhuang Qingxin
Wan

Hyperlipemia

Jiangzhi Ling Jiaowan

Xiaoshuan Zaizao Wan

Xiaoshuan Tongluo Pian

Maian Chongji

Yigan Ling Pian

Coronary Heart Disease

Huoxin Wan

Yixin Wan

Huanxin Dan

Subing Di Wan

Fufang Danshen Pian

Fufang Danshen Zhusheye

Baoxin Wan

Suxiao Jiuxin Wan

Xinke Shu Pian

Jiexin Tong Pian

Guanxin Suhe Wan

Shuxin Jiangya Pian

Honghua Zhusheye

Maile Tong

Yufeng Ningxin Pian

Huatuo Zaizao Wan

Guanxin Tongmai Ling Pian

Cerebrovascular Accident

Angong Niuhuang Wan

Renshen Zaizao Wan

Dahuo Luo Wan

Tianma Wan

Zaizao Wan

Niuhuang Jiangya Pian

Jufang Niuhuang Qingxin Wan

Epilepsy

Mengshi Guntan Wan

Yixianfeng Wan

Yangxian Wan

Baijin Wan

Cizhu Wan

Jufang Zhibao Dan

Jufang Niuhuang Qingxin Wan

Zhusha Anshen Wan

Cerebral Thrombosis

Xiaoshuan Zaizao Wan

Xiaoshuan Tongluo Pian

Mailuo Tong

Guanxin Tongmai Ling

Acute Gastriculcer

Libi Ling Pian

Yinnhuang Pian

Gegen Qinlian Pian

Sixiao Wan

Zhishi Daozhi Wan

Sijun Zi Wan

Baohe Wan

Liuhe Dingzhong Wan

Qingwei Baoan Wan

Yande Ping Jiaonang

Qianliguang Pian

Shayao

Yiyuan San

Xingjun San

Wuji Wan

Xiaoban Xia Heji

Chronic Gastric Uler

Muxiang Shunqi Wan

Pingwei Wan

Renshen Jianpi Wan

Xiangsha Yangwei Wan

Gipi Wan

Baohe Wan

Anwei Wan

Liangfu Pian

Kaixiong Shunqi Wan

Jiuqi Niantong Wan

Lanji Wan

Yuanhu Zhitong Pian

Sanren Heji

Gastroduodenal Ulcer

Sheling Baizhu San

Xiangsha Liujun Wan

Fuzi Lizhong Wan

Zuojin Wan

Shugan Wan

Neurosis

Anshen Buxin Wan

Jiannao Bushen Wan

Neurasthenia

Tianwang Buxin Dan

Zhusha Anshen Wan

Zhenzhong Dan

Bozi Yangxin Wan

Anshen Buxin Wan

Naoling Su

Jiannao Bushen Wan

Jiannao Wan

Zhigan Cao Heji

Renshen Guipi Wan

Cizhu Wan

Lingzhi Tangjiang

Wuwei Zi Chongji

Xiangsha Liujun Wan

Xiaojian Zhong Heji

Huangqi Jianzhong Wan

Xiaoyao Wan

Lutai Gao

Buzhong Yiqi Wan

Danggui Buxue Jing

Qingchun Bao

Shuangbao Su

Renshen Jing

Renshen Fengwangjiang

Hyperthermy Heliosis

Huoxiang Zhengqishui

Qushu Wan

Qingshu Yiqi Wan

Shuzheng Wan

Rendan

Shushi Zhengqi Wan

Qingliang Dan

Jinyin Hua Lu

Shengmai Yin Koufuye

Shidi Shui

Rheumatioc Muscle Fiber Inflamation

Dahuo Luo Wan
Xiaohuo Luo Wan
Zhenjiang Gaoyao
Fengshi Qutong Gao
Fengshi Zhitong Gao
Yanghe Jiening Gao

Wuli Bahan San
Xijian Wan
Jiufen San
Fufang Danggui Zhusheye
Qufeng Shujin Wan
Kanli Sha

Rheumatic Arthritis

Guogong Jiu
Xiaoluo Tong
Xiaohuo Luo Wan
Tianma Wan
Duhuo Jisheng Wan
Mugua Wan
Zhenjiang Gaoyao
Shangshi Baozhen Gao
Shangshi Zhitong Gao

Fengshi Zhitong Gao
Yanghe Jiening Gao
Jinbu Huan Gaoyao
Fengliao Xing Yaojiu
Shujin Huoluo Jiu
Qufeng Shujin Wan
Fufang Danggui Zhusheye
Jiufen San
Kanli Sha

Hyperosteogeny

Guci Pian
Guzh Zengsheng Wan
Guci Wan
Guxian Wan

Guci Xiaotong Ye
Dahuo Luo Dan
Xiaohuo Luo Dan
Xijian Wan

Pyogenic Infection

Kangjun Xiaoyan Pian
Zicao Gao
Qianli Guang Pian

Niuhuang Jiedu Pian
YiLi Zu

Chanshu Wan

Badu Gao

Fracture

Dieda Wan

Zhenggu Shui

Zhonghua Dieda Wan

Shenyang Hongyao

Qili San

Jiegu San

Guzhe Cuoshang San

Shenjin Dan

Traumatic Bleeding

Yunnan Baiyao

Huaijiao Wan

Sanqi Pian

Phlegmon

Xiaojin Wan

Chansu Wan

Zhizi Jinhua Wan

Badu Gao

Eczema

Ermiao Wan

Jingfang Baidu Wan

Ruyi Jinhua San

Jinji Chongji

Oncoma

Xihuang Wan

Xingxiao Wan

Pianzi Huang

Yadan Ziru Zhusheye

Xinhuang Pian

Gongjing Ai Pian

Hekui Zhusheye

Hougujun Pian

Menoxenia

Jixue Teng Pian

Yimu Wan

Wuji Baifeng Wan

Xiaoyao Wan

Babao Kunshun Wan
Qizhi Xiangfu Wan
Fuke Tiaojing Wan
Aifu Nuangong Wan
Nujin Dan
Danggui Yangxue Wan
Bazhen Yimu Wan
Danggui Jinggao Pian

Fukang Ning Pian
Qianjin Zhidai Wan
Chanhou Shentong Pian
Shaofu Zhuyu Wan
Tiaojing Zhibao Wan
Jinji Chongji
Shixiao San

Amenorrhoea

Danggui Yangxue Wan
Fuke Tongjing Wan

Dahuang Zhechong Wan

Leucorrhoea

Baidai Wan
Nüjin Dan
Qianjin Zhidai Wan
Wuji Baifeng Wan

Aifu Nuangong Wan
Wenjing Wan
Gujing Wan

Dysmenorrhoea

Yueju Wan
Liangfu Wan
Tongjing Wan
Wenjing Wan
Jiuqi Niantong Wan
Yuanhu Zhitong Pian
Qizhi Xiangfu Wan
Danggui Jingao Pian

Yimu Wan
Yimu Caogao
Shixiao San
Bazhen Yimu Wan
Tiaojing Zhibao Wan
Shaofu Zhuyu Wan
Jinji Chongji

Infertility

LutaiGao

Lujiao Jiao

Chufeng Jing

Ajiao

Habitual Abortion

Antai Wan

Baotai Wan

Shandong Ajiao Gao

Dysfunctional Uterine Bleeding

Renshen Guipi Wan

Ajiao

Nüjin Dan

Wuji Baifeng Wan

Shihui San

Heye Wan

Constipation

Maren Wan

Wuren Runchang Wan

Zhishi Daozhi Wan

Sixiao Wan

Glaucoma

Shihu Yeguang Wan

Huanglian Yanggan Wan

Qiju Dihuang Wan

Cataract

Zhangyanming Pian

Huanglian Yanggan Wan

Shihun Yieguan Wan

Qiju Dihuang Wan

Pheumonia

Baihe Gujin Wan

Zhishou Dingchuan Wan

Maxing Zhike Tangjiang

Fenghan Ganmao Chongji

Xiling Jiedu Pian

Yinqiao Jiedu Pian

Lingqiao Jiedu Pian

Kangjun Xiaoyan Pian

Fufang Daqingye Zhusheye

Sanren Heji

Yinhuang Pian

Qianliguang Pian

Kongxian Dan

Bronchial Asthma

Zhihou Qingguo Wan

Qingfei Yihuo Wan

Zhisou Dingchuan Wan

Fuling Wan

Xiaoqinglong Heji

Zhikechuan Reshen Pian

Baihua Dingchuan Wan

Xianzhuli Koufuye

Dingchuan Wan

Tanchuan Wan

Chuanshuning

Hailong Gajie Jing

Aiyeyou Qiwuji

· Shuzhijiangqi Wan

Chronic Trachitis

Ermu Ningsou Wan

Erchen Wan

Juhong Wan

Luohanguo Chongji

Chuanbei Pipa Zhike
    Tangjiang

Fufang Chuanbeijing Pian

Tanke Jing

Xiaokechuan

Banxia Lu

Yupingfeng Wan

Qingwen Jiedu Wan

Laiyangli Zhike Tangjiang

Suzi Jiangqi Wan

Zhisou Dingchuan Wan

Chuanshu Pian

Mengshi Guntan Wan

Whooping Cough

Bairike Pian

Shedan Chenpi Mo

Shedan Chuanbei Mo

Sexual Neurasthenia

Zhibao Sanbian Wan

Guiling Ji

Hailong Gajie Jing

Huanshao Dan

Quanlu Wan

Nanbao

Sanshen Wan

HaiMa Bushen Wan

Bushenning Pian

Suoyang Gujing Wan

Hailong Jiao

Erxian Gao

Lujiao Jiao

Chufeng Jing

Lutai Gao

Renshen Jing

5

常用中成药

序

　　《英汉实用中医药大全》即将问世，吾为之高兴。

　　歧黄之道，历经沧桑，永盛不衰。吾中华民族之强盛，由之。世界医学之丰富和发展，亦由之。然而，世界民族之差异，国别之不同，语言之障碍，使中医中药的传播和交流受到了严重束缚。当前，世界各国人民学习、研究、运用中医药的热潮方兴未艾。为使吾中华民族优秀文化遗产之一的歧黄之道走向世界，光大其业，为世界人民造福，徐象才君集省内外精英于一堂，主持编译了《英汉实用中医药大全》。是书之问世将使海内外同道欢呼雀跃。

　　世界医学发展之日，当是歧黄之道光大之时。

　　吾欣然序之。

中华人民共和国卫生部副部长

兼国家中医药管理局局长

世界针灸学会联合会主席

中国科学技术协会委员

中华全国中医学会副会长

中国针灸学会会长

胡熙明

1989 年 12 月

序

中华民族有同疾病长期作斗争的光辉历程，故而有自己的传统医学——中国医药学。中国医药学有一套完整的从理论到实践的独特科学体系。几千年来，它不但被完好地保存下来，而且得到了发扬光大。它具有疗效显著、副作用小等优点，是人们防病治病，强身健体的有效工具。

任何一个国家在医学进步中所取得的成就，都是人类共同的财富，是没有国界的。医学成果的交流比任何其他科学成果的交流都应进行得更及时，更准确。我从事中医工作30多年来，一直盼望着有朝一日中国医药学能全面走向世界，为全人类解除病痛疾苦做出其应有的贡献。但由于用外语表达中医难度较大，中国医药学对外传播的速度一直不能令人满意。

山东中医学院的徐象才老师发起并主持了大型系列丛书《英汉实用中医药大全》的编译工作。这个工作是一项巨大工程，是一种大型科研活动，是一个大胆的尝试，是一件新事物。对徐象才老师及与其合作的全体编译者夜以继日地长期工作所付出的艰苦劳动，克服重重困难所表现出的坚韧不拔的毅力，以及因此而取得的重大成绩，我甚为敬佩。作为一个中医界的领导者，对他们的工作给予全力支持是我应尽的责任。

我相信《英汉实用中医药大全》无疑会在中国医学史和世界科学技术史上找到它应有的位置。

中华全国中医学会常务理事
山东省卫生厅副厅长

张奇文

1990年3月

出 版 前 言

　　中国医药学是我中华民族优秀文化遗产之一，建国以来由于党和国家对待中医药采取了正确的政策，使中医药理论宝库不断得到了发掘整理，取得了巨大的成绩。当前，世界各国人民对中国医药学的学习和研究热潮日益高涨，为促进这一热潮更加蓬勃的发展，为使中国医药学能更好地为全人类解除病痛服务，就必须促进中医中药在世界范围内的传播和交流，而要使这一传播和交流进行得更及时、更准确，就必须首先排除语言障碍。因此，编译一套英汉对照的中医药基本知识的书籍，供国内外学习、研究中医药时使用，已成为国内外医药学界和医药学教育界许多人士的迫切需要。

　　多年来，在卫生部门的号召下，在"中医英语表达研究"方面，已经作出了一些可喜的成绩。本书《英汉实用中医药大全》的编辑出版就是在调查上述研究工作的历史和现状的基础上，继续对中医药英语表达作较系统、较全面的研究，以适应中国医药学对外传播交流的需要。

　　这部"大全"的版本为英汉对照，共有 21 个分册，一个分册介绍论述中国医药学的一个分科。在编著上注意了中医药汉文稿的编写特色，在内容上注意了科学性、实用性、全面性和简明易读。汉文稿的执笔撰写者主要是有 20 年以上实践经验的教授、副教授、主任医师和副主任医师。各分册汉文稿撰写成后，均经各学科专家逐一审订。各分册英文主译、主审主要是国内既懂中医又懂英语的权威人士，还有许多中医院校的英语教师及医药卫生部门的专业翻译人员。英译稿脱稿后，经过了复审、终审，有些译稿还召开全国 22 所院校和单位人员参加的英译稿统稿定稿研讨会，对英译稿进行细致的研讨和推敲，对如何较全面、较系统、较准确地用英语表达中国医药学进行了探讨，从而推动整个译文达到较高水平，因此，这部"大全"可供中医院校高年级学生作为泛读教材使用。

这部"大全"的编纂得到了国家教育委员会、国家中医药管理局、山东省教育委员会、山东省卫生厅等各部门有关领导的支持。在国家教委高等教育司的指导下，成立了《英汉实用中医药大全》编译领导委员会。还得到了全国许多中医院校和中药生产厂家领导的支持。

希望这部"大全"的出版，对中医院校加强中医英语教学，对国内卫生界培养外向型中医药人才，以及在推动世界各国人民对中医药的学习和研究方面，都将产生良好的影响。

高等教育出版社

1990 年 3 月

前　言

　　《英汉实用中医药大全》是一部以中医基本理论为基础，以中医临床为重点，较为全面系统、简明扼要、易读实用的中级英汉学术性著作。它的主要读者是：中医药院校高年级学生和中青年教师，中医院的中青年医生和中医药科研单位的科研人员，从事中医对外函授工作的人员和出国讲学或行医的中医人员，西学中人员，来华学习中医的外国留学生和各类进修人员。

　　由于中国医药学为我中华民族之独有，因此，英译便成了本《大全》编译工作的重点。为确保译文能准确表达中医的确切含义，我们邀集熟悉中医的英语人员、医学专业翻译人员、懂英语的中医药人员及至医古文人员于一堂，共同翻译、共同对译文进行研讨推敲的集体翻译法，这样，就把众人之长融进了译文质量之中。然而，即使这样，也难确保译文都能尽如人意。汉文稿虽反映了中国医药学的精髓和概貌，但也难能十全十美。我衷心地盼望读者能提出批评和建议，以便《大全》再版时修改。

　　参加本《大全》编、译、审工作的人员达 200 余名，他们来自全国 28 个单位，其中有山东、北京、上海、天津、南京、浙江、安徽、河南、湖北、广西、贵阳、甘肃、成都、山西、长春等 15 所中医学院，还有中国中医研究院，山东省中医药研究所等中医药科研单位。

　　山东省教育委员会把本《大全》的编译列入了科研计划并拨发了科研经费，山东省卫生厅和一些中药生产厂家也给了很大支持，济南中药厂的资助为编译工作的开端提供了条件。

　　本《大全》的编译成功是全体编译审者集体劳动的结晶，是各有关单位主管领导支持的结果。在《大全》各分册即将陆续出版之际，我诚挚地感谢全体编译审者的真诚合作，感谢许多专家、教授、各级领导和生产厂家的热情支持。

愿本《大全》的出版能在培养通晓英语的中医人才和使中医早日全面走向世界方面起到我所期望的作用。

主编　徐象才

于山东中医学院

1990 年 3 月

目　录

说　明

　　《常用中成药》是《英汉实用中医药大全》的第5分册。

　　本分册的编写采用了现代药物学的分类方法，并特别指明了每种成药的西医适应症。全册分18章，共介绍常用中成药449种。为方便读者查阅，还在书后附有两个索引。

　　中成药是一类疗效确切，副作用小、服用方便的中草药制剂，是中医药学的重要组成部分。本分册的编译旨在使它生翅远飞，走出国门，为世界人民的健康事业服务。但编译此种书籍尚属首次，不足之处在所难免。欢迎国内外读者指正。

　　为使英文稿达到要求，曾在原稿的基础上进行过全面的重译。另有一些女士们、先生们曾对翻译工作做出过贡献，其中包括孙祥燮，寻建英，李军林、陈清、郭洪祝。在此，对他们一并表示感谢。

编者

1 中枢神经系统药物

1.1 抗癫痫药

白 金 丸

〔药物组成〕 郁金 70% 白矾 30%

〔功能与主治〕 开郁豁痰，安神镇惊。用于痰壅内闭，惊痫抽风，狂燥不安，神志不清。

〔用法与用量〕 口服，1 次 0.3 g，1 日 1 次。

〔剂型与规格〕 水丸，每 150 粒重 3 g

〔附注〕 处方来源于清·王洪绪《外科证治全生集》。

本品具有安神除烦，调节中枢神经系统功能，抗癫痫的作用。临床适用于癫痫、抽搐、狂燥不安，神志不清。

羊 痫 疯 丸

〔药物组成〕 郁金 白矾 芥子 橘红 大黄 黄芩 黄连 黄柏 栀子 神曲 磁石 沉香

〔功能与主治〕 清热化痰，镇惊安神。用于痰涎壅盛，牙关紧闭，昏迷不省，角弓反张。

〔用法与用量〕 口服，日一次，小儿 1-4 岁，1 次 1.5 g；5-7 岁，1 次 3 g；成人 1 次 9 g，1 日 1 次。

〔剂型与规格〕 水丸，每 50 粒重 3 g

〔附注〕 本品具有解热、镇静、解痉、抗癫痫的作用。临床适用于癫痫、羊痫疯等。

孕妇及久病体弱者忌服。

医 痫 丸

〔药物组成〕　　生白附子 4.3%　天南星 8.6%　半夏 8.6%　猪牙皂 43.2%　白矾 13%　僵蚕 8.6%　蜈蚣 0.2%　全蝎 1.7%　乌梢蛇 8.6%　雄黄 1.3%　朱砂 1.7%

〔功能与主治〕　　祛风化痰，定痫止搐。用于癫痫抽搐，时发时止。

〔用法与用量〕　　口服，1 次 3 g，1 日 2 次，小儿酌减。

〔剂型与规格〕　　水丸，每包重 3 g

〔附注〕　　本品具有安定、解痉、抗癫痫的作用。临床适用于癫痫、抽搐。

本品与羊痫疯丸比较，其解痉抗抽搐作用较强，但抗昏迷作用不如羊痫疯丸。

孕妇忌服。

1.2　抗精神病药

礞石滚痰丸

〔药物组成〕　　金礞石 10%　沉香 5%　黄芩 42.5%　熟大黄 42.5%

〔功能与主治〕　　降水逐痰。用于实热顽痰，多为癫狂惊悸，或咳喘痰稠，大便秘结。

〔用法与用量〕　　口服，1 次 6-12 g，1 日 1 次。

〔剂型与规格〕　　水丸，每 20 粒重 1 g

〔附注〕　　本品具有祛痰，抗精神病作用。临床适用于实热顽痰型精神分裂症，慢性支气管炎，肺气肿合并感染，癫痫等。

孕妇忌用。

竹沥达痰丸

〔药物组成〕 竹沥 青礞石 橘红 半夏 大黄 黄芩 沉香 生姜 甘草

〔功能与主治〕 清火豁痰，顺气平喘。用于痰热上壅，喘急昏迷，顽痰交结，烦闷癫狂，痰多等。

〔用法与用量〕 口服，1次6～9g，1日1～2次。

〔剂型与规格〕 水丸，每袋重18g

〔附注〕 本品具有祛痰，抗精神病的作用。临床适用于精神分裂症(实热顽痰型)。

1.3 镇惊、催眠药

天王补心丹

〔药物组成〕 丹参3.5% 当归7% 石菖蒲3.5% 党参3.5% 茯苓3.5% 五味子7% 麦冬7% 天冬7% 地黄28.2% 玄参3.5% 远志3.5% 酸枣仁7% 柏子仁7% 桔梗3.5% 甘草3.5% 朱砂1.4%

〔功能与主治〕 滋阴养血，补心安神。用于心阴不足，心悸健忘，失眠多梦，大便干燥。

〔用法与用量〕 口服，1次1丸，1日2次。

〔剂型与规格〕 蜜丸，每丸重9g

〔附注〕 处方来源于元·危亦林《世医得效方》。

本品具有安定，滋养强壮，调节中枢神经系统及机体器官功能等作用。临床适用于神经衰弱，风湿性心脏病，甲状腺机能亢进，更年期综合症(属阴虚血亏，阴虚火旺者)，心悸、失眠、多梦、健忘，口舌生疮等。

朱砂安神丸

〔药物组成〕 朱砂 21.4% 黄连 32.2% 当归 21.4% 生地 21.4% 甘草 3.6%

〔功能与主治〕 镇惊安神，清心养血。用于心火亢盛，心血受损之心神不安，烦躁不眠，胸中烦热，夜寐多梦。

〔用法与用量〕 口服，1 次 1 丸，1 日 1—2 次。

〔剂型与规格〕 蜜丸，每丸重 9 g

〔附注〕 处方来源于明·龚廷贤《寿世保元》。

本品具有安定除烦，调节中枢神经系统功能的作用。临床适用于心火亢盛，心血不足型烦躁，心悸，失眠，神经衰弱，精神抑郁，癫痫等。

不宜与溴化钾、溴化钠、碘化钠同服。

枕 中 丹

〔药物组成〕 龟板 25% 龙骨 25% 石菖蒲 25% 远志 25%

〔功能与主治〕 滋阴降火，镇心安神。用于心血虚弱，思虑过度，阴虚火旺，心悸怔忡，头晕失眠，遗精盗汗。

〔用法与用量〕 口服，1 次 1 丸，1 日 1—2 次。

〔剂型与规格〕 蜜丸，每丸重 9 g

〔附注〕 处方来源于唐·孙思邈《千金要方》。

本品具有安定、调节中枢神经系统及植物神经系统功能的作用。临床适用于神经衰弱，心悸失眠，记忆力减退以及遗精盗汗等。

柏子养心丸

〔药物组成〕 柏子仁 3.2% 党参 3.2% 黄芪 12.8% 川芎 12.8% 当归 12.8% 茯苓 25.6% 远志 3.2% 酸枣仁

3.2%　肉桂 3.2%　甘草 1.3%　半夏曲 12.8%　五味子 3.2%
朱砂 2.7%

〔功能与主治〕　补气养血，益智安神。用于心血不足，虚火上升引起的心悸气短，失眠健忘，精神不振，自汗盗汗。

〔用法与用量〕　口服，1 次 1 丸，1 日 2 次。

〔剂型与规格〕　蜜丸，每丸重 9 g

〔附注〕　处方来源于明·王肯堂《证治准绳》。
本品临床适用于神经衰弱之心悸气短，失眠健忘，精神不振，自汗盗汗等。

安神补心丸

〔药物组成〕　丹参 27%　五味子 13.5%　石菖蒲 9%　安神膏 50.5%

〔功能与主治〕　养心安神。用于心悸、失眠、健忘、头晕耳鸣。

〔用法与用量〕　口服，1 次 15 粒，1 日 3 次。

〔剂型与规格〕　水丸，15 粒重 2 g

〔附注〕　本品具有安定、调节中枢神经系统功能，滋养升血等作用。临床适用于神经衰弱(属心血不足者)，神经官能症，症见失眠，健忘，烦躁不宁，头晕目眩者。

脑 灵 素 片

〔药物组成〕　黄精　淫羊藿　苍耳子　麦冬　远志　红参　酸枣仁　五味子　龟板　枸杞子　鹿茸　茯苓　大枣肉　熟地黄　鹿角胶

〔功能与主治〕　补气血，养心肾，健脑安神。用于健忘失眠，头晕心悸，身倦无力，体虚自汗，阳萎遗精，精神紊乱。

〔用法与用量〕　口服，1 次 2-3 片，1 日 2-3 次。

〔剂型与规格〕　糖衣片，每片(基片)重 0.3 g

〔附注〕 本品具有滋养作用，能调节机体各器官的机能，尤以中枢神经系统为显著。临床适用于神经衰弱，精神病，慢性肾炎、贫血、慢性肝炎、糖尿病等。

五味子冲剂

〔药物组成〕 五味子100%

〔功能与主治〕 益气补肾，镇静安眠。用于肾气虚弱，心烦不眠，神疲乏力。

〔用法与用量〕 开水冲服，1次10 g，1日3次。

〔剂型与规格〕 冲剂，每袋重10 g

〔附注〕 本品临床适用于神经衰弱，心肌劳损，疲劳过度，失眠等。

牛黄清脑片

〔药物组成〕 玄参6.6% 黄芩6.6% 金银花2.8% 甘草6.6% 板兰根6.5% 蒲公英9.5% 天花粉6.6% 大黄4.8% 连翘3.9% 石决明1.4% 石膏6.6% 雄黄7.3% 赭石6.6% 冰片0.7% 朱砂0.2% 麦冬6.6% 栀子3.9% 生地黄4.8% 葛根3.9% 苦胆膏0.3% 黄连0.7% 珍珠0.3% 磁石2.8%

〔功能与主治〕 清热解毒，清脑安神。用于头身高热，头晕脑胀，言语狂躁，舌干眼花，咽喉肿痛，小儿内热惊风抽搐。

〔用法与用量〕 口服，1次2-4片，1日3次，神经官能症者可适当增量或遵医嘱，小儿酌减。

〔剂型与规格〕 糖衣片，每片(基片)重0.34 g

〔附注〕 本品具有安定、解痉、抗菌消炎、镇痛、抗休克及降低血压等作用。临床适用于高血压症，神经官能症，神经性头痛，失眠及高烧之头晕、烦躁、发烧抽搐等。

小儿体弱或低血压者慎用。孕妇忌服。

健脑补肾丸

〔药物组成〕 人参 3.5% 鹿茸 0.8% 狗肾 1.6% 肉桂 3.5% 金牛草 1.4% 牛蒡子 2% 金樱子 1.4% 杜仲 (炭)4.2% 川膝藤 4.2% 金银花 3% 连翘 2.8% 蝉蜕 2.8% 山药 5.6% 远志 4.9% 酸枣仁 4.2% 砂仁 4.9% 当归 4.2% 龙骨 4.1% 牡蛎 4.9% 茯苓 9.7% 白术 4.9% 桂枝 4.1% 白芍 4.1% 朱砂 5.2% 豆蔻4.1% 甘草 3.2%

〔功能与主治〕 健脑益气，补肾填精。用于健忘失眠，头晕目眩，耳鸣心悸，腰膝酸软，肾亏遗精。

〔用法与用量〕 口服，1 次 15 粒，1 日 2 次。

〔剂型与规格〕 水丸，每 20 粒重 1 g

〔附注〕 本品具有改善大脑功能，镇静、降压等作用。临床适用于神经衰弱、慢性肾炎、贫血、神经官能症等。

健 脑 丸

〔药物组成〕酸枣仁 19.4% 肉苁蓉 9.7% 枸杞子 9.7% 益智仁 9.7% 五味子 7.3% 柏子仁 7.3% 胆南星 4.8% 远志 4.8% 天竺黄 4.8% 九节菖蒲 4.8% 龙齿 4.8% 琥珀 4.8% 当归3.6% 朱砂 4.5%

〔功能与主治〕 补脑安神，宁心益智。用于怔忡健忘，头目眩晕，心悸不安，烦躁失眠。

〔用法与用量〕 口服，1 次 20 粒，1 日 2 次。

〔剂型与规格〕 水丸，每瓶装 200 粒

〔附注〕 本品具有安定、调整中枢神经系统功能，调整血压作用。临床适用于用脑过度、神经衰弱，失眠健忘，头目眩晕，心悸烦躁等。

灵 芝 糖 浆

〔药物组成〕 灵芝子实体 46.2% 灵芝菌丝体 38.5% 枇杷叶 7.7% 薄荷脑 0.008% 桔梗 7.7%

〔功能与主治〕 利肝健脾，益气平喘，镇惊降压。用于急性黄疸型肝炎，高血压，神经衰弱，喘息性气管炎。

〔用法与用量〕 口服，1 次 15-20 ml，1 日 3 次，小儿酌减。

〔剂型与规格〕 糖浆剂，每瓶装 500 ml

〔附注〕 本品能提高机体免疫功能，增强机体抗病能力，并能降低血脂，调整血压，调节中枢神经系统功能，安定除烦，且能抗过敏，止咳平喘。临床适用于急性黄疸性肝炎，克山病，高血压，神经衰弱，喘息性气管炎等。

磁 朱 丸

〔药物组成〕 磁石（煅）28.6% 朱砂 14.3% 六神曲（炒）57.1%

〔功能与主治〕 镇心安神，明目。用于心肾阴虚，心阳偏亢，心悸失眠，耳鸣耳聋，视物昏花，烦躁不安。

〔用法与用量〕 口服，1 次 3g，1 日 2 次。

〔剂型与规格〕 水丸，每包装 18 g

〔附注〕 本品具有调节中枢神经系统功能，改善脑血管供血状况，安定除烦等作用。临床适用于神经衰弱，心悸，失眠，耳鸣耳聋，癫痫，焦虑症等。

2 心血管系统药物

2.1 抗冠心病、心绞痛药

活 心 丸

〔药物组成〕 人参 牛黄等

〔功能与主治〕 清心安神，镇静开窍。用于胸痹，真心痛，胸闷气短，心悸。

〔用法与用量〕 口服，1 次 1～2 丸，1 日 3 次。

〔剂型与规格〕 小水丸，每丸重 20 mg

〔附注〕 本品具有调整心律，提高心脏功能，改善微循环，扩张冠状动脉和脑血管，提高心肌抗缺血能力，消除心绞痛，增加脑血流量等作用。临床适用于冠心病及各种心脏病引起的心绞痛，心肌缺血和慢性心功能不全，脑动脉硬化引起的脑缺血综合症。

孕妇及妇女月经期慎用。

益 心 丸

〔药物组成〕 人参 牛黄 蟾酥 珍珠 冰片 田三七等

〔功能与主治〕 益气强心，芳香开窍，活血化瘀。用于真心痛，厥心痛，胸闷气短，心悸。

〔用法与用量〕 舌下含化，1 次 1～2 丸，1 日 1～2次。

〔剂型与规格〕 水丸，每瓶装 20 丸

〔附注〕 本品具有扩张冠状动脉，调节心律，提高心肌抗缺氧能力，增强心肌收缩力等作用。临床适用于冠心病，心绞痛，心律失常，心功能不全等。

经 332 例临床观察，本品对心绞痛患者总有效率达 85.4%，对心电图有改变的慢性冠脉供血不足患者，总有效率为 82.7%。

孕妇忌服，妇女月经期慎用。

环 心 丹

〔药物组成〕 三七　人参　珍珠等

〔功能与主治〕 活血化瘀，通脉活络。用于真心痛，胸闷，气短，心悸。

〔用法与用量〕 口服，1 次 2 粒，1 日 2～3 次；急性发作时嚼碎含化，每次 3～4 粒。

〔剂型与规格〕 半浓缩丸，每 10 粒重 0.25 g

〔附注〕 本品具有扩张冠状动脉，增加冠脉血流量，改善微循环，降低心肌耗氧量，调整心率，提高心肌抗缺血，抗缺氧能力，缓解心绞痛等作用。临床适用于冠心病，心绞痛，心律失常，心肌梗塞等。

发热、哮喘发作、出血者及孕妇禁用。

生脉饮口服液

〔药物组成〕 人参 25%　麦冬 50%　五味子 25%

〔功能与主治〕 益气复脉，养阴生津。用于气阴两伤，心悸气短，脉微虚汗，久病体虚。

〔用法与用量〕 口服，1 次 10 ml，1 日 3 次。

〔剂型与规格〕 口服液，每支装 10 ml

〔附注〕 处方来源于金·李杲《内外伤辨惑论》。

本品具有调整机体各器官机能，提高抗病能力，调整心律，加强心肌收缩力，提高心脏输出量，降低心肌耗氧量，调整血压，抗休克，强心，以及扩张冠状动脉，增加冠脉流量等作用。临床适用于冠心病，肺心病，风湿性心脏病，并可用于心律不齐，心脏神经官能症，低血压以及中暑，慢性支气管炎，肺结核等。

保 心 丸

〔药物组成〕　苏合香脂　蟾酥　牛黄　肉桂　冰片　人参

〔功能与主治〕　芳香开窍，理气止痛，活血化瘀。用于真心痛，厥心痛，胸闷气短，心悸等。

〔用法与用量〕　口服，1 次 1～2 粒，1 日 3 次。

〔剂型与规格〕　微丸，每 300 粒重 1 g

〔附注〕　本品具有扩张冠状动脉，改善心肌供血状况，降低心肌耗氧量，提高心肌耐缺氧能力，缓解心绞痛的作用。临床适用于冠心病，各种原因引起的心绞痛、胸闷等。

据报道，本品口服后 50 秒钟起效，大部分在 5 分钟以内起效。持续作用时间最短 30 分钟，最长 24 小时，大部分在 11 小时左右。

个别人服后有口干、头胀或有轻度的唇、舌麻木感。个别特异体质服后有荨麻疹者慎用。孕妇忌用。

速效救心丸

〔药物组成〕　川芎　冰片等

〔功能与主治〕　活血化瘀，芳香开窍，理气止痛。用于真心痛，胸闷，气短，心悸。

〔用法与用量〕　含服，1 次 4～6 粒，1 日 3 次，急性发作时 10～15 粒。

〔剂型与规格〕　滴丸，每瓶装 40 粒。

〔附注〕　本品具有扩张冠状动脉，增加冠脉血流量，减慢心率，降低心肌耗氧量，改善微循环的作用。临床适用于冠心病，心绞痛、胸闷等。既可做为冠心病长期用药，又可做为急救药使用。

脉 络 通 片

〔药物组成〕 丹参 麦门冬 三七 郁金 黄芩 钩藤 夏枯草 木香 降香 槐米 人参 琥珀 甘松 代赭石 黄连 石菖蒲 牛黄 檀香 甘草 冰片 珍珠

〔功能与主治〕 行气化瘀，通脉活络。用于胸痹，胸闷气短，胸背引痛。

〔用法与用量〕 口服，1次4片，1日2～3次。

〔剂型与规格〕 片剂，每片重 0.4 g

〔附注〕 本品具有扩张冠状动脉，增加冠脉血流量，改善微循环，降低血脂及血液粘度等作用。临床适用于冠心病心绞痛，高血压，脑血管栓塞，心肌梗塞，动脉粥样硬化等。

冠心苏合丸

〔药物组成〕 苏合香 7.4% 冰片 15.4% 炙乳香 15.4% 檀香 30.9% 青木香 30.9%

〔功能与主治〕 芳香开窍，宽胸，理气，止痛。用于胸痹，真心痛，心悸气短。

〔用法与用量〕 含化或咬碎后吞服，1次1丸，1日3次，也可发病时服用。

〔剂型与规格〕 蜜丸，每丸重 3 g

〔附注〕 本品具有扩张冠状动脉，增加冠脉血流量，降低心肌耗氧量等作用。临床适用于气滞寒郁型冠心病，心绞痛，胸闷等。与苏合香丸相比，本品突出了扩冠，降低心肌耗氧量的作用，但抗昏迷作用不及苏合香丸。

本品不宜与溴化钾、溴化钠、碘化钠同服。

愈风宁心片

〔药物组成〕 葛根 100%

〔功能与主治〕 解肌退热，生津透疹，升阳止泻。用于真心痛，厥心痛，胸痹以及肝阳上亢所至的眩晕。

〔用法与用量〕 口服，1 次 5 片，1 日 3 次。

〔剂型与规格〕 片剂，每片重 0.25 g

〔附注〕 本品系葛根的醇提取物制剂，主要有效成分为葛根总黄酮。

药理实验表明：葛根总黄酮能扩张冠状动脉和脑血管，增加冠脉及脑血流量，降低血管阻力，减少心肌耗氧量，对抗垂体后叶素引起的冠脉血管痉挛，改善心肌代谢，并有降低血压的作用。临床适用于冠心病，高血压，并可做为治疗美尼尔氏综合症的眩晕、耳鸣用药。

解 心 痛 片

〔药物组成〕 香附 25%　瓜蒌 50%　淫羊藿 25%

〔功能与主治〕 宽胸理气，通脉止痛。用于真心痛，厥心痛，胸痹，胸闷。

〔用法与用量〕 口服，1 次 6～8 片，1 日 3 次。

〔剂型与规格〕 糖衣片，每片(基片)重约 0.28 g

〔附注〕 本品能显著增加冠状动脉血流量，对抗肾上腺素性心律失常，降低心肌耗氧量，增强心肌耐缺氧能力，改善心电图症状，并有明显的镇静催眠作用。临床适用于冠心病，心绞痛，心律失常。

复方丹参片

〔药物组成〕 丹参 22.5%　三七 75%　冰片 2.5%

〔功能与主治〕 活血化瘀，芳香开窍，理气止痛。用于真心痛，厥心痛，胸闷，心悸，气短。

〔用法与用量〕　口服，1次3片，1日3次。

〔剂型与规格〕　片剂，每片重 0.25 g

〔附注〕　本品具有扩张冠状动脉，增加冠脉血流量，降低心肌耗氧量，缓解心绞痛，降低血脂等作用。临床适用于冠心病，心绞痛等属气滞血瘀者。

据报道：用本品治疗 377 例心绞痛患者，总有效率 85.6%。

本品不宜与胃舒平合用。

心 可 舒 片

〔药物组成〕　山楂31.9%　丹参31.9%　葛根31.9%
三七粉2.2%　木香粉2.1%

〔功能与主治〕　活血散瘀，舒心降压。用于真心痛，厥心痛，胸闷，气短，心悸。

〔用法与用量〕　口服，1次4片，1日3次。

〔剂型与规格〕　糖衣片，每片(基片)重 0.25 g

〔附注〕　本品具有扩张冠状动脉，改善心功能及微循环，降低三酸甘油酯及胆固醇浓度，降低血液粘度，改变血液流变性。临床适用于慢性冠状动脉供血不足，心功能不全等。

苏 冰 滴 丸

〔药物组成〕　苏合香脂33.3%　冰片66.7%

〔功能与主治〕　芳香开窍，理气止痛。用于真心痛，厥心痛，胸闷等。

〔用法与用量〕　口服，1次2～4粒，1日3次，也可发病时立即吞服或含化。

〔剂型与规格〕　滴丸，每瓶装30粒

〔附注〕　本品处方系"苏合香丸"方经抗冠心病药理筛选而成，突出了原方抗冠心病，心肌梗塞及抗休克的作用。

本品具有扩张冠状动脉，增加冠脉血流量，降低心肌耗氧量，增加脑血流量，抗休克的作用。临床适用于冠心病心绞痛。

本品对胃有一定的刺激作用，胃病患者慎用。

冠心通脉灵片

〔药物组成〕　当归 5.9%　丹参 14.7%　何首乌 9.8% 桃仁 3.9%　红花 3.9%　郁金 5.9%　黄精 9.8%　葛根 14.7%　血竭 3.3%　没药 3.3%　延胡索 5.9%　冰片 0.6%　乳香 3.3%　鸡血藤 14.7%

〔功能与主治〕　活血行瘀。用于真心痛，胸闷，气短，心悸。

〔用法与用量〕　口服，1 次 5 片，1 日 3 次。

〔剂型与规格〕　糖衣片，每片(基片)重 0.3 g

〔附注〕　本品具有扩张冠状动脉血管，改善心脏供血，降低心肌耗氧量的作用，并能降低血脂及血液粘度，扩张脑动脉，改善脑供血状况。临床适用于冠状动脉供血不足，心绞痛，脑血栓等。

复方丹参注射液

〔药物组成〕　丹参 90.9%　降香 9.1%

〔功能与主治〕　活血通经，行气止痛。用于真心痛，厥心痛，胸闷等。

〔用法与用量〕　肌肉注射，1 日 2 次，1 次 2 ml；静脉滴注遵医嘱。

〔剂型与规格〕　注射剂，每支装 2 ml

〔附注〕　药理实验表明，丹参，降香均具改善心肌收缩力，扩张冠状动脉，增加冠脉流量，减慢心率，明显改善心脏功能的作用，丹参尚能降低血液粘稠度，改善微循环。本品临床适用于冠心病，心肌梗塞。

丹参注射液具有与本品类似的作用，但改善微循环，降低心肌耗氧量的作用不及本品。

2.2 抗高血压药

牛黄降压片

〔药物组成〕　牛黄等

〔功能与主治〕　清心化痰，镇静降压。用于肝阳上亢，头目眩晕，痰火壅盛，昏迷口禁，肢体麻木，半身不遂，口眼㖞斜。

〔用法与用量〕　口服，1 次 1～2 片，1 日 2 次。

〔剂型与规格〕　蜜丸，每丸重 1.6 g

〔附注〕　本品具有降低血压，调整中枢神经系统功能，镇静等作用。临床适用于肝阳上亢及痰火壅盛型高血压，脑血管意外等。

腹泻者忌服。

脑 立 清 丸

〔药物组成〕　赭石 18.4%　磁石 10.5%　清半夏 10.5%　酒曲 10.5%　熟酒曲 10.5%　牛膝 10.5%　珍珠母 5.3%　薄荷脑 2.6%　冰片 2.6%　鲜猪胆汁 18.4%

〔功能与主治〕　重镇潜阳，醒脑安神。用于阴虚阳亢，头晕目眩，中风，口眼㖞斜。

〔用法与用量〕　口服，1 次 10 粒，1 日 2 次。

〔剂型与规格〕　水丸，每 10 粒重 1 g

〔附注〕　本品具有扩张周围毛细血管，降低血压，解热镇痛的作用。临床适用于Ⅰ、Ⅱ型高血压(阴虚阳亢型)，脑血管痉挛。

舒心降压片

〔药物组成〕　丹参11.8%　郁金5.9%　菊花7.8%　红花5.9%　槐米7.8%　石菖蒲5.9%　槲寄生9.8%　葛根11.8%　桃仁7.8%　柏子仁7.8%　钩藤11.8%　牛膝5.9%

〔功能与主治〕　活血化瘀，舒心降压。用于头晕目眩，头痛脑胀，真心痛，厥心痛。

〔用法与用量〕　口服，1次6～8片，1日3次。

〔剂型与规格〕　片剂，每片重0.3g

〔附注〕　本品能扩张冠状动脉和周围血管，降低血压，血脂，减小血液粘度，延长血小板聚集时间。临床适用于原发性高血压，冠心病，动脉硬化等。

复方罗布麻片

〔药物组成〕　罗布麻　防己　野菊花等

〔功能与主治〕　清热利水，平肝安神。用于肝阳上亢，头晕目眩，头痛脑胀。

〔用法与用量〕　口服，1次2片，1日3次。

〔剂型与规格〕　片剂，每片重0.1g

〔附注〕　本品具有降低血压，扩张周围毛细血管及利尿作用。临床适用于轻、中度高血压症，可减轻其头痛，头晕，失眠等症状，对患有胃溃疡，慢性鼻炎及抑郁症的高血压患者也可应用。

杜仲降压片

〔药物组成〕　杜仲　黄芩　钩藤　夏枯草　益母草

〔功能与主治〕　镇肝熄风。用于肝阳上亢，头目眩晕，头痛脑胀。

〔用法与用量〕　口服，1次5片，1日3次。

〔剂型与规格〕　片剂，每片重0.3g

〔附注〕　本品具有扩张毛细血管，利尿，降低血压的作用。临床适用于轻、中度高血压。

孕妇忌服。

降 压 平 片

〔药物组成〕　夏枯草10.5%　黄芩10.5%　槲寄生10.5%　葛根10.5%　珍珠母10.5%　槐花10.5%　生地黄5.4%　菊花10.5%　淡竹叶10.5%　地龙10.5%　薄荷冰0.01%

〔功能与主治〕　平肝熄风。用于肝阳上亢，头晕，目眩。

〔用法与用量〕　口服，1次4片，1日3次。

〔剂型与规格〕　糖衣片，每片(基片)重0.3g

〔附注〕　本品具有降低血脂浓度，降低血液粘度，扩张周围毛细血管，降血压等作用。临床适用于高血压症，并可预防动脉硬化。

罗布麻降压片

〔药物组成〕　罗布麻　泽泻　夏枯草　珍珠母

〔功能与主治〕　平肝降压，镇静安神，强心利尿。用于肝阳上亢，头目眩晕。

〔用法与用量〕　口服，1次2~4片，1日3次。

〔剂型与规格〕　片剂，每片重0.3g

〔附注〕　本品临床适用于轻、中度高血压。

2.3　降血脂药

降脂灵胶丸

〔药物组成〕　蒲黄　菜子油

〔功能与主治〕　降低血清胆固醇和甘油三酯。用于高脂血症。

〔用法与用量〕　口服，1次5粒，1日3次。

〔剂型与规格〕　胶丸，每粒重0.25 g

〔附注〕　本品具有降血脂作用。临床适用于高脂血症及冠心病的预防。

消栓通络片

〔药物组成〕　三七8%　川芎15.9%　黄芪23.9%　郁金8%　桂枝8%　山楂8%　木香4%　泽泻8%　槐米4%　丹参12%　冰片0.3%

〔功能与主治〕　活血化瘀，温经通络。用于中风，不醒人事，精神呆滞，舌质发硬，言语迟涩，发音不清，手足发凉。

〔用法与用量〕　口服，1次8片，1日3次。

〔剂型与规格〕　糖衣片，每片(基片)重0.4 g

〔附注〕　本品能够降低血清胆固醇，三酸甘油酯，β-脂蛋白的浓度，降低血液粘度，减小血小板的聚集性，能扩张心脑血管，改善脑血管硬化患者的脑供血状况，并有一定的降压作用。临床适用于高脂血症，脑血管硬化，脑血栓等引起的精神呆滞。

脉安冲剂

〔药物组成〕　山楂50%　麦芽50%

〔功能与主治〕 降血脂，防止动脉粥样硬化。用于高脂血症。

〔用法与用量〕 口服，1次20g，1日2次。

〔剂型与规格〕 冲剂，每袋装20 g

〔附注〕 本品具有降低血脂，三酸甘油酯，胆固醇，β-脂蛋白浓度，降低血液粘度，扩张冠状动脉，改善心脑功能，降低心肌耗氧量，并能调整血压，促进排尿等作用。临床适用于高脂血症。

2.4 脑血管病用药

再 造 丸

〔药物组成〕 蕲蛇肉 全蝎 地龙 僵蚕 牛黄等

〔功能与主治〕 祛风化痰，活血通络。用于中风，口眼喎斜，半身不遂，手足麻木，疼痛拘挛，语言蹇塞。

〔用法与用量〕 口服，1次1丸，1日2次。

〔剂型与规格〕 蜜丸，每丸重9 g

〔附注〕 本品具有调节机体代谢，改善机体功能，促进微循环，滋养神经的作用。临床适用于脑血管意外后遗症，并可预防高血压和脑血管意外。

孕妇禁用。

人参再造丸

〔药物组成〕 乌梢蛇 槲寄生 威灵仙 全蝎 葛根麻黄 白芷 大黄 人参等

〔功能与主治〕 舒筋活血，祛风化痰。用于中风，口眼歪斜，言语不清，手足拘挛，半身不遂。

〔用法与用量〕 口服，1次1丸，1日2次。

〔剂型与规格〕 蜜丸，每丸重10 g

〔附注〕 本品具有改善微循环，调节机体功能，促进机体代谢及滋养强壮作用。临床适用于脑血管意外后遗症恢复期。

本品与再造丸相比，加强了滋补和改善微循环的作用，更适用于久病、体虚者。

孕妇忌服。

消栓再造丸

〔药物组成〕 川芎 丹参 三七 天麻 白花蛇 安息香 苏合香 人参 沉香等

〔功能与主治〕 活血化瘀，祛风通络，补气养血。用于中风，口眼㖞斜，半身不遂。

〔用法与用量〕 口服，1 次 1～2 丸，1 日 2 次。

〔剂型与规格〕 蜜丸，每丸重 9 g

〔附注〕 本品具有降低血脂及血液粘度，改善微循环及脑血管供血状况的作用，并能抗血小板凝聚，对已凝聚的血小板有解聚作用。临床适用于脑血栓形成，脑栓塞，高脂血症。

红花注射液

〔药物组成〕 红花 100%

〔功能与主治〕 活血化瘀。用于中风，口眼㖞斜，半身不遂以及胸痹，真心痛。

〔用法与用量〕 静脉滴注，1 次 15 ml，用 10% 葡萄糖注射液 250～500 ml 稀释。[1 日 1 次，15～20 天为 1 疗程；治疗冠心病。]静脉滴注，1 次 5～20 ml，方法同上；治疗脉管炎，肌肉注射，1 次 2.5～5 ml，1 日 1～2 次。

〔剂型与规格〕 注射剂，每支装 5 ml

〔附注〕 本品具有扩张冠状动脉，增加冠脉流量，降低血液粘度，改善微循环等作用。临床适用于闭塞性脑血管病，冠心病，心肌梗塞，脉管炎等。

局方牛黄清心丸

〔药物组成〕　牛黄　羚羊角　冰片　黄芩　白蔹　雄黄　柴胡　麦门冬　白芍　当归　肉桂　干姜　大豆黄卷　防风　桔梗　神曲　杏仁等

〔功能与主治〕　清心化痰，镇惊祛风。用于痰涎壅盛，神志不清，头晕目眩，癫痫惊风，痰迷心窍。

〔用法与用量〕　口服，1次1丸，1日1次。

〔剂型与规格〕　蜜丸，每丸重3g

〔附注〕　处方来源于宋·陈师文《太平惠民和剂局方》。

本品具有镇静解痉，解热，改善微循环及降压作用。临床适用于脑血管痉挛，脑溢血后遗症，癫痫等。

孕妇忌服。

华佗再造丸

〔药物组成〕　（略）

〔功能与主治〕　舒筋活络，祛风养血。用于中风，半身不遂，口眼㖞斜，手足拘挛，言语不清，胸痹等。

〔用法与用量〕　口服，1次1～2丸，1日1～2次。

〔剂型与规格〕　蜜丸，每丸重3g

〔附注〕　本品具有调整机体机能，改善微循环，扩张冠状动脉，增加冠脉血流量，提高心脏抗缺氧能力，滋养等作用，并能降低血胆固醇及甘油三酯的浓度，降低血液粘度，改善脑血管血循环。临床适用于脑溢血，脑血栓，脑血管痉挛等脑血管疾病及冠心病，心绞痛，心功能不全等心血管疾病。

据报道：本品对脑血管疾病总有效率 94.2%，对心血管疾病总有效率 93.2%。

3 呼吸系统药物

3.1 祛痰、镇咳药

茯 苓 丸

〔药物组成〕 茯苓 33.3% 半夏 16.7% 枳壳 8.3% 风化硝 41.7%

〔功能与主治〕 祛湿化痰，通络止痛。用于脾胃虚弱，筋脉拘急，四肢麻痛等。

〔用法与用量〕 口服，1 次 5～9 g，1 日 2 次。

〔剂型与规格〕 浓缩丸，每袋装 18 g

〔附注〕 处方来源于明·王肯堂《证治准绳》。

本品临床适用于慢性支气管炎，哮喘以及风湿性肌纤维炎，神经炎等。

便溏者忌服。

二母宁嗽丸

〔药物组成〕 生石膏 16% 栀子 9.6% 茯苓 8% 枳实 5.6% 知母 12% 桑白皮 8% 黄芩 9.6% 瓜蒌子 8% 甘草 1.6% 贝母 12% 桔皮 8% 五味子 1.6%

〔功能与主治〕 清热化痰，顺气止嗽。用于肺热咳嗽，痰盛气促。

〔用法与用量〕 口服，1 次 2 丸，1 日 2 次。

〔剂型与规格〕 蜜丸，每丸重 9 g

〔附注〕 处方来源于明·龚信《古今医鉴》。

本品具有抑菌、消炎等作用。临床适用于慢性支气管炎，肺脓肿等。

肺结核患者忌服。

百合固金丸

〔药物组成〕 百合 7.6% 熟地黄 22.9% 麦门冬 11.5% 川贝母 7.6% 玄参 6.1% 地黄 15.3% 当归 7.6% 白芍 7.6% 桔梗 6.2% 甘草 7.6%

〔功能与主治〕 养肺润燥、止咳。用于肺肾阴虚咳喘，咽痛失血及虚劳骨蒸，午后潮热，口干小便赤。

〔用法与用量〕 口服，1 次 1 丸，1 日 1~2 次。

〔剂型与规格〕 蜜丸，每丸重 9 g

〔附注〕 处方来源于清·汪昂《医方集解》。

本品具有抑菌消炎、解热、止咳、止血及滋养强壮作用。临床适用于肺结核、肺炎、咽炎、百日咳、咯血等。

止嗽青果丸

〔药物组成〕 川贝母 3.4% 百合 4.5% 黄芩 8.9% 石膏 3.4% 青果 5.6% 桑白皮 8.9% 白果 22.3% 麻黄 17.9% 杏仁 1.7% 款冬花 8.9% 清半夏 8.9% 马兜铃 2.2% 甘草 3.4%

〔功能与主治〕 清热化痰，止咳平喘。用于咳嗽，痰多气喘，口苦咽干，老人哮喘。

〔用法与用量〕 口服，1 次 1 丸，1 日 2 次。

〔剂型与规格〕 蜜丸，每丸重 9 g

〔附注〕 本品具有镇咳祛痰，平喘的作用。临床适用于慢性支气管炎，支气管哮喘等。

肺结核，痰多呼吸困难者忌服。

清肺抑火丸

〔药物组成〕 黄芩 20% 栀子 14.1% 大黄 17.1%

黄柏 5.7%　　苦参 8.3%　　天花粉 10.4%　　知母 8.3%　　桔梗 10.4%　　前胡 5.7%

〔功能与主治〕　　清热通便，止咳化痰。用于咳嗽痰盛，咽喉肿痛，口干舌燥，大便秘结。

〔用法与用量〕　　口服，1 次 1 丸，1 日 2 次。

〔剂型与规格〕　　蜜丸，每丸重 9 g

〔附注〕　　处方来源于明·龚廷贤《寿世保元》。

本品具有祛痰、止咳、平喘、抑菌、消炎作用。临床适用于慢性支气管炎，支气管扩张，肺结核，肺脓肿，肺寄生虫病，支气管肿瘤等。

感冒所致咳嗽慎用。

尚有同名片剂、水丸、膏滋，药物组成，功用同上。

二 陈 丸

〔药物组成〕　　姜半夏 34.5%　　陈皮 34.5%　　茯苓 20.7%　　甘草 10.3%

〔功能与主治〕　　祛痰化湿，和胃调气。用于咳嗽痰多而粘，胸腹胀满，恶心呕吐，头眩心悸等。

〔用法与用量〕　　口服，1 次 1 丸，1 日 2 次。

〔剂型与规格〕　　蜜丸，每丸重 6 g

〔附注〕　　处方来源于宋·陈师文《太平惠民和剂局方》。

本品具有抑菌、消炎、止咳、促进呼吸道分泌，有利于排痰，以及健胃助消化作用，临床适用于慢性支气管炎，咳嗽多痰并伴有厌食，吐酸烧心等胃肠症状者，慢性肠胃炎兼有咳嗽多痰者。

橘 红 丸

〔药物组成〕　　橘红 11.1%　　陈皮 7.4%　　法半夏 5.6%

石膏 7.4%　　浙贝母 7.4%　　栝蒌皮 7.4%　　紫菀 5.6%　　款冬花 3.7%　　苦杏仁 7.4%　　紫苏子 5.6%　　桔梗 5.6%　　麦门冬 7.4%　　地黄 7.4%　　茯苓 7.4%　　甘草 3.6%

〔功能与主治〕　　清肺祛湿，止嗽化痰。用于咳嗽痰盛，呼吸气促，口苦咽干，胸中痞满，饮食无味。

〔用法与用量〕　　口服，1 次 2 丸，1 日 2 次。

〔剂型与规格〕　　蜜丸，每丸重 6 g

〔附注〕　　处方来源于明·龚信《古今医鉴》。

本品具有抑菌、消炎、祛痰、扩张支气管平滑肌等作用。临床适用于急、慢性支气管炎，多痰咳嗽，呼吸气促，口干，厌食等。

感冒发烧者忌用。

尚有同名冲剂、药物组成、功用同上。

清气化痰丸

〔药物组成〕　　胆南星 16.7%　　黄芩 11.1%　　瓜蒌仁 11.1%　　枳实 11.1%　　桔红 11.1%　　姜半夏 16.7%　　杏仁 11.1%　　茯苓 11.1%

〔功能与主治〕　　清肺止嗽，降逆化痰。用于咳嗽喘促，胸膈痞闷，恶心呕吐。

〔用法与用量〕　　口服，1 次 6-9 g，1 日 2 次。

〔剂型与规格〕　　药汁丸，每袋装 18 g

〔附注〕　　处方来源于明·张介宾《景岳全书》。

本品具有抑菌、消炎、扩张支气管平滑肌解除其痉挛，并能增加呼吸道分泌，以便痰液排出。临床适用于慢性支气管炎、痰多、便秘、尿黄者。

风寒咳嗽和干咳无痰者忌用。

控涎丸

〔药物组成〕　白芥子 33.3%　甘遂 33.3%　红大戟 33.3%

〔功能与主治〕　攻泄痰饮，消水解毒。用于痰饮咳喘胁痛，胸腔积水。

〔用法与用量〕　口服，1 次 1-3 g，1 日 1-2 次。

〔剂型与规格〕　水丸，每袋装 6 g

〔附注〕　处方来源于宋·陈言《三因极·病证方论》。

本品具有抑菌、消炎、祛痰和较强的利尿作用。临床适用于咳喘胸痛，胸腹水肿，四肢水肿，支气管炎，肺炎，慢性淋巴结炎、颈项淋巴结核、骨结核，肝硬化腹水，渗出性胸膜炎，晚期血吸虫病腹水等。

孕妇及体弱患者忌用。

尚有同名糊丸、蜜丸，药物组成，功用同上。

通宣理肺丸

〔药物组成〕　麻黄 9.2%　紫苏叶 14%　前胡 9.3%　杏仁 7%　桔梗 9.3%　陈皮 9.3%　半夏 7%　茯苓 9.3%　枳壳 9.3%　黄芩 9.3%　甘草 7%

〔功能与主治〕　宣肺止咳。用于外感风寒咳嗽，发热恶寒，头痛无汗，肢体酸痛。

〔用法与用量〕　口服，1 次 2 丸，1 日 2-3 次。

〔剂型与规格〕　蜜丸，每丸重 6 g

〔附注〕　处方来源于明·王肯堂《证治准绳》。

本品具有解热、抗菌、消炎、镇咳作用。临床适用于流行性感冒，支气管炎等。

尚有同名片剂，药物组成，功用同上。

罗汉果冲剂

〔药物组成〕 罗汉果100%

〔功能与主治〕 清热润肺，祛痰止咳。用于肺热痰多，咳嗽喘息。

〔用法与用量〕 口服，1次1包，1日2~3次。

〔剂型与规格〕 冲剂，每包装15 g

〔附注〕 本品具有解热、消炎、抑菌、祛痰止咳作用，并具有提高机体免疫能力和滋养强壮作用。临床适用于感冒咳嗽、喉痛、失音，急、慢性支气管炎等。

川贝枇杷止咳冲剂

〔药物组成〕 枇杷叶 桔梗 川贝母 薄荷脑 苦杏仁等

〔功能与主治〕 镇咳祛痰。用于咳嗽痰多，喘促气逆，口干舌燥。

〔用法与用量〕 口服，1次1袋，1日3次，小儿酌减。

〔剂型与规格〕 冲剂，每袋重10 g

〔附注〕 本品能刺激咽头粘膜及胃粘膜反射性引起呼吸道粘膜产生分泌亢进，稀释并排除储于支气管和气管中的痰液，产生祛痰镇咳作用。临床适用于支气管哮喘，支气管炎，慢性咽喉炎。

养阴清肺膏

〔药物组成〕 地黄 24.7% 玄参 19.8% 麦门冬 14.8% 川贝母 9.9% 牡丹皮 9.9% 当归 9.9% 薄荷 6.2% 甘草 4.8%

〔功能与主治〕 养阴清肺、利咽。用于阴虚咳嗽，口渴咽干，失音声哑，痰中带血，咽喉肿痛。

〔用法与用量〕　口服，1 次 15 g，1 日 2 次。

〔剂型与规格〕　膏滋，大瓶装 60 g，小瓶装 30 g

〔附注〕　处方来源于清·郑梅涧《重楼玉钥》。

药理试验表明，本品对白喉杆菌有较好的抑制作用，体外对白喉毒素有很高的"中和能力"。临床适用于感冒咳嗽、白喉、咽炎、扁桃体炎，尤其对急性扁桃体炎，效果更好。

尚有同名丸剂，药物组成，功用同上。

二　冬　膏

〔药物组成〕　天门冬 50%　麦门冬 50%

〔功能与主治〕　润肺生津止渴。用于咳嗽、烦渴、咽喉疼痛，声哑失音，痰中带血。

〔用法与用量〕　口服，1 次 15 g，1 日 2 次。

〔剂型与规格〕　膏滋，每瓶装 60 g

〔附注〕　处方来源于清·张璐《张氏医通》。

本品具有抑菌、消炎，增加呼吸道分泌，以及止血作用。临床适用于百日咳、咽炎，并可作为肺结核病的配合治疗药。

感冒咳嗽患者忌服。

复方百部止咳糖浆

〔药物组成〕　百部 16.7%　黄芩 16.7%　苦杏仁 8.3%　陈皮 16.7%　桔梗 8.3%　桑白皮 8.3%　麦冬 4.2%　天南星 4.2%　知母 4.2%　枳壳 8.3%　甘草 4.1%

〔功能与主治〕　清肺止咳。用于肺热咳嗽，痰黄粘稠。

〔用法与用量〕　口服，1 次 10~20 ml，1 日 2~3 次，小儿酌减。

〔剂型与规格〕　糖浆剂，每瓶装 100 ml

〔附注〕 本品临床适用于上呼吸道感染咳嗽，小儿百日咳等。

润肺补膏

〔药物组成〕 莱阳梨清膏 党参等

〔功能与主治〕 益气润肺，止咳化痰。用于肺燥久咳，咽干音哑。

〔用法与用量〕 口服，1 次 15 g，1 日 2 次。

〔剂型与规格〕 膏滋剂，每瓶装 250 g

〔附注〕 本品具有祛痰健胃作用，能增进新陈代谢，帮助消化，促进乳糜吸收。临床适用于慢性支气管炎，支气管哮喘，老年性支气管哮喘等。

川贝止咳糖浆

〔药物组成〕 川贝母 28.3% 枇杷叶 64.7% 苦杏仁精 1.5% 薄荷脑 0.1% 桔梗 5.4%

〔功能与主治〕 润肺祛痰、止咳。用于感冒引起的咳嗽，气急喘息。

〔用法与用量〕 口服，1 次 10 ml，1 日 3 次，小儿酌减。

〔剂型与规格〕 糖浆剂，每瓶装 100 ml

〔附注〕 本品具有祛痰，镇咳作用，能增加呼吸道分泌，促进痰液排出。临床适用于上呼吸道感染及支气管疾病所致的咳嗽，痰多等。

莱阳梨止咳糖浆

〔药物组成〕 莱阳梨清膏 66.3% 北沙参流浸膏 5.1% 桔梗流浸膏 6.3% 远志流浸膏 3.3% 百合流浸膏 2.5% 杏仁水 3.8% 麻黄提取液 12.7%

〔功能与主治〕 止咳祛痰。用于伤风感冒，咳嗽痰多。

〔用法与用量〕 口服，1 次 10 ml，1 日 4 次，小儿酌减。

〔剂型与规格〕 糖浆剂，每瓶装 100 ml

〔附注〕 本品具有镇咳祛痰作用。临床适用于感冒咳嗽，痰多，急、慢性支气管炎。

尚有同名冲剂，药物组成，功用同上。

麻杏止咳糖浆

〔药物组成〕 麻黄 15.5%　苦杏仁 15.5%　生石膏 43.1%　薄荷 15.5%　甘草 10.4%

〔功能与主治〕 清热宣肺，止咳平喘。用于咳嗽、痰多、咳逆气急。

〔用法与用量〕 口服，1 次 10 ml，1 日 3 次，小儿酌减。

〔剂型与规格〕 糖浆剂，每瓶装 100 ml

〔附注〕 本品具有解热消炎、止咳、平喘作用。临床适用于感冒头痛发热，急性支气管炎，大叶性肺炎，小儿支气管肺炎，猩红热，荨麻疹，急性结合膜炎，支气管哮喘等。

半 夏 露

〔药物组成〕 生半夏 14.2%　桔皮酊 29.6%　枳壳 7.4%　枇杷叶 8.5%　远志 9.1%　紫菀 8.5%　麻黄 5.7%　薄荷油 0.5%　杏仁水 10.8%　桔梗 5.7%

〔功能与主治〕 止咳化痰。用于咳嗽痰多，喘促气逆等。

〔用法与用量〕 口服，1 次 10 ml，1 日 3 次。

〔剂型与规格〕 糖浆剂，每瓶装 100 ml

〔附注〕 本品具有抑菌、消炎、止咳、祛痰的作用。临床适用于各种咳嗽、痰多、支气管炎等。

尚有同名冲剂，药物组成，功用同上。

杏仁止咳糖浆

〔药物组成〕　杏仁水 10.6%　远志流浸膏 6.1%　桔梗流浸膏 5.3%　百部流浸膏 5.3%　陈皮流浸膏 3.9%　甘草流浸膏 3.9%　砂糖 64.9%

〔功能与主治〕　化痰止咳。用于咳嗽痰多，气促喘息。

〔用法与用量〕　口服，1 次 15 ml，1 日 3～4 次，小儿酌减。

〔剂型与规格〕　糖浆剂，每瓶装 100 ml

〔附注〕　本品具有镇咳祛痰作用。临床适用于感冒咳嗽、喉炎、咽炎，急、慢性支气管炎。

小青龙合剂

〔药物组成〕　麻黄 12.5%　桂枝 12.5%　白芍 12.5%　干姜 12.5%　细辛 6.2%　五味子 12.5%　半夏 18.8%　甘草 12.5%

〔功能与主治〕　解表祛痰，止咳平喘。用于外感风寒，发热无汗，喘咳痰稀。

〔用法与用量〕　口服，1 次 15～20 ml，1 日 3 次，用时摇匀。

〔剂型与规格〕　合剂，每瓶装 100 ml

〔附注〕　处方来源于汉·张仲景《伤寒论》。

本品具有解热、镇痛、祛痰、止咳、平喘作用。临床适用于慢性支气管炎，支气管哮喘，老年性肺气肿及合并上呼吸道感染、流感等。

炙甘草合剂

〔药物组成〕　炙甘草 9%　桂枝 6%　生姜 9%　大枣 12.1%　胡麻仁 9%　阿胶 9%　人参 6%　麦冬 9%　生地黄 30.9%

〔功能与主治〕　益气滋阴，补血复脉。用于虚热咳嗽，气虚血少，心悸等。

〔用法与用量〕　口服，1 次 15~20 ml，1 日 3 次。

〔剂型与规格〕　合剂，每瓶装 500 ml

〔附注〕　本品具有解热消炎、止咳作用，能提高机体免疫能力，调节机体代谢与器管功能，促进机体造血机能等。临床适用于肺结核，肺气肿，心律不齐，神经衰弱。

鲜竹沥口服液

〔药物组成〕　鲜竹沥　鱼腥草　枇杷叶　制半夏　生姜等

〔功能与主治〕　清热化痰。用于肺热咳嗽痰多，气喘胸闷，中风舌强等。

〔用法与用量〕　口服，1 次 15~30 ml，1 日 2~3 次。

〔剂型与规格〕　口服液，每瓶装 30 ml

〔附注〕　本品具有解热，镇咳、祛痰作用。临床适用于感冒咳嗽、气管炎、支气管哮喘，高热抽搐等。

痰 咳 净

〔药物组成〕　杏仁　桔梗　甘草　龙脑　远志

〔功能与主治〕　止咳、祛痰。用于气促喘息，多痰、咳嗽。

〔用法与用量〕　口腔或舌下含服，1 日 3~6 次，成人 1 次 0.2 g，小儿酌减。

〔剂型与规格〕 散剂，每盒装 6 g

〔附注〕 药理试验表明，本品扩张支气管平滑肌，解除其痉挛而起到镇咳、平喘的作用，同时增加呼吸道分泌，以便痰液易于排出。抑菌试验表明：本品对咽喉部常见的致病菌有较强的抑菌作用，故有较好的消炎效果。临床适用于急、慢性支气管炎、支气管哮喘、肺气肿、咽喉炎等。

临床验证 300 多例，均认为本药是一种新型快速排痰、镇咳药。

孕妇慎用。

蛇胆陈皮末

〔药物组成〕 蛇胆汁 0.02%　陈皮 94.1%　地龙炭 1.9%　朱砂 1.9%　僵蚕 1.9%　琥珀 0.2%

〔功能与主治〕 祛风除痰，镇惊定喘。用于风热发狂，精神不安，咳嗽喘促。

〔用法与用量〕 口服，1 次 0.6 g，1 日 2-3 次，两岁以下儿童减半。

〔剂型与规格〕 散剂，每瓶装 0.6 g

〔附注〕 本品具有解热、镇咳、祛痰作用。临床适用于感冒咳嗽，小儿百日咳，小儿上呼吸道感染等。

据报道：本品临床治疗 59 例百日咳，平均 7-10 天为 1 疗程，总有效率为 94.9%。

蛇胆川贝末

〔药物组成〕 蛇胆汁 14.2%　川贝母 85.8%

〔功能与主治〕 清肺止咳化痰。用于肺热咳嗽，痰多。

〔用法与用量〕 口服，1 次 0.3-0.6 g，1 日 2-3 次。小儿酌减。

〔剂型与规格〕 散剂，每瓶装 0.6 g

〔附注〕 本品具有镇咳、祛痰、消炎作用。临床适用于感冒咳嗽，小儿百日咳等。

桃 花 散

〔药物组成〕 石膏 43.9%　贝母 3.4%　半夏 43.9%
朱砂 8.8%

〔功能与主治〕 清热祛痰，止嗽定喘。用于肺热、咳嗽、喘息。

〔用法与用量〕 口服，1 次 1 袋，1 日 2 次。3 岁以下儿童酌减。

〔剂型与规格〕 散剂，每袋装 1 g

〔附注〕 本品具有扩张支气管平滑肌，解除支气管平滑肌痉挛及祛痰作用。临床适用于肺炎，急、慢性支气管炎等。

紫花杜鹃片

〔药物组成〕 紫花杜鹃 100%

〔功能与主治〕 止咳祛痰。用于咳嗽喘息。

〔用法与用量〕 口服，1 次 5 片，1 日 3 次。

〔剂型与规格〕 片剂，每片重 0.25 g

〔附注〕 本品为紫花杜鹃浸膏片，具有祛痰镇咳作用。临床适用于慢性支气管炎。

据报道：用本品治疗老年慢性支气管炎 2921 例，1-2 个疗程(10-20 天)，有效率 90.2%。

尚有同名胶囊，药物组成，功用同上。

3.2　平喘药

复方川贝精片

〔药物组成〕 川贝母 35.8%　盐酸麻黄碱 0.5%　陈皮

13.4%　法半夏 10.8%　远志 7.6%　桔梗 13.4%　五味子 7.6%　甘草 10.9%

〔功能与主治〕　止咳化痰，润肺平喘。用于风寒痰喘咳嗽，气促喘息。

〔用法与用量〕　口服，1 次 3-6 片，1 日 3 次。小儿酌减。

〔剂型与规格〕　糖衣片，每片(基片)重 0.25 g(相当于原药材 0.5 g)

〔附注〕　本品具有抑菌、消炎、祛痰、扩张支气管平滑肌，解除支气管平滑肌痉挛作用。临床适用于急、慢性支气管炎，咳嗽、痰多等。

高血压、心脏病、冠状动脉硬化患者及孕妇忌服。

止咳喘热参片

〔药物组成〕　热参 100%

〔功能与主治〕　平喘止咳，祛痰。用于喘息胸闷、痰多、咳嗽。

〔用法与用量〕　口服，1 次 1-2 片，1 日 3 次。

〔剂型与规格〕　片剂，每片含莨菪碱 0.12 mg

〔附注〕　本品具有显著的平喘作用，能抑制气管及支气管粘膜腺体分泌，使痰量减少，并能缓解支气管痉挛。临床适用于支气管哮喘，各型慢性支气管炎。

青光眼病人和孕妇忌用。

尚有同名气雾剂，药物组成，功用同上。

喘　舒　片

〔药物组成〕　升华硫　大黄　黄芩提取物等。

〔功能与主治〕　平喘止咳，温肾纳气。用于肾虚气喘，喘息胸闷。

〔用法与用量〕 口服，1次2片，1日3次。小儿酌减。

〔剂型与规格〕 糖衣片，每片(基片)重0.35 g

〔附注〕 本品具有镇咳，平喘作用。临床适用于支气管哮喘，肺气肿、慢性气管炎，尤适用于喘息型气管炎。

牡荆油胶丸

〔药物组成〕 牡荆100%

〔功能与主治〕 平喘、镇咳、祛痰。用于气急喘息，痰多、咳嗽。

〔用法与用量〕 口服，1次1丸，重者2丸，1日3次。

〔剂型与规格〕 胶丸，每丸含油1.7 mg

〔附注〕 本品具有平喘、镇咳、祛痰的作用，临床适用于支气管扩张症，慢性支气管炎和急性肺脓肿等的对症治疗。

芸香油滴丸

〔药物组成〕 芸香油100%

〔功能与主治〕 平喘、镇咳。用于咳嗽、痰多、气急喘息。

〔用法与用量〕 口服，1次4-6丸，1日3次，饭后服。

〔剂型与规格〕 肠溶丸，每丸含芸香油0.2 ml

〔附注〕 本品具有平喘、镇咳、扩张支气管平滑肌的作用。临床适用于喘息型慢性支气管炎和支气管哮喘等。

尚有同名片剂，药物组成，功用同上。

艾叶油气雾剂

〔药物组成〕　艾叶油100%

〔功能与主治〕　平喘、止咳、祛痰。用于咳嗽、痰多、气急喘息。

〔用法与用量〕　鼻吸及口吸入，1次喷吸2~3下，1日3次。

〔剂型与规格〕　气雾剂，每瓶装14 ml，含艾叶油3 ml

〔附注〕　本品具有松弛支气管平滑肌，解除支气管痉挛的作用，并有一定的镇咳、祛痰、抑菌和抗过敏作用。临床适用于支气管哮喘、支气管炎、口腔有白色念珠菌感染的患者。

尚有同名胶囊剂，药物组成，功用同上。

百花定喘丸

〔药物组成〕　百合7.1%　款冬花3.7%　石膏3.7%　天花粉7.1%　黄芩7.1%　牡丹皮7.1%　北沙参3.7%　天门冬7.1%　麦门冬7.1%　五味子3.7%　麻黄7.1%　桔梗7.1%　紫菀7.1%　苦杏仁7.1%　前胡7.1%　陈皮7.1%　薄荷冰0.01%

〔功能与主治〕　清热止咳，化痰定喘。用于风热所致的咳嗽，气喘，咽干口渴。

〔用法与用量〕　口服，1次1丸，1日2次。

〔剂型与规格〕　蜜丸，每丸重9 g

〔附注〕　处方来源于清·吴仪洛《成方切用》。

本品具有平喘、止咳、祛痰的作用。临床适用于支气管炎、肺炎、肺气肿等。

感冒引起的气喘，咳嗽不宜使用。

尚有同名片剂。药物组成，功用同上。

蛤蚧定喘丸

〔药物组成〕　蛤蚧 0.4%　鳖甲 9%　黄连 5.1%　黄芩 9%　石膏 9%　麦门冬 9%　百合 13.5%　紫菀 13.5%　栝蒌子 9%　紫苏子 4.5%　苦杏仁 9%　甘草 9%

〔功能与主治〕　滋阴清肺，止咳定喘。用于虚劳久咳，气短发热，自汗盗汗，胸满郁闷，不思饮食。

〔用法与用量〕　口服，1 次 1 丸，1 日 2 次。

〔剂型与规格〕　蜜丸，每丸重 9 g

〔附注〕　本品具有平喘、止咳、抑菌、消炎、扩张支气管的作用。临床适用于肺结核，老年支气管哮喘和慢性支气管炎等。

止嗽定喘丸

〔药物组成〕　麻黄 25%　杏仁 25%　生石膏 25%　甘草 25%

〔功能与主治〕　润肺化痰，止嗽定喘。用于风热引起的咳嗽气喘。

〔用法与用量〕　口服，1 次 6 g，1 日 2 次。

〔剂型与规格〕　水丸，每袋装 18 g

〔附注〕　处方来源于汉·张仲景《伤寒论》。

本品具有平喘、止咳、祛痰、消炎等作用。临床适用于急性支气管炎，哮喘性支气管炎，大叶性肺炎，小儿肺炎以及麻疹并发肺炎。

苏子降气丸

〔药物组成〕　苏子 10.6%　法半夏 10.6%　厚朴 10.6%　前胡 10.6%　桔皮 10.6%　沉香 7.4%　当归 7.4%　生姜 10.6%　红枣 10.6%　甘草 11.4%

〔功能与主治〕 降气平喘，温肾纳气。用于咳嗽喘促，胸膈满闷，头目昏眩，饮食少思，大便秘结，肢体浮肿等。

〔用法与用量〕 口服，1 次 3~6 g，1 日 2 次，空腹服。

〔剂型与规格〕 水丸，每袋装 18 g

〔附注〕 处方来源于宋·陈师文《太平惠民和剂局方》。

本品具有平喘、止咳、祛痰及抑菌消炎作用。临床适用于支气管哮喘，慢性支气管炎，肺气肿等。

定 喘 丸

〔药物组成〕 白果 31.3%　苦杏仁 6.3%　款冬花 11.3%　炙桑白皮 11.3%　黑苏子 7.5%　麻黄 11.3%　制半夏 11.3%　炒黄芩 6.3%　甘草 3.4%

〔功能与主治〕 定喘、平气。用于久咳虚喘，胸闷气短，喉中痰鸣。

〔用法与用量〕 口服，1 次 2 丸，1 日 2 次

〔剂型与规格〕 蜜丸，每丸重 6 g。

〔附注〕 本品具有平喘、止咳作用，能扩张支气管，解除支气管痉挛，改善肺功能。临床适用于各种疾病引起的肺功能障碍，慢性支气管炎，支气管哮喘等。

痰 喘 丸

〔药物组成〕 前胡　杏仁　细辛　桑叶　党参　半夏曲　桂花　贝母　紫菀　紫苏子　桔红　海浮石　桔梗　旋复花　甘草　远志　茯苓　款冬花　五味子　石膏　白芍　白前　射干　百部　黄芩　葶苈子　麻黄　大枣　薤白　马兜铃　海蛤　青黛　鲜姜　枇杷叶

〔功能与主治〕 散风祛痰，止咳定喘。用于肺热咳嗽，痰多喘息，胸膈胀满。

〔用法与用量〕　口服，1 次 6 g，1 日 2 次。小儿酌减。

〔剂型与规格〕　水丸，每 5 丸重约 1 g

〔附注〕　本品具有平喘、止咳祛痰，解热的作用。临床适用于上呼吸道感染咳嗽，支气管痿缩，支气管炎，支气管哮喘等。

消咳喘糖浆

〔药物组成〕　满山红 100%

〔功能与主治〕　平喘、止咳、祛痰。用于感冒咳嗽，气促喘息。

〔用法与用量〕　口服，1 次 7-10 ml，1 日 3 次。小儿酌减。

〔剂型与规格〕　糖浆剂，每瓶装 100 ml

〔附注〕　本品具有平喘、镇咳、祛痰作用。临床适用于单纯型慢性支气管炎，感冒咳嗽等。

尚有同名滴丸、胶囊，药物组成、功用同上。

4 消化系统药物

4.1 健胃、助消化药

附子理中丸

〔药物组成〕   附子 15.4%   党参 30.8%   白术 23.0%   干姜 15.4%   甘草 15.4%

〔功能与主治〕   温中散寒，健脾助阳。用于脾胃虚寒，阳虚较甚，下利不止，腹痛呕吐，手足厥冷。

〔用法与用量〕   口服，蜜丸 1 次 1 丸；水丸 1 次 6 g，1 日 2～3 次。

〔剂型与规格〕   蜜丸，每丸重 9 g；水丸，每 20 粒重 1 g

〔附注〕   处方来源于宋·陈师文《太平惠民和剂局方》。

本品具有健胃，消炎，增强胃肠活动功能的作用。临床适用于脾胃虚寒型急、慢性胃肠炎，消化不良，术后胃肠功能紊乱，胃及十二指肠溃疡，急慢性痢疾，胃扩张，胃下垂，溃疡性结肠炎，肠结核以及神经衰弱等。

尚有同名片剂，药物组成、功用同上。

木香顺气丸

〔药物组成〕   香附 7.5%   醋炙香附 7.5%   乌药 7.5%   陈皮 7.5%   莱菔子 7.5%   枳壳 7.5%   茯苓 7.5%   木香 7.5%   山楂 7.5%   麦芽 7.5%   槟榔 5.7%   青皮 5.7%   甘草 5.7%   六神曲 7.5%

〔功能与主治〕   顺气消食，宽中和胃。用于气滞不舒，胸脘痞闷，腹胀疼痛，胃呆食少，大便不爽。

〔用法与用量〕 口服，1 次 3～6 g，1 日 2～3 次。

〔剂型与规格〕 水丸，每 20 粒重 1 g

〔附注〕 处方来源于清·沈金鳌《沈氏尊生书》。

本品具有健胃，保肝，调节胃肠功能的作用。临床适用于气滞型慢性胃炎，慢性肠炎，慢性肝炎，早期肝硬化，消化不良等。

尚有同名片剂，药物组成、功用同上。

开胸顺气丸

〔药物组成〕 槟榔 24.5% 牵牛子 32.5% 陈皮 8.2% 厚朴 8.2% 木香 6.1% 三棱 8.2% 猪牙皂 4.1% 莪术 8.2%

〔功能与主治〕 消积化滞，行气止痛。用于停食停水，气郁不舒，胸胁胀满，胃脘疼痛。

〔用法与用量〕 口服，1 次 3～9 g，1 日 1～2 次。

〔剂型与规格〕 水丸，每 20 粒重 1 g

〔附注〕 处方来源于明·龚廷贤《寿世保元》。

本品具有健胃，调节胃肠功能的作用。临床适用于慢性胃炎，慢性肠炎，慢性肝炎等。

孕妇及年老体弱者忌服。

尚有同名片剂，药物组成、功用同上。

香砂六君丸

〔药物组成〕 木香 7.8% 砂仁 8.9% 党参 11.1% 茯苓 22.2% 白术 22.2% 陈皮 8.9% 半夏 11.1% 甘草(蜜炙)7.8%

〔功能与主治〕 健脾，理气，消胀，和胃。用于脾胃气虚，脘腹胀满，食少便溏，嗳气呕秽。

〔用法与用量〕 口服，1 次 6～9 g，1 日 2～3 次。

〔剂型与规格〕 水丸，每 20 粒重 1 g

〔附注〕 处方来源于宋·陈师文《太平惠民和剂局方》。

本品具有健胃，消炎，镇吐，调节胃肠活动功能的作用。临床适用于气虚性胃溃疡，十二指肠溃疡，胃扩张，慢性胃炎，慢性腹泻，胃肠功能紊乱，神经衰弱，胃肠型感冒等。

尚有同名片剂、合剂，药物组成、功用同上。

大 山 楂 丸

〔药物组成〕　山楂 77.0%　麦芽 11.5%　六神曲 11.5%

〔功能与主治〕　消食化滞，健胃和中。用于饮食停滞，脘腹胀满，水谷不化。

〔用法与用量〕　口服，1 次 1～2 丸，1 日 1～3 次，小儿减半。

〔剂型与规格〕　蜜丸，每丸重 9 g

〔附注〕　本品具有健胃，助消化作用。临床适用于单纯性消化不良，胃肠功能紊乱等。

不宜与碳酸氢钠，氢氧化铝，胃舒平，氨茶碱同服。

尚有同名冲剂，药物组成、功用同上。

平 胃 丸

〔药物组成〕　苍术 29.6%　甘草 11.1%　厚朴 18.6%　陈皮 11.1%　六神曲 29.6%

〔功能与主治〕　燥湿健脾，行气和胃。用于脾胃不和，脘腹胀满，恶心呕吐，大便溏薄。

〔用法与用量〕　口服，1 次 6 g，1 日 2 次。

〔剂型与规格〕　水丸，每 20 粒重 1 g

〔附注〕　处方来源于宋·陈师文《太平惠民和剂局方》。

本品具有健胃，增强胃肠活动功能的作用。临床适用于胃酸过多，慢性胃炎，胃无力或胃下垂，胃肠神经官能症，急性胃炎以及支气管哮喘等。

据报道，本品可治疗嘴下唇生疮，腹股沟发炎，霍乱病。

尚有同名片剂，药物组成、功用同上。

人参健脾丸

〔药物组成〕　人参 13.3%　山楂 10%　麦芽 13.3%　六神曲 16.8%　白术 13.3%　陈皮 13.3%　枳实 20%

〔功能与主治〕　补气健脾，理气消食。用于脾胃虚弱，饮食不消，胸脘痞满，气短乏力，肠鸣腹胀，大便溏泄。

〔用法与用量〕　口服，水丸 1 次 4 g，蜜丸 1 次 1 丸，1 日 2～3 次。

〔剂型与规格〕　水丸，每 20 粒重 1 g；蜜丸，每丸重 6 g

〔附注〕　处方来源于清·汪昂《医方集解》。

本品具有健胃，调节胃肠活动功能的作用。临床适用于脾虚型慢性肠胃炎，慢性肝炎，肠功能紊乱，结肠过敏，肠结核等。

香砂养胃丸

〔药物组成〕　香附 7.6%　甘草 3.2%　藿香 7.6%　枳实 7.6%　白术 10.9%　陈皮 10.9%　半夏 10.9%　茯苓 10.9%　木香 7.6%　砂仁 7.6%　豆蔻 7.6%　厚朴 7.6%

〔功能与主治〕　健脾养胃，理气化湿，行气宽胸。用于脾胃虚弱，两胁胀满，胃脘作痛，呕吐嘈杂，面色萎黄，四肢倦怠。

〔用法与用量〕　口服，1 次 9 g，1 日 2 次。

〔剂型与规格〕　水丸，每 50 粒重 3 g

〔附注〕　处方来源于明·龚廷贤《寿世保元》。

本品具有健胃，消炎，镇痛作用。临床适用于慢性胃炎，十二指肠溃疡，并可作为慢性肝炎的辅助治疗药物。

尚有同名片剂、冲剂，药物组成，功用同上。

四 君 子 丸

〔药物组成〕　党参 28.6%　茯苓 28.6%　白术 28.6%　甘

草 14.2%

〔功能与主治〕 补气，健脾，养胃。用于脾胃气虚，胃纳不佳，食少便溏。

〔用法与用量〕 口服，1 次 3～6 g，1 日 3 次。

〔剂型与规格〕 水丸，每 50 粒重 3 g

〔附注〕 处方来源于宋·陈师文《太平惠民和剂局方》。

本品具有健胃，助消化，增强机体免疫功能的作用。临床适用于脾胃气虚型慢性胃肠炎，胃无力，胃下垂，贫血和其他慢性消耗性疾病。

尚有同名合剂、冲剂，药物组成、功用同上。

六合定中丸

〔药物组成〕 广藿香 1.5% 紫苏叶 1.5% 香薷 1.5% 木香 3.3% 檀香 3.3% 厚朴 4.4% 枳壳 4.4% 陈皮 4.4% 桔梗 4.4% 甘草 4.4% 茯苓 4.4% 木瓜 4.4% 白扁豆 1.5% 山楂 4.4% 六神曲 17.4% 麦芽 17.4% 稻芽 17.4%

〔功能与主治〕 祛暑除湿，和中消食。用于夏伤暑湿，宿食停滞，寒热头痛，胸闷恶心，吐泻腹痛。

〔用法与用量〕 口服，1 次 3～6 g，1 日 2～3 次。

〔剂型与规格〕 水丸，每 50 粒重 3 g；蜜丸，每丸重 6 g

〔附注〕 处方来源于《古今医方集成》。

本品具有健胃，镇吐，解暑作用。临床适用于夏季胃肠型感冒，流行性腹泻，急性胃肠炎等。

本品与藿香正气水比较，藿香正气水偏重于治疗吐泻腹痛较急，暑湿较重者。

启 脾 丸

〔药物组成〕 人参 12% 茯苓 12% 白术 12% 甘草 6% 莲子 12% 陈皮 6% 山楂 6% 山药 12% 麦芽 6%

泽泻 6%　六神曲 10%

〔功能与主治〕　健脾和胃，消食止泻。用于脾胃虚弱，腹痛腹胀，呕吐泄泻。

〔用法与用量〕　口服，1 次 1 丸，1 日 2～3 次，小儿酌减。

〔剂型与规格〕　蜜丸，每丸重 3 g

〔附注〕　处方来源于明·李梴《医学入门》。

本品具有健胃，助消化，增强胃肠活动的作用。临床适用于慢性胃肠炎，慢性腹泻，消化不良以及其他慢性消耗性疾病。

尚有同名片剂，药物组成、功用同上。

香砂枳术丸

〔药物组成〕　木香 16.7%　砂仁 16.7%　枳实 16.7%　白术 50%

〔功能与主治〕　健胃醒脾，理气宽胸。用于脾虚食积，气滞不畅，脘腹胀闷，呕恶吞酸。

〔用法与用量〕　口服，1 次 9 g，1 日 1～2 次。

〔剂型与规格〕　水丸，每 20 粒重 1 g

〔附注〕　本品具有健胃，调节胃肠活动的作用。临床适用于年老体弱和小儿之消化不良，胃下垂，慢性胃炎等。

越 鞠 丸

〔药物组成〕　香附 20%　川芎 20%　栀子 20%　苍术 20%　六神曲 20%

〔功能与主治〕　理气解郁，宽中除满。用于气、血、痰、火、湿、食诸郁，胸脘痞闷，嗳气不舒，吞酸呕吐。

〔用法与用量〕　口服，1 次 6～9 g，1 日 2 次。

〔剂型与规格〕　水丸，每 50 粒重 3 g

〔附注〕 处方来源于元·朱震亨《丹溪心法》。

本品具有健胃，调节胃肠活动的作用。临床适用于消化不良，胃潴留，胃肠神经官能症等慢性胃肠道疾病和慢性肝炎，胆囊炎，痛经，精神抑郁症等。

体弱者慎用。

保 和 丸

〔药物组成〕 山楂 37.3%　六神曲 12.5%　半夏 12.5% 茯苓 12.5%　陈皮 6.3%　连翘 6.3%　莱菔子 6.3%　麦芽 6.3%

〔功能与主治〕 消食，导滞，和胃。用于食积停滞，脘腹胀满，嗳气厌食，呕吐泄泻。

〔用法与用量〕 口服，1 次 6～9 g，1 日 2 次，小儿酌减。

〔剂型与规格〕 水丸，每 50 粒重 3 g

〔附注〕 处方来源于元·朱震亨《丹溪心法》。

本品具有健胃，助消化作用。临床适用于消化不良，慢性胃炎，急性胃肠炎等。

小儿夜半咳嗽痰多，兼见厌食，腹胀者，用本品治疗效果显著。

尚有同名片剂，药物组成、功用同上。

沉香化气丸

〔药物组成〕 沉香 3.8%　木香 7.4%　广藿香 14.8%　香附 7.4%　砂仁 7.4%　陈皮 7.4%　莪术 14.8%　六神曲 14.8%　麦芽 14.8%　甘草 7.4%

〔功能与主治〕 理气疏肝，消积和胃。用于脾胃气滞，脘腹胀满，胸膈痞闷，不思饮食，嗳气泛酸。

〔用法与用量〕 口服，1 次 3～6 g，1 日 2 次。

〔剂型与规格〕 水丸，每 50 粒重 3 g

〔附注〕 本品具有调节胃肠活动功能，健胃作用。临床适用于气滞型胃肠功能紊乱及消化不良等。

尚有同名片剂，药物组成、功用同上。

左 金 丸

〔药物组成〕 黄连85.7% 吴茱萸14.3%

〔功能与主治〕 泻火疏肝，和胃降逆。用于肝火犯胃，胸脘胀痛，呕吐吞酸，口苦嘈杂，大便热泻。

〔用法与用量〕 口服，1次3～6g，1日2次。

〔剂型与规格〕 水丸，每50粒重3g

〔附注〕 处方来源于元·朱震亨《丹溪心法》。

本品具有抗菌消炎，制酸，镇吐作用。临床适用于急慢性胃炎，胃酸过多，胃及十二指肠溃疡，菌痢，腹膜炎等。

九气拈痛丸

〔药物组成〕 香附13.8% 木香3.5% 高良姜3.5% 陈皮6.9% 莪术27.4% 郁金6.9% 延胡索13.8% 槟榔6.9% 五灵脂13.8% 甘草3.5%

〔功能与主治〕 理气，活血，止痛。用于脘腹满闷，胸胁胀痛，呕吐酸水，痛经。

〔用法与用量〕 口服，1次6～9g，1日2次。

〔剂型与规格〕 水丸，每20粒重1g

〔附注〕 处方来源于明·龚廷贤《鲁府禁方》。

本品具有调节胃肠功能及抗炎镇痛作用。临床适用于慢性胃炎，急性胃肠炎，慢性肝炎，痛经等属于寒郁气滞者。

孕妇禁用。

清胃保安丸

〔药物组成〕 白术5.6% 陈皮5.6% 六神曲5.6% 麦

芽 5.6%　青皮 5.6%　茯苓 5.6%　枳壳 5.6%　甘草 5.6%　枳实 5.6%　砂仁 5.6%　厚朴 5.6%　槟榔 5.6%　酒曲 11%　山楂 22%

〔功能与主治〕　健脾和胃，消食化滞。用于食积停滞，脘腹胀闷。

〔用法与用量〕　口服，1 次 1 丸，不满周岁小儿 1／2～1／3 丸，1 日 2 次。

〔剂型与规格〕　蜜丸，每丸重 6 g

〔附注〕　本品具有健胃，助消化作用。临床适用于单纯性消化不良，慢性胃肠炎等。

沉香化滞丸

〔药物组成〕　沉香 8.8%　香附 70.6%　砂仁 8.8%　甘草 11.8%

〔功能与主治〕　理气化滞，消食健脾。用于胸膈胀满，气滞腹痛。

〔用法与用量〕　口服，1 次 6 g，1 日 2 次。

〔剂型与规格〕　水丸，每 50 粒重 3 g

〔附注〕　处方来源于明·龚廷贤《万病回春》。

本品具有调节胃肠活动及健胃作用。临床适用于气滞型慢性胃炎，慢性肝炎、胃肠神经官能症等。

戊 己 丸

〔药物组成〕　黄连 46.2%　白芍 46.2%　吴茱萸 7.6%

〔功能与主治〕　泄肝火，和脾胃。用于肝脾不和，胃痛吞酸，腹痛泄泻，小儿疳积。

〔用法与用量〕　口服，1 次 3～6 g，1 日 2 次。

〔剂型与规格〕　水丸，每 20 粒重 1 g

〔附注〕　处方来源于宋·陈师文《太平惠民和剂局方》。

本品具有抗菌消炎，健胃，止泻作用。临床适用于胃炎，急性胃肠炎，痢疾，小儿消化不良性腹泻等属于肝脾不和者。

肚 痛 丸

〔药物组成〕 豆蔻8.5% 干姜16.9% 砂仁8.5% 荜茇3.4% 厚朴8.5% 罂粟壳3.4% 肉桂8.5% 枳实16.9% 木香16.9% 乌药8.5%

〔功能与主治〕 温中散寒，理气止痛。用于停寒气滞，腹中冷痛，胸胁胀闷，呕逆吐酸。

〔用法与用量〕 口服，1次3g，1日2次。

〔剂型与规格〕 水丸，每20粒重1g

〔附注〕 本品具有健胃，制酸，镇痛作用。临床适用于脾胃虚寒型慢性胃炎，萎缩性胃炎，肠痉挛等。

小半夏合剂

〔药物组成〕 制半夏62.5% 生姜37.5%

〔功能与主治〕 止呕，降逆。用于胃气上逆，恶心呕吐。

〔用法与用量〕 口服，1次10～15ml，1日3次。

〔剂型与规格〕 合剂，每瓶装100ml

〔附注〕 本品具有调节植物神经功能，健胃作用。临床适用于慢性胃肠炎，妊娠呕吐等。

4.2 抗溃疡药

安 胃 片

〔药物组成〕 延胡索12.6% 白矾50% 海螵蛸37.4%

〔功能与主治〕 健脾和胃，温中止痛。用于脘腹胀痛，嗳气泛酸，恶心呕吐或大便溏薄。

〔用法与用量〕 口服，1次5～7片，1日3～4次。

〔剂型与规格〕 片剂，每片重 0.6 g

〔附注〕 本品具有制酸，镇痛，促进溃疡愈合作用。临床适用于胃及十二指肠溃疡，慢性胃炎，胃酸过多等。

良 附 丸

〔药物组成〕 高良姜 50%　香附 50%

〔功能与主治〕 温中和胃，理气止痛。用于肝郁气滞，胃脘寒痛，胸闷不舒，喜温喜按。

〔用法与用量〕 口服，1 次 3～6 g，1 日 2 次。

〔剂型与规格〕 水丸，每 20 粒重 1 g

〔附注〕 处方来源于《良方集腋》。

本品具有消炎，镇痛作用。临床适用于肝郁气滞、脾胃虚寒型慢性胃炎，胃溃疡，十二指肠球部溃汤，慢性肝炎，胃神经官能症，肋间神经痛，痛经等。

元胡止痛片

〔药物组成〕 延胡索 66.6%　白芷 33.4%

〔功能与主治〕 活血散瘀，理气止痛。用于气血瘀滞，脘腹胀痛，头痛，瘀血痛经。

〔用法与用量〕 口服，1 次 4～6 片，1 日 3 次。

〔剂型与规格〕 糖衣片，每片重约 0.35 g

〔附注〕 本品具有消炎，镇痛作用。临床适用于急慢性胃炎，肠炎，胃溃疡，痛经，头痛等属于气血瘀滞者。

小建中合剂

〔药物组成〕 饴糖 37.1%　桂枝 11.1%　白芍 22.2%　甘草 7.4%　生姜 11.1%　大枣 11.1%

〔功能与主治〕 温中补虚，缓急止痛。用于脾胃虚寒，脘腹胀痛，喜温喜按，嘈杂吞酸，食少心悸。

〔用法与用量〕 口服，1 次 20～30 ml，1 日 3 次，用时摇匀。

〔剂型与规格〕 合剂，每瓶装 100 ml

〔附注〕 处方来源于汉·张仲景《伤寒论》。

本品具有健胃，制酸，保护胃肠粘膜的作用。临床适用于脾胃虚寒型胃溃疡，十二指肠溃疡，肠痉挛等。也可用于慢性肝炎，慢性腹膜炎，鼻炎，鼻出血，肺气肿，前列腺肥大以及神经衰弱，再生不良性贫血等。

黄芪建中丸

〔药物组成〕 黄芪 36.4%　肉桂 18.2%　白芍 36.4%　甘草 9.0%

〔功能与主治〕 补气散寒，健胃和中。用于脾胃虚寒，脘腹胀痛，喜温喜按，自汗盗汗，四肢倦怠。

〔用法与用量〕 口服，1 次 1 丸，1 日 2～3 次。

〔剂型与规格〕 蜜丸，每丸重 9 g

〔附注〕 处方来源于汉·张仲景《金匮要略》。

本品具有抗炎，促进溃疡愈合作用。临床适用于脾胃虚寒型胃及十二指肠溃疡，寒性脓疡，慢性肝炎，慢性腹膜炎，神经衰弱，植物神经紊乱等。

猴 菇 菌 片

〔药物组成〕 猴菇菌 100%

〔功能与主治〕 健脾和胃，解郁止痛。用于胃脘疼痛，胸腹胀满，呕逆嘈杂，嗳气吞酸。

〔用法与用量〕 口服，1 次 3～4 片，1 日 3 次。

〔剂型与规格〕 糖衣片，每片(基片)重约 0.25 g

〔附注〕 本品具有制酸，镇痛，增强机体免疫功能的作用。临床适用于胃及十二指肠溃疡，萎缩性胃炎，慢性胃炎，亦可用于胃癌，食管癌等消化道癌症的辅助治疗。

据报道，猴菇菌中含多糖类物质，对肿瘤细胞有明显的抑制作用，还可以提高细胞免疫功能，缩小肿块和延长生存时间。

胃 特 灵 片

〔药物组成〕　延胡索　白矾等

〔功能与主治〕　温中和胃，消胀止痛。用于脘腹胀满，吞酸嘈杂，恶心呕吐，不思饮食。

〔用法与用量〕　口服，1次4～6片，1日3次。

〔剂型与规格〕　糖衣片，每片(基片)重约0.25 g

〔附注〕　本品具有制酸，镇痛作用。临床适用于胃及十二指肠溃疡，慢性胃炎等。

4.3　缓泻药

四 消 丸

〔药物组成〕　大黄 22.3%　猪牙皂 3.7%　牵牛子14.8%　槟榔 14.8%　香附 14.8%　五灵脂 14.8%

〔功能与主治〕　消水化痰，行气消食，导滞通便。用于一切气食痰水，停积胸脘，腹胀痞满，大便秘结。

〔用法与用量〕　口服，1次1.5～3 g，1日2次。

〔剂型与规格〕　水丸，每20粒重1 g

〔附注〕　本品具有解痉，镇痛，缓泻作用。临床适用于急性胃肠炎，胃肠痉挛，幽门梗阻，肠梗阻之实症便秘。

孕妇忌服。

槟榔四消丸

〔药物组成〕　槟榔 13.8%　牵牛子 27.6%　香附 13.8%　猪牙皂 3.4%　五灵脂 13.8%　大黄 27.6%

〔功能与主治〕 消食导滞，利水消胀。用于停食停水，水谷不化，倒饱嘈杂，呕吐吞酸，大便秘结。

〔用法与用量〕 口服，蜜丸1次9g，水丸1次6g，1日2～3次。

〔剂型与规格〕 蜜丸，每丸重9g；水丸，每20粒重1g

〔附注〕 处方来源于《古今医方集成》。

本品具有健胃，泻下作用。临床适用于消化不良，便秘等实证。

体质虚弱者慎用。

清 宁 丸

〔药物组成〕 大黄64.5% 绿豆2.7% 车前草2.7% 白术2.7% 黑豆2.7% 半夏2.7% 香附2.7% 桑叶2.7% 桃枝0.4% 牛乳5.4% 厚朴2.7% 麦芽2.7% 陈皮2.7% 侧柏叶2.7%

〔功能与主治〕 泻热导滞，清理肠胃。用于饮食停滞，胸胁胀满，咽喉肿痛，口舌生疮，目赤牙痛，大便秘结。

〔用法与用量〕 口服，1次1丸，1日1～2次。

〔剂型与规格〕 蜜丸，每丸重9g

〔附注〕 处方来源于清·《银海指南》。

本品具有抗菌消炎，缓泻作用。临床适用于急性牙周炎，急性结膜炎，便秘等。

孕妇忌服。

烂 积 丸

〔药物组成〕 三棱3.8% 槟榔3.8% 枳实11.4% 青皮7.6% 山楂11.4% 牵牛子19% 大黄19% 陈皮11.4% 莪术7.6% 红曲2.5% 滑石2.5%

〔功能与主治〕 消食破积，除胀通便。用于食滞积聚，胸闷胀满，腹痛吞酸，大便秘结。

〔用法与用量〕　口服，小儿 1 次 30 粒，1 日 2 次，成人酌增。

〔剂型与规格〕　水丸，每 20 粒重 1 g

〔附注〕　本品具有泻下作用。临床适用于慢性胃炎，消化不良，小儿消耗性疾病等。

尚有同名片剂，药物组成、功用同上。

枳实导滞丸

〔药物组成〕　枳实 13.9%　大黄 27.8%　黄连 8.3%　黄芩 8.3%　六神曲 13.9%　白术 13.9%　茯苓 8.3%　泽泻 5.6%

〔功能与主治〕　消积导滞，清利湿热。用于食积湿热，胸脘痞满，下痢后重或泄泻腹痛，或大便秘结，小便黄赤。

〔用法与用量〕　口服，1 次 6～9 g，1 日 2 次。

〔剂型与规格〕　水丸，每 50 粒重 3 g

〔附注〕　处方来源于金·李杲《内外伤辨惑论》。

本品具有抗菌消炎，缓泻作用。临床适用于痢疾初期，或急性肠胃炎，便秘等湿热症。

痢疾后期体质虚弱者，不宜使用。

木香槟榔丸

〔药物组成〕　木香 4.3%　槟榔 4.3%　枳壳 4.3%　陈皮 4.3%　青皮 4.3%　香附 13%　三棱 4.3%　莪术 4.3%　黄连 4.3%　黄柏 13%　大黄 13%　牵牛子 17.9%　芒硝 8.7%

〔功能与主治〕　行气导滞，泻热通便。用于胃肠积滞，脘腹胀痛，大便秘结，或赤白痢疾，里急后重。

〔用法与用量〕　口服，1 次 3～6 g，1 日 2～3 次。

〔剂型与规格〕　水丸，每 50 粒重 3 g

〔附注〕　处方来源于清·汪昂《医方集解》。

本品具有抗菌消炎，泻下作用。临床适用于急性肠炎，急性细菌性痢疾初期，消化不良等。

孕妇禁用。

麻 仁 丸

〔药物组成〕 火麻仁 20% 苦杏仁 10% 大黄 20% 枳实 20% 厚朴 10% 白芍 20%

〔功能与主治〕 润肠通便。用于肠胃燥热，大便秘结，脘腹胀满，腹中疼痛。

〔用法与用量〕 口服，1 次 1 丸，1 日 1～2 次。

〔剂型与规格〕 蜜丸，每丸重 9 g

〔附注〕 处方来源于汉·张仲景《伤寒论》。

本品具有缓泻作用，能促进肠管蠕动。临床适用于习惯性便秘，痔疮便秘，肛裂等。

孕妇及体虚便秘者不宜使用。

不宜与酶制剂同服。

尚有同名合剂，药物组成、功用同上。

五仁润肠丸

〔药物组成〕 火麻仁 7.1% 桃仁 7.1% 郁李仁 2.1% 柏子仁 3.5% 松子仁 2.1% 地黄 28.4% 陈皮 28.4% 熟大黄 7.1% 肉苁蓉 7.1% 当归 7.1%

〔功能与主治〕 滋阴养血，润肠通便。用于素体肾气虚弱，津亏血燥引起的腰脊酸痛，大便燥结，腹胀便秘。

〔用法与用量〕 口服，1 次 1 丸，1 日 2 次。

〔剂型与规格〕 蜜丸，每丸重 9 g

〔附注〕 本品具有缓泻作用。临床适用于年老体弱性便秘，产后，术后体虚之便秘。

4.4 止泻药

四 神 丸

〔药物组成〕 肉豆蔻 15.4% 吴茱萸 7.7% 补骨脂 30.7% 大枣 15.4% 五味子 15.4% 生姜 15.4%

〔功能与主治〕 温肾暖脾，固肠止泻。用于脾肾虚寒，五更泄泻，便溏腹痛，腰膝酸冷。

〔用法与用量〕 口服，1 次 9 g，1 日 1～2 次，睡前服。

〔剂型与规格〕 水丸，每 50 粒重 3 g

〔附注〕 处方来源于明·张介宾《景岳全书》。

本品具有消炎、利尿、止泻作用。临床适用于虚寒性慢性肠炎，肠结核，溃疡性、过敏性结肠炎等。

香 连 丸

〔药物组成〕 黄连 80% 木香 20%

〔功能与主治〕 清热化湿，行气止痛。用于热痢赤白，里急后重，腹痛泄泻，四肢倦怠。

〔用法与用量〕 口服，1 次 3—6 g，1 日 2～3 次，小儿酌减。

〔剂型与规格〕 水丸，每 30 粒重 1 g

〔附注〕 处方来源于宋·陈师文《太平惠民和剂局方》。

本品具有抗菌消炎作用。临床适用于急性菌痢，慢性肠炎，尤对发热腹泻的控制较明显，也可治疗由单纯性消化不良引起的各种病症。

不宜与酶制剂同服。

痢 必 灵 片

〔药物组成〕 苦参 55.6% 白芍 27.8% 木香 16.6%

〔功能与主治〕 清热燥湿，涩肠止痢。用于热毒壅盛，腹痛腹胀，里急后重，食少便溏。

〔用法与用量〕 口服，1次8片，1日3次，儿童酌减。

〔剂型与规格〕 糖衣片，每片重约0.25 g

〔附注〕 本品具有抗菌消炎作用。临床适用于细菌性痢疾，慢性肠炎，胃肠炎等。对于上述病症服用抗生素等药物效果不佳，或有副作用者，用本品效果显著。

黄芩素铝胶囊

〔药物组成〕 黄芩100%

〔功能与主治〕 清热解毒，涩肠止痢。用于热毒血痢，腹痛泄泻，里急后重，食少便溏。

〔用法与用量〕 口服，1次2～4粒，1日2～3次。

〔剂型与规格〕 胶囊剂，每粒装0.2 g

〔附注〕 本品为黄芩提取物的铝螯合物制剂。具有抑菌，消炎，止泻作用。临床适用于急、慢性肠炎，细菌性痢疾等。

4.5 利胆药

利 胆 片

〔药物组成〕 大黄9.5% 黄芩4.8% 金银花9.5% 木香15.9% 金钱草9.5% 茵陈9.5% 柴胡9.5% 白芍9.5% 芒硝3.3% 知母9.5% 大青叶9.5%

〔功能与主治〕 疏肝利胆，清热解毒，排石止痛。用于湿热郁滞，肝气郁结，黄疸。

〔用法与用量〕 口服，1次4～6片，1日3次。

〔剂型与规格〕 糖衣片，每片重约0.23 g

〔附注〕 本品具有利胆、排石、消炎作用。临床适用于急慢性胆道感染，胆囊炎，肝、胆管结石，胆石症合并感染，以及上述症状不能手术者。

实验证明，本品可增加胆汁分泌，松弛胆道口括约肌，达到引流胆汁的作用。

利胆排石片

〔药物组成〕　金钱草 22.7%　茵陈 22.7%　黄芩 6.8%　木香 6.8%　郁金 6.8%　大黄 11.4%　槟榔 11.4%　枳实 4.5%　芒硝 2.4%　厚朴 4.5%

〔功能与主治〕　清热解毒，利胆排石。用于湿热交蒸，腹痛腹胀，胸胁满闷。

〔用法与用量〕　口服，排石 1 次 6～10 片，1 日 2 次；炎症 1 次 4～6 片，1 日 2 次。

〔剂型与规格〕　片剂，每片重 0.25 g

〔附注〕　本品临床适用于胆道结石，胆道感染，胆囊炎等。本品尤长于排石，对胆结石疗效明显。

孕妇禁用。

消炎利胆片

〔药物组成〕　穿心莲 33.3%　苦术 33.3%　溪黄草 33.3%

〔功能与主治〕　清热解毒，疏肝利胆。用于肝胆湿热，胸腹胀痛。

〔用法与用量〕　口服，1 次 6 片，1 日 3 次。

〔剂型与规格〕　糖衣片，每片(基片)重约 0.3 g

〔附注〕　本品具有消炎，镇痛作用，可促进胆汁分泌。临床适用于急性胆囊炎，胆道炎及肝胆结石并发感染等。

胆石通胶囊

〔药物组成〕　茵陈　黄芩　金钱草　溪黄草　柴胡　枳壳等

〔功能与主治〕 疏肝利胆，清热解毒。用于肝胆湿热，腹痛腹胀。

〔用法与用量〕 口服，1次4～6粒，1日3次。

〔剂型与规格〕 胶囊剂，每粒装0.5 g

〔附注〕 本品具有消炎、利胆、排石作用。临床适用于胆石症，胆囊炎，胆道炎。

4.6 肝脏辅助药

龙胆泻肝丸

〔药物组成〕 龙胆14.3% 柴胡14.3% 栀子7.1% 黄芩7.1% 车前子7.1% 泽泻14.3% 当归7.1% 木通7.1% 甘草7.1% 地黄14.3%

〔功能与主治〕 清肝胆实火，清利肝胆经湿热。用于肝胆实火上逆，胁痛口苦，头晕目赤，耳鸣耳聋，肝经湿热下注，尿赤涩痛，湿热带下。

〔用法与用量〕 口服，1次3～6 g，1日2次。

〔剂型与规格〕 水丸，每20粒重1 g

〔附注〕 处方来源于清·吴谦《医宗金鉴》。

本品具有抗菌，消炎，利尿作用。临床适用于急性结膜炎，急性中耳炎，急性黄疸性肝炎，急性胆囊炎，以及急性肾盂肾炎，膀胱炎，尿道炎，急性盆腔炎，外阴炎，睾丸炎，前列腺炎，带状疱疹等。

尚有同名片剂，药物组成，功用同上。

舒肝和胃丸

〔药物组成〕 姜半夏5.5% 甘草5.5% 青皮5.5% 陈皮5.5% 厚朴5.5% 白芍5.5% 草豆蔻5.5% 乌药5.5% 六神曲5.5% 郁金5.5% 枳壳5.5% 当归5.5% 槟榔

5.5%　砂仁 3.5%　番泻叶 3.5%　柴胡 3.5%　山楂 18.0%

〔功能与主治〕　舒肝和胃。用于胸胁胀满，嘈杂吐酸，恶心呕吐。

〔用法与用量〕　口服，1 次 9 g，1 日 2 次。

〔剂型与规格〕　每 20 粒重 1 g

〔附注〕　本品具有抗炎、利胆、保护损伤的肝细胞作用。临床适用于慢性肝炎，胆囊炎等。

舒　肝　丸、

〔药物组成〕　川楝子 13.2%　延胡索 8.6%　白芍 10.4%　片姜黄 8.6%　木香 6.9%　沉香 8.6%　豆蔻仁 5.2%　砂仁 6.9%　厚朴 5.2%　陈皮 6.9%　枳壳 8.6%　茯苓 8.6%　朱砂 2.3%

〔功能与主治〕　舒肝解郁，理气止痛。用于肝郁气滞，胸胁胀满，胃脘疼痛，嘈杂呕吐，嗳气泛酸。

〔用法与用量〕　口服，1 次 1 丸，1 日 2～3 次。

〔剂型与规格〕　蜜丸，每丸重 6 g

〔附注〕　处方来源于明·朱天壁方。

本品具有消炎镇痛，保护肝脏功能的作用。临床适用于慢性胃炎，胃溃疡及十二指肠球部溃疡，慢性肝炎，慢性肝管炎，慢性胰腺炎及肝郁气滞型神经官能症。可用于门脉高压症及腹部手术后胃肠功能紊乱。

孕妇慎用。

云芝肝泰冲剂

〔药物组成〕　云芝 100%

〔功能与主治〕　舒肝解郁，导滞和胃。用于肝郁气滞，两胁胀痛，恶心呕吐，吞酸嘈杂。

〔用法与用量〕　口服，1 次 1 袋，1 日 2～3 次。

〔剂型与规格〕 冲剂，每袋重 5 g

〔附注〕 本品为多孔菌科真菌云芝的子实体提取物，有效成分为葡聚多糖。

药理实验表明，本品具有增强机体免疫功能，保护肝细胞，增加肝糖元，降低转氨酶作用。

临床适用于乙型肝炎，迁延性肝炎，慢性活动性肝炎。对慢性气管炎亦有较好疗效。本品对肝癌早期 AFP(胎甲蛋白)阳性患者有明显的转阴效果，可用于肝癌的预防和治疗，以及消化道实体瘤术后防转移。

强 肝 丸

〔药物组成〕 当归 白芍 丹参 郁金 黄芪 党参 茵陈 板兰根 山药等

〔功能与主治〕 补脾养血，益气解郁，利湿清热。用于脾肾两虚，肝郁气滞，胁痛胀满，恶心呕吐。

〔用法与用量〕 口服，1 次 2 丸，1 日 2 次。

〔剂型与规格〕 蜜丸，每丸重 9 g

〔附注〕 本品具有增强机体免疫机能，保护肝细胞作用，临床适用于慢性肝炎，早期肝硬化，脂肪肝，中毒性肝炎等。

鸡 骨 草 丸

〔药物组成〕 鸡骨草 牛黄 胆汁等

〔功能与主治〕 清肝利胆，清热解毒。用于胸胁胀痛，吞酸嗳气，恶心呕吐。

〔用法与用量〕 口服，1 次 4 粒，1 日 3 次。

〔剂型与规格〕 胶囊剂，每粒装 0.5 g

〔附注〕 本品具有消炎、镇痛、抗病毒作用。临床适用于急慢性肝炎，胆囊炎等。

健 肝 片

〔药物组成〕 萱草根 13.3%　板兰根 20%　茵陈 33.3%　丹参 20%　大枣 13.3%

〔功能与主治〕 清热利湿。用于湿热黄疸，两胁胀痛，胸脘痞满，恶心呕吐，吞酸嘈杂。

〔用法与用量〕 口服，1 次 8～10 片，1 日 2 次，小儿酌减。

〔剂型与规格〕 片剂，每片重约 0.5 g

〔附注〕 本品具有消炎、镇痛、抗病毒作用。临床适用于慢性肝炎、急性黄疸性肝炎等。

五仁醇胶囊

〔药物组成〕 五味子 100%

〔功能与主治〕 清热解毒，舒肝止痛。用于脘腹胀满，胁痛嗳气，吞酸呕吐。

〔用法与用量〕 口服，1 次 2～4 粒，1 日 2～3 次。

〔剂型与规格〕 胶囊剂，每粒含五味子乙素 10 mg

〔附注〕 本品具有降低谷丙转氨酶的作用。临床适用于慢性、迁延性肝炎等。

茵陈五苓丸

〔药物组成〕 茵陈 15.9%　赤茯苓 7.8%　猪苓 7.8%　泽泻 7.8%　白术 7.8%　苍术 7.8%　陈皮 3.9%　厚朴 7.8%　枳椇子 7.8%　黄芩 7.8%　山楂 7.8%　六神曲 3.9%　甘草 6.1%

〔功能与主治〕 清热利湿，健脾消胀。用于肝胆湿热所致脘腹胀满，面目身黄，恶心食少，小便短赤。

〔用法与用量〕 口服，1 次 6～9 g，1 日 2～3 次，小儿酌减。

〔剂型与规格〕　　水丸，每 50 粒重 3 g

〔附注〕　　处方来源于汉·张仲景《金匮要略》。

本品具有对抗多种毒物对肝细胞的影响，改善肝功能，降低转氨酶和黄疸指数的作用。临床适用于急性黄疸性肝炎，中毒性肝炎，肾炎等。

忌油腻食物。

复 肝 宁 片

〔药物组成〕　　金银花　板兰根　牡丹皮

〔功能与主治〕　　清热解毒，舒肝理脾。用于肝脾不和，胸胁胀痛，不思饮食，恶心呕吐。

〔用法与用量〕　　口服，1 次 6 片，1 日 3 次。

〔剂型与规格〕　　糖衣片，每片重约 0.3 g

〔附注〕　　本品具有抗病毒、降低转氨酶作用。临床适用于乙型肝炎，迁延性肝炎，慢性活动性肝炎，肝硬化。尤其对慢性乙肝表面抗原阳性者效果较好。

益 肝 灵 片

〔药物组成〕　　水飞蓟种子 100%

〔功能与主治〕　　舒肝解郁，消胀止痛。用于肝胆湿热，胸胁痞满，恶心呕吐。

〔用法与用量〕　　口服，1 次 4～6 片，1 日 2～3 次。

〔剂型与规格〕　　糖衣片，每片含水飞蓟素 38.5 mg

〔附注〕　　本品为水飞蓟种子的提取物水飞蓟素的制剂。具有改善肝功能，对抗多种毒物对肝脏的影响作用。临床适用于慢性肝炎，慢性活动性肝炎，早期肝硬变，高脂血症，中毒性肝炎等。

5 血液和造血系统药物

5.1 升血药

阿 胶

〔药物组成〕 驴皮89.3% 冰糖5.9% 豆油3.0% 黄酒1.8%

〔功能与主治〕 滋阴润燥，补血止血。用于血虚、心悸、咯血、崩漏，胎动下血等。

〔用法与用量〕 口服，1次3~9g，溶化兑服，1日1次。

〔剂型与规格〕 胶剂，每盒装500g

〔附注〕 本品具有增加红细胞数及血红蛋白含量，预防血液粒细胞减少，促进中性粒细胞绝对值增多，加速失血性的贫血恢复等作用。临床适用于一般性贫血，白细胞减少症，功能性子宫出血，再生障碍性贫血。

新 阿 胶

〔药物组成〕 猪皮97.2% 豆油1.1% 冰糖1.3% 黄酒0.4%

〔功能与主治〕 滋阴，补血，止血。用于血虚。肺痨咯血，产前产后血虚，身体虚弱，月经不调等。

〔用法与用量〕 口服，1次5~15g，打碎加到煎好的汤剂中溶化后服，或用温开水(黄酒)燉化服，1日1次。

〔剂型与规格〕 胶剂，每盒装500g

〔附注〕 本品能加速失血性的贫血恢复，明显的增加红细胞及血红蛋白含量；有预防血液粒细胞减少的作用。临床适用于一般性的贫血，痰中带血，白细胞减少，月经失调，产前产后贫血等。

复方阿胶浆

〔药物组成〕　阿胶　人参　熟地　山楂等

〔功能与主治〕　益气养血，调和脾胃。用于心悸气短、倦怠乏力，头晕失眠，少气懒言等虚劳证。

〔用法与用量〕　口服，1 次 20 ml，1 日 3 次，1 个月为 1 个疗程。小儿酌减。

〔剂型与规格〕　煎膏剂，每瓶装 250 ml

〔附注〕　本品具有提高机体的免疫能力，调节中枢神经系统，及机体各脏器功能，促进食物的消化和吸收，改善造血功能，止血等作用。临床适用于白细胞减少症，缺铁性贫血，失血性贫血等。

山东阿胶膏

〔药物组成〕　阿胶 25%　党参 20%　白术 10%　黄芪 20%　枸杞子 10%　白芍 5%　甘草 10%

〔功能与主治〕　养血止血，补虚润燥。用于气血不足，虚痨咳嗽，肺萎吐血，妇女崩漏，胎动不安。

〔用法与用量〕　口服，1 次 20～25 g，1 日 3 次。

〔剂型与规格〕　煎膏剂，每瓶装 250 g

〔附注〕　本品具有增强机体的抵抗能力，改善血液循环及营养状况，调节神经系统功能等作用。临床适用于缺铁性、营养不良性贫血，白血病，先兆流产或习惯性流产等。

黄 明 胶

〔药物组成〕　本品为牛皮经煎煮浓缩制成的固体胶。

〔功能与主治〕　滋阴润燥，养血止血。用于体虚便秘，肾虚遗精，吐血，呕血，胎漏，崩漏等。

〔用法与用量〕　烊化兑服，1 次 10 g，1 日 1～2 次。

〔剂型与规格〕　胶剂，每盒重 500 g

〔附注〕　本品具有改善全身脏器功能，调节机体代谢，增加血液的红细胞数和血红蛋白量和止血等作用。临床适用于一般性贫血，各种出血，心烦失眠，先兆流产或习惯性流产等。

人参归脾丸

〔药物组成〕　人参 15.3%　当归 10.7%　黄芪 10.7%　龙眼肉 10.7%　木香 3.1%　远志 3.8%　酸枣仁 10.7%　茯苓 10.7%　白术 10.7%　甘草 13.6%

〔功能与主治〕　健脾安神，益气补血。用于心脾两虚，气血不足，心悸失眠，经血过多。

〔用法与用量〕　口服，1 次 9 g，1 日 2～3 次。

〔剂型与规格〕　蜜丸，每丸重 9 g

〔附注〕　处方来源于宋·严用和《济生方》

临床适用于神经衰弱，再生障碍性贫血，功能性子宫出血，血小板减少性紫癜，胃、十二指肠溃疡出血等。

尚有同名片剂，药物组成、功用同上。

健血冲剂

〔药物组成〕　黄芪　太子参　棉花根等

〔功能与主治〕　养血益气，去瘀生新。用于气虚衰弱，气虚血滞，四肢麻木等。

〔剂型与规格〕　冲剂，每袋重 18 g

〔附注〕　本品具有改善机体造血机能，升高血液白细胞及血色素浓度，促进机体免疫功能的作用。临床适用于放疗或化疗引起的白细胞减少症，以及接触有机溶剂引起的职业性和原因不明的白细胞减少症。

升 血 膏

〔药物组成〕　熟地黄　黄芪　当归　代赭石等

〔功能与主治〕　益气养血。用于心肝血虚，唇甲苍白，眩晕，心悸等。

〔用法与用量〕　口服，1～3岁1次10～15 g；4～7岁1次25 g，1日2次。

〔剂型与规格〕　膏剂，每瓶装250 g

〔附注〕　本品临床适用于各种贫血症。

鸡 血 藤 片

〔药物组成〕　鸡血藤100%

〔功能与主治〕　补血活血，舒筋通络。用于风湿痹痛，腰膝酸痛，关节不利及血虚眩晕等。

〔用法与用量〕　口服，1次4片，1日3次。

〔剂型与规格〕　片剂，每片重0.25 g

〔附注〕　本品临床适用于各种贫血、白细胞减少症及风湿性关节炎、类风湿性关节炎、月经失调等。

孕妇忌服。

5.2　止血药

云 南 白 药

〔药物组成〕　略

〔功能与主治〕　活血，止血。用于跌打损伤，各种出血，月经不调，产后瘀血等。

〔用法与用量〕　口服，1次0.2～0.3 g，1日2～3次。外敷于伤口处。

〔附注〕　本品临床适用于内、外伤出血、吐血，鼻出血，跌打损伤等。

国外报导：从本品中分离到两种细胞毒皂甙具有抑癌活性。

孕妇忌服。

三 七 片

〔药物组成〕　三七100%

〔功能与主治〕　散瘀止血，消肿止痛。用于跌打损伤，瘀血肿痛，吐血，衄血，便血及产后血瘀腹痛。

〔用法与用量〕　口服，1次3～5片，1日1～2次；外用，剥去糖衣，研细敷患处。

〔剂型与规格〕　糖衣片，每片(基片)含三七粉0.3 g。

〔附注〕　本品临床适用于外伤血瘀肿痛，产后下腹腹痛，各种出血等。

孕妇忌服。

尚有同名散剂，药物组成、功用同上。

荷 叶 丸

〔药物组成〕　荷叶炭27.6%　大蓟4.1%　小蓟4.1%　黄芩5.5%　地黄8.3%　棕板8.3%　茅根8.3%　焦枝子5.5%　香墨0.7%　知母5.5%　玄参8.3%　白芍5.5%　当归2.8%　藕节5.5%

〔功能与主治〕　清热凉血，祛瘀止血。用于阴虚血热的各种出血症，咳血、吐血、尿血、便血、崩漏等。

〔用法与用量〕　口服，1次1丸，1日2次。

〔剂型与规格〕　蜜丸，每丸重6 g

〔附注〕　本品临床适用肾炎尿血，功能性子宫出血等。

十 灰 散

〔药物组成〕　大蓟10%　小蓟10%　侧柏叶10%　白茅

根 10%　茜草 10%　大黄 10%　棕榈皮 10%　牡丹皮 10%
荷叶 10%　枝子 10%

〔功能与主治〕　凉血止血。用于吐血，咯血等出血。

〔用法与用量〕　口服，1 次 6～9 g，1 日 2 次。

〔剂型与规格〕　散剂，每袋装 18 g

〔附注〕　处方来源于元·葛可久《十药神书》。

本品临床适用于各种内伤出血，吐血，肺痨咯血，功能性子
宫出血等。

脏　连　丸

〔药物组成〕　黄连 3.6%　黄芩 21.4%　赤芍 3.7%　当归
7.1%　槐米 10.7%　阿胶 7.1%　槐角 14.3%　地榆炭 14.3%
荆芥穗 7.1%　地黄 10.7%

〔功能与主治〕　清热止血。用于便血，肛门坠痛，痔疮下
血肿痛。

〔用法与用量〕　口服，1 次 1 丸，1 日 2 次。

〔剂型与规格〕　蜜丸，每丸重 9 g

〔附注〕　处方来源于明·陈实功《外科正宗》。

本品临床适用于痔疮红肿灼痛，肛裂，肛乳头炎，便秘带
血。

6　泌尿系统药物

6.1　利尿药

十　枣　丸

〔药物组成〕　黑枣肉　甘遂　红大戟　芫花

〔功能与主治〕　攻逐水饮。用于水饮积滞，腹水肿胀，胁下疼痛，喘逆气急，胃脘痞硬，头痛目眩，或胸背掣痛。

〔用法与用量〕　空腹口服，1 次 2-3 g，1 日 1~2 次。

〔剂型与规格〕　水丸，每 10 粒重 1 g

〔附注〕　处方来源于汉·张仲景《伤寒论》。

本品具有较强的利尿作用。临床适用于肝硬化，血吸虫病等所致的腹水，渗出性胸膜炎。

体弱及孕妇忌服。禁食食盐。

舟　车　丸

〔药物组成〕　牵牛子 34.6%　大黄 17.2%　甘遂 8.6%　陈皮 8.6%　红大戟 8.6%　木香 4.3%　芫花 8.6%　轻粉 0.9%　青皮 8.6%

〔功能与主治〕　行气逐水，用于水肿浮胀，胸腹胀满，停饮喘急，大便秘结，小便短少。

〔用法与用量〕　口服，1 次 3 g，1 日 1 次。

〔剂型与规格〕　水丸，每袋装 3 g

〔附注〕　处方来源于明·张介宾《景岳全书》。

本品具有较强的利尿作用。临床适用于急、慢性肾炎，肝硬化、晚期血吸虫病腹水。

体弱者慎用，孕妇忌服。不可久服，以防中毒。服药期间应进低盐饮食或忌盐。

忌与甘草同用。

五 苓 散

〔药物组成〕　白术 18.8%　茯苓 18.8%　泽泻 31.1%　猪苓 18.8%　肉桂 12.5%

〔功能与主治〕　温阳化气，利湿行水。用于水饮停蓄所致水肿，小便不利，呕逆泄泻，渴不思饮及诸湿肿满。

〔用法与用量〕　口服，1 次 6～9 g，1 日 2 次。

〔剂型与规格〕　散剂，每袋装 9 g

〔附注〕　处方来源于汉·张仲景《伤寒论》。

本品具有利尿作用，临床适用于急性肾炎、心脏病所致的水肿，肝硬化腹水，营养不良性水肿，也可用于腹部手术后因排尿功能受抑制，膀胱括约肌痉挛引起的尿潴留，以及急性胃肠炎，传染性肝炎，泌尿系感染等。

三 仁 合 剂

〔药物组成〕　苦杏仁 16.7%　厚朴 6.7%　白豆蔻 6.7%　通草 6.7%　淡竹叶 6.5%　滑石 20%　薏苡仁 20%　姜半夏 16.7%

〔功能与主治〕　宣化畅中，清热利湿。用于湿温初起，邪留气分，尚未化燥，暑温夹湿，头痛身重，胸闷不饥，午后身热，舌白不渴。

〔用法与用量〕　口服，1 次 20～30 ml，1 日 3 次。用时应摇匀。

〔剂型与规格〕　合剂，每瓶装 500 ml

〔附注〕　处方来源于清·吴鞠通《温病条辨》。

本品具有利尿，解热，抗菌作用。临床适用于肾盂肾炎，肠伤寒，慢性膀胱炎，支气管肺炎，不明原因发热，术后肠粘连，急性胃肠炎。

二　妙　丸

〔药物组成〕　苍术 50%　黄柏 50%

〔功能与主治〕　燥湿清热。用于湿热下注所致足膝部疮疡，流火，带下，绣球风，臁疮。

〔用法与用量〕　口服，1 次 6～9 g，1 日 2 次。

〔剂型与规格〕　水丸，每 50 粒重 3 g

〔附注〕　处方来源于元·朱震亨《丹溪心法》。

本品具有利尿，抗菌，抗病毒，消炎作用。临床适用于足膝部外科感染，下肢丹毒，白带，阴囊湿疹，臁疮。

肾炎四味片

〔药物组成〕　黄芪　石韦等

〔功能与主治〕　活血化瘀，清热解毒，补肾益气。用于面色惨白，精神萎靡，疲乏无力，头痛眩晕，耳鸣，恶心呕吐，周身浮肿，尿少或尿闭。

〔用法与用量〕　口服，1 次 8 片，1 日 3 次，3 个月为 1 疗程，饭后服用，儿童酌减。

〔剂型与规格〕　片剂，每片重 0.6 g

〔附注〕　本品临床适用于慢性肾小球肾炎，肾功能不全失代偿期及尿毒症。

服用期忌用激素，环磷酰胺，氮芥等药物。

缩　泉　丸

〔药物组成〕　益智仁 33.3%　山药 33.3%　乌药 33.3%

〔功能与主治〕　温补肾阳，固涩缩尿。用于虚寒尿频，小儿遗尿。

〔用法与用量〕　口服，1 次 6～9 g，1 日 2 次。

〔剂型与规格〕　水丸，每 500 粒重 31 g

〔附注〕　处方来源于宋·陈自明《妇人良方大全》。

本品具有减少尿量，减少小便次数，调整泌尿系统神经功能等作用。临床适用于肾阳虚寒型多尿，遗尿症，小便失禁，小便次数增多等。对糖尿病亦有一定疗效。

6.2　排石药

八 正 合 剂

〔药物组成〕　车前子 12.5%　木通 12.5%　甘草梢 12.5%　萹蓄 12.5%　瞿麦 12.5%　滑石 12.5%　栀子 12.5%　大黄 12.5%

〔功能与主治〕　清热，利尿，通淋。用于湿热内蕴所致热淋，石淋，血淋，小便涩痛，刺痛，频数，淋沥不畅，或癃闭不通，小腹胀急，目赤咽干。

〔用法与用量〕　口服，1 次 15～20 ml，1 日 3 次。

〔剂型与规格〕　合剂，每瓶装 500 ml

〔附注〕　处方来源于宋·陈师文《太平惠民和剂局方》。

本品具有解热，利尿，抗菌作用。临床适用于泌尿系结石，急、慢性肾炎，肾盂肾炎，急，慢性膀胱炎，尿道炎，及产妇、手术后尿潴留。

体质虚弱及孕妇不宜用。

分清五淋丸

〔药物组成〕　车前子 5.5%　大黄 16.4%　关木通 11%　黄芩 11%　滑石 11%　猪苓 5.5%　泽泻 5.5%　黄柏 5.5%　萹蓄 5.5%　栀子 5.5%　瞿麦 5.5%　知母 5.5%　茯苓 5.5%　甘草 1.1%

〔功能与主治〕　泻热通淋，利尿止痛。用于膀胱湿热所致尿急，尿频，尿道涩痛，淋沥不畅，小腹停水胀满，大便秘结。

〔用法与用量〕 口服，1 次 6～9 g，1 日 2～3 次。

〔剂型与规格〕 水丸，每 50 粒重 3 g

〔附注〕 处方来源于宋·陈师文《太平惠民和剂局方》。

本品具有解热，利尿，抗菌作用。临床适用于膀胱炎，尿道炎，急性前列腺炎，泌尿系结石，急性肾炎，急性肾盂肾炎及丝虫病。

孕妇慎用。

石 淋 通 片

〔药物组成〕 广金钱草 100%

〔功能与主治〕 清湿热，利尿，排石。用于湿热蕴结下焦之淋症。

〔用法与用量〕 口服，1 次 5 片，1 日 3 次。

〔剂型与规格〕 片剂，每片重 0.21 g(含干浸膏 0.12 g)

〔附注〕 本品为广金钱草的浸膏片，具有利尿，消炎，利胆，排石作用。临床适用于泌尿系结石，泌尿系感染，胆道结石，胆囊炎，黄疸性肝炎，肝硬化腹水，肾炎水肿，小儿营养障碍性疾病。

三 金 片

〔药物组成〕 金樱根 金刚刺 海金砂 雷公根 肖野牡丹

〔功能与主治〕 清热解毒，利尿通淋。用于湿热蕴结下焦，小便频数短涩，淋沥刺痛，欲出未尽，小腹拘急，或痛引腰腹。

〔用法与用量〕 口服，1 次 5 片，1 日 3～4 次。

〔剂型与规格〕 片剂，每片重 0.5 g

〔附注〕 本品具有利尿，解热，抗菌，消炎作用。临床适用于急、慢性肾盂肾炎，慢性肾盂肾炎急性发作，急性膀胱炎、尿路感染。

排 石 冲 剂

〔药物组成〕　　金钱草　忍冬藤　滑石　甘草　木通　车前子　石韦　徐长卿　瞿麦　冬葵子

〔功能与主治〕　　利水通淋，排石。用于湿热蕴结下焦之淋症。

〔用法与用量〕　　口服，1 次 20 g，1 日 3 次。

〔剂型与规格〕　　冲剂，每袋装 20 g

〔附注〕　　本品具有利尿，排石，消炎镇痛作用。临床适用于肾结石，输尿管结石，膀胱结石之泌尿系统结石症。

7 影响生长代谢机能药物

7.1 抗甲状腺药

海 藻 丸

〔药物组成〕 海藻 94.3% 盐梅 5.7%

〔功能与主治〕 软坚散结。用于瘰疬瘿瘤,坚硬肿痛。

〔用法与用量〕 口服,1 次 9 g,1 日 2 次。

〔剂型与规格〕 水丸,每 50 粒重 3 g

〔附注〕 处方来源于明·王肯堂《证治准绳》。

本品具有软化血管,缩小甲状腺肿的作用。临床适用于甲状腺肿大,甲状腺瘤,结核性结节炎等。

夏 枯 草 膏

〔药物组成〕 夏枯草 80.8% 当归 1.7% 甘草 1% 桔梗 1% 白芍 1.7% 红花 0.7% 陈皮 1% 昆布(漂)1% 川芎 1% 玄参 1.7% 香附 3.3% 浙贝母 1.7% 僵蛹 1.7% 乌药 1.7%

〔功能与主治〕 清火散结,消肿止痛。用于痰热蕴结引起的瘰疬结核,瘿瘤肿痛。

〔用法与用量〕 口服,1 次 9~15 g,1 日 2 次。

〔剂型与规格〕 膏滋,每瓶重 60 g

〔附注〕 本品具有促进甲状腺功能,抗菌,利尿作用。临床适用于单纯性甲状腺肿,慢性淋巴结炎,淋巴结核,腮腺炎等。

7.2 降血糖药

消 渴 丸

〔药物组成〕 黄芪 天花粉 生地黄等

〔功能与主治〕 滋肾养阴，益气生津。用于多饮，多尿，多食，消瘦，体倦乏力之消渴症。

〔用法与用量〕 口服，初次 5 丸，以后递增至 10 丸，1 日 3 次，至出现疗效后减为 1 日 2 次。

〔剂型与规格〕 水丸，每丸重 0.25 g

〔附注〕 本品具有显著的降血糖作用，并能改善糖尿病患者的症状。临床适用于轻、中度以及稳定型的糖尿病。

肝炎患者慎服，对严重肾机能不全，少年糖尿病，酮体糖尿，妊娠期糖尿病，糖尿性昏迷等症不宜应用。服用本品时严禁加服优降糖制剂。

玉 泉 丸

〔药物组成〕 五味子 生地黄 麦冬 茯苓 黄芪 天花粉 葛根 乌梅等

〔功能与主治〕 养阴滋肾，生津止渴，清热除烦，益气和中。用于消渴症，多饮多食，消瘦无力。

〔用法与用量〕 口服，1 次 9 g，1 日 4 次，1 个月为 1 疗程。

〔剂型与规格〕 水丸，每 10 粒重 1.5 g

〔附注〕 本品具有明显的降血糖、降尿糖作用。临床适用于因胰岛功能减退而引起物质代谢紊乱，中、轻型糖尿病。

消 渴 平 片

〔药物组成〕 人参 1.1% 黄连 1.1% 天花粉 26.9% 天冬 2.7% 黄芪 26.9% 丹参 8.0% 枸杞子 6.5% 沙苑子

8.0%　　葛根 8.0%　　知母 5.4%　　五倍子 2.7%　　五味子 2.7%

〔功能与主治〕　　益气养阴，清热泻火，益肾缩尿。用于消渴症，烦热多尿，阴液亏耗。

〔用法与用量〕　　口服，1 次 6～8 片，1 日 3 次，1 个月为 1 疗程。

〔剂型与规格〕　　半薄膜衣片，每片重约 0.28 g

〔附注〕　　本品具有降血糖，降血脂作用，并可改善肝、肾功能。临床适用于非胰岛素依赖型糖尿病。

8 抗菌、抗病毒药物

安宫牛黄丸

〔药物组成〕 牛黄 郁金 黄连 黄芩 栀子 水牛角浓缩粉 珍珠 冰片等

〔功能与主治〕 清热解毒，开窍安神。用于热性病，邪入心包，高热惊厥，神昏谵语狂躁不安或舌塞肢厥。

〔用法与用量〕 口服，1次1丸，3岁以下小儿1次1／4丸，4～6岁1次1／2丸，或遵医嘱。

〔剂型与规格〕 蜜丸，每丸重3g

〔附注〕 处方来源于清·吴鞠通《温病条辨》。

本品具有抗菌，抗病毒，解痉，镇静，解热作用。临床适用于乙型脑炎，流行性脑脊髓膜炎，中毒性痢疾，尿毒症，脑血管意外，中毒性肝炎，肝昏迷，神经系统感染引起的高热，昏迷，抽搐等。

孕妇慎用

局方至宝丹

〔药物组成〕 水牛角浓缩粉 玳瑁 琥珀 安息香 牛黄 冰片等

〔功能与主治〕 清热解毒，祛痰开窍。用于瘟病，痰热内闭，神昏谵语，痉厥抽搐，小儿急惊。

〔用法与用量〕 口服，1次1丸，小儿减半。

〔剂型与规格〕 蜜丸，每丸重3g

〔附注〕 处方来源于宋·陈师文《太平惠民和剂局方》。

本品临床适用于乙型脑炎，流行性脑脊髓膜炎，斑疹伤寒等急性传染病高热、昏迷者，以及中毒性脑病，脑出血，败血症，肝昏迷，癫痫等。

身体虚弱及高血压患者禁用。

紫雪丹

〔药物组成〕 石膏 寒水石 滑石 磁石 玄参 木香 沉香 升麻 甘草等。

〔功能与主治〕 清热解毒，镇惊开窍。用于热邪内陷，高热烦躁，神昏谵语，惊风抽搐，尿赤便闭。

〔用法与用量〕 口服，1次1.5～3 g，1日2次，周岁小儿1次0.3 g，5岁以内小儿每增1岁，递增0.3 g，1日1次。

〔剂型与规格〕 散剂，每瓶装1.5 g

〔附注〕 处方来源于宋·陈师文《太平惠民和剂局方》。

本品临床适用于斑疹伤寒，麻疹等急性发疹性疾病及乙型脑炎，流行性脑脊髓膜炎所致的高热、昏迷等。

孕妇禁用。

牛黄解毒片

〔药物组成〕 牛黄0.6% 雄黄6.4% 石膏25.7% 大黄25.7% 黄芩19.2% 桔梗12.8% 冰片3.2% 甘草6.4%

〔功能与主治〕 清热解毒，散风止痛。用于火热内感，咽喉肿痛，牙龈肿痛，口舌生疮，目赤耳鸣。

〔用法与用量〕 口服，大片1次2片，小片1次3片，1日2～3次。

〔剂型与规格〕 片剂，小片每片重0.4 g，大片每片重0.6 g

〔附注〕 处方来源于明《辨证准绳妇幼集》。

本品具有抗菌消炎，镇痛作用。临床适用于急性咽喉炎，急性扁桃体炎，牙周炎，流行性腮腺炎等。

孕妇忌服。不宜与酶制剂同服。

清瘟解毒丸

〔药物组成〕　大青叶 8.3%　连翘 6.3%　玄参 8.3%　天花粉 8.3%　桔梗 6.3%　牛蒡子 8.3%　羌活 6.3%　防风 4.2%　葛根 8.3%　柴胡 4.2%　黄芩 8.3%　白芷 4.2%　川芎 4.2%　赤芍 4.2%　淡竹叶 8.3%　甘草 2%

〔功能与主治〕　清瘟解毒。用于外感时疫，憎寒壮热，头痛无汗，口渴咽干，疟腮，大头瘟。

〔用法与用量〕　口服，1 次 2 丸，1 日 2 次。

〔剂型与规格〕　蜜丸，每丸重 9 g

〔附注〕　处方来源于《真方汇录》。

本品临床适用于上呼吸道感染，急性支气管炎，肺炎等。

孕妇慎服。

万氏牛黄清心丸

〔药物组成〕　牛黄 1.7%　朱砂 10.2%　黄连 33.9%　黄芩 20.3%　栀子 20.3%　郁金 13.6%

〔功能与主治〕　清热解毒，镇惊安神。用于邪热内闭，烦躁不安，神昏谵语，小儿高热惊厥。

〔用法与用量〕　口服，1 次 2 丸，1 日 2～3 次。

〔剂型与规格〕　蜜丸，每丸重 1.5 g

〔附注〕　处方来源于万密斋《痘疹世医心法》。

本品临床适用于原发性高血压，尿毒症昏迷，肝昏迷等。

银翘解毒片

〔药物组成〕　金银花 17.9%　连翘 17.9%　薄荷 10.7%　荆芥 7.2%　淡豆豉 8.9%　牛蒡子 10.7%　桔梗 10.7%　淡竹叶 7.2%　甘草 8.9%

〔功能与主治〕　清热解毒。用于风热感冒，发热头痛，咳嗽口干，咽喉肿痛。

〔用法与用量〕 口服，1次4片，1日2～3次。

〔剂型与规格〕 片剂，每片含药1 g

〔附注〕 处方来源于清·吴鞠通《温病条辨》。

本品具有抗菌，抗病毒，利尿作用。临床适用于风热型感冒，流行性感冒，上呼吸道感染，流行性腮腺炎，急性支气管炎，肺炎等。

西羚解毒片

〔药物组成〕 薄荷 荆芥穗 连翘 金银花 牛蒡子 淡竹叶 淡豆豉 桔梗 甘草 羚羊角 冰片等

〔功能与主治〕 解表清热。用于感冒发热，头痛咳嗽，咽喉肿痛。

〔用法与用量〕 口服，1次4片，1日3次。

〔剂型与规格〕 片剂，每片重约0.25 g

〔附注〕 本品临床适用于风热型感冒，上呼吸道感染，急性支气管炎，肺炎等。

西羚感冒片

〔药物组成〕 羚羊角 忍冬藤 野菊花 北豆根等。

〔功能与主治〕 清热解毒。用于伤风感冒，头痛咳嗽，咽喉肿痛。

〔用法与用量〕 口服，1次3～4片，1日3次。

〔剂型与规格〕 片剂，每片重约0.3 g

〔附注〕 本品临床适用于上呼吸道感染，急性支气管炎，肺炎等。

羚翘解毒片

〔药物组成〕 金银花 17.1% 连翘 17.1% 桔梗 11.4%

牛蒡子 11.4%　薄荷 11.4%　淡竹叶 8.5%　荆芥穗 8.5%　淡豆豉 7.1%　羚羊角 0.4%　甘草 7.1%

〔功能与主治〕　疏风解表，清热解毒。用于感冒初起，发热恶寒，四肢酸软，头痛咳嗽，咽喉肿痛。

〔用法与用量〕　口服，1次4～6片，1日3次。

〔剂型与规格〕　片剂，每片重约0.3 g

〔附注〕　本品临床适用于风热型感冒发热，上呼吸道感染，肺炎等。

连翘败毒丸

〔药物组成〕　连翘 7.3%　金银花 7.3%　大黄 7.3%　栀子 5.5%　黄芩 5.5%　木通 5.5%　蒲公英 5.5%　地丁 5.5%　天花粉 3.3%　玄参 5.5%　浙贝母 5.5%　赤芍 5.5%　桔梗 5.5%　防风 5.5%　白芷 5.5%　蝉蜕 3.3%　白藓皮 5.5%　甘草 5.5%

〔功能与主治〕　清热解毒，消肿止痛。用于疮疡初起，红肿疼痛，疮疖溃烂，灼热流脓，丹毒疮疹，疥癣痛痒。

〔用法与用量〕　口服，1次9 g，1日2次。

〔剂型与规格〕　水丸，每50粒重3 g

〔附注〕　处方来源于明·王肯堂《证治准绳》。
本品临床适用于各种皮肤化脓性炎症，皮癣，脚气等。

黄连上清丸

〔药物组成〕　大黄 10.8%　黄芩 10.8%　赤芍 10.8%　栀子 6.7%　连翘 6.7%　当归 6.7%　川芎 6.7%　薄荷 6.7%　荆芥 6.7%　菊花 5.4%　天花粉 5.4%　桔梗 2.8%　玄参 2.8%　黄连 2.8%　黄柏 5.4%　甘草 2.8%

〔功能与主治〕　清火散风，通便泻热。用于胃肠实热引起的头昏耳鸣，牙龈肿痛，口舌生疮，咽喉肿痛，暴发火眼，便秘溺赤等。

〔用法与用量〕　口服，1 次 9 g，1 日 1 次。

〔剂型与规格〕　水丸，每 50 粒重 3 g

〔附注〕　处方来源于明·龚廷贤《万病回春》。

本品具有抗炎，镇痛，解热作用。临床适用于急性咽喉炎，急性腮腺炎，牙周炎，各种传染性眼病。

孕妇忌服。

牛黄上清丸

〔药物组成〕　牛黄 0.3%　薄荷 4.8%　菊花 6.4%　荆芥穗 2.6%　白芷 2.6%　川芎 2.6%　栀子 8%　黄连 2.6%　黄柏 1.6%　黄芩 8%　大黄 12.9%　连翘 8%　赤芍 2.6%　当归 8%　地黄 10.3%　桔梗 2.6%　石膏 12.9%　冰片 1.6%　甘草 1.6%

〔功能与主治〕　清热泻火，散风止痛。用于头痛眩晕，目赤耳鸣，咽喉肿痛，口舌生疮，牙龈肿痛，大便燥结。

〔用法与用量〕　口服，1 次 1 丸，1 日 2 次。

〔剂型与规格〕　蜜丸，每丸重 6 g

〔附注〕　处方来源于明·李梴《医学入门》。

本品具有抗炎，解热，镇痛作用。临床适用于风热型感冒，上呼吸道感染，牙周炎等。

川芎茶调散

〔药物组成〕　川芎 16.3%　白芷 8.2%　羌活 8.2%　细辛 4.1%　防风 6.1%　薄荷 32.7%　荆芥 16.3%　甘草 8.1%

〔功能与主治〕　疏风止痛。用于风邪头痛，恶寒发烧，鼻塞等。

〔用法与用量〕　口服，1 次 3~6 g，1 日 2 次。

〔剂型与规格〕　散剂，每袋装 30 g

〔附注〕　处方来源于宋·陈师文《太平惠民和剂局方》。

本品具有消炎，镇痛作用。临床适用于风寒型感冒，鼻炎，鼻窦炎，神经性头痛。

桑菊感冒片

〔药物组成〕　桑叶 21.2%　菊花 8.4%　薄荷油 0.1%　苦杏仁 16.9%　桔梗 16.9%　连翘 12.8%　芦根 16.9%　甘草 6.8%

〔功能与主治〕　疏风清热，宣肺止咳。用于风热感冒初起，头痛，咳嗽，口干，咽痛。

〔用法与用量〕　口服，1 次 4～8 片，1 日 2～3 次。

〔剂型与规格〕　片剂，每片重 0.6 g

〔附注〕　处方来源于清·吴鞠通《温病条辨》。

本品临床适用于风热型感冒，上呼吸道感染，支气管炎，肺炎，急性扁桃体炎。

复方大青叶注射液

〔药物组成〕　大青叶 44.5%　金银花 22.2%　羌活 11.1%　拳参 11.1%　大黄 11.1%

〔功能与主治〕　清瘟解毒。用于瘟病发烧，咳嗽气喘，咽喉肿痛。

〔用法与用量〕　肌肉注射，每次 2～4 ml，1 日 1～2 次。

〔剂型与规格〕　注射剂，每支装 2 ml

〔附注〕　本品临床适用于流行性感冒，流行性脑脊髓膜炎，流行性腮腺炎，病毒性肺炎，上呼吸道感染等。

感冒解热冲剂

〔药物组成〕　麻黄 8.1%　菊花 8.1%　白术 8.1%　羌活 8.1%　防风 8.1%　生姜 5.4%　石膏 27.1%　葛根 16.2%　钩

藤 10.8%

〔功能与主治〕 疏风清热。用于伤风感冒，恶寒发烧，四肢酸痛，头晕头痛。

〔用法与用量〕 口服，1 次 1～2 包，1 日 3 次。

〔剂型与规格〕 冲剂，每包装 15 g

〔附注〕 本品临床适用于上呼吸道感染，流行性感冒，支气管炎，无名热等。

牛黄消炎丸

〔药物组成〕 牛黄 9.7% 大黄 19.2% 天花粉 19.2% 青黛 7.7% 蟾酥 5.8% 雄黄 19.2% 珍珠母 19.2%

〔功能与主治〕 清热解毒，消肿止痛。用于咽喉肿痛，疔、痈、疮、疖等。

〔用法与用量〕 口服，1 次 10 粒，1 日 3 次；外用，研末调敷患处。

〔剂型与规格〕 水丸，每 60 粒重 0.3 g

〔附注〕 本品临床适用于上呼吸道感染，多发性脓肿，咽喉炎等。

感冒清热冲剂

〔药物组成〕 荆芥穗 16.9% 薄荷 5.1% 防风 8.5% 柴胡 8.5% 紫苏叶 5.1% 葛根 8.5% 桔梗 5.1% 苦杏仁 6.8% 白芷 5.1% 苦地丁 16.9% 芦根 13.5%

〔功能与主治〕 疏风散寒，解表清热。用于风寒感冒，头痛发热，恶寒身痛，鼻流清涕，咳嗽咽干。

〔用法与用量〕 口服，1 次 12 g，1 日 2 次。

〔剂型与规格〕 冲剂，每袋装 12 g

〔附注〕 本品临床适用于感冒，上呼吸道感染(风寒型)等。

防风通圣丸

〔药物组成〕　防风 3.8%　荆芥穗 1.9%　薄荷 3.8%　麻黄 3.8%　大黄 3.8%　芒硝 3.8%　栀子 1.9%　滑石 22.6%　桔梗 7.5%　石膏 7.5%　川芎 3.8%　当归 3.8%　白芍 3.8%　黄芩 7.5%　连翘 3.8%　甘草 15%　白术 1.9%

〔功能与主治〕　解表通里，清热解毒。用于外寒内热，表里俱实，恶寒壮热，头痛咽干，小便短赤，大便秘结，瘰疬初起，风疹湿疮。

〔用法与用量〕　口服，1 次 6 g，1 日 2 次。

〔剂型与规格〕　水丸，每 50 粒重 3 g

〔附注〕　处方来源于金·刘完素《宣明论方》。

本品临床适用于感冒发热，皮肤化脓性感染，荨麻疹，肥胖症，高血压症等。

九味羌活丸

〔药物组成〕　羌活 15%　防风 15%　苍术 15%　细辛 5%　川芎 10%　白芷 10%　黄芩 10%　地黄 10%　甘草 10%

〔功能与主治〕　解表除湿。用于恶寒发热，无汗，头痛口干，肢体酸痛。

〔用法与用量〕　口服，1 次 6～9 g，1 日 2～3 次。

〔剂型与规格〕　水丸，每 500 粒重 31 g

〔附注〕　处方来源于元·王好古《此事难知》。

本品临床适用于风寒型感冒，流感，上呼吸道感染，风湿性关节炎等。

银　黄　片

〔药物组成〕　金银花膏 56%　黄芩素 44%

〔功能与主治〕　清热解毒。用于疮疖痈肿，痢疾，丹毒，咽喉肿痛。

〔用法与用量〕 口服，1次4~6片，1日4次。

〔剂型与规格〕 片剂，每片含绿原酸不低于18 mg、黄芩甙不低于36 mg

〔附注〕 本品具有抗菌消炎，抗病毒，利尿作用。临床适用于上呼吸道感染，急性肠炎，菌痢，肺炎等。

感 冒 冲 剂

〔药物组成〕 忍冬藤31.6% 板兰根22.6% 前胡10.1% 桔梗10.1% 葛根10.1% 甘草10.1% 牛蒡子5.1% 薄荷脑0.3%

〔功能与主治〕 清热解毒，宣肺止咳。用于风热感冒，头痛咳嗽，咽喉肿痛。

〔用法与用量〕 口服，1次1~2袋，1日3次，小儿酌减。

〔剂型与规格〕 冲剂，每袋(块)重15 g

〔附注〕 本品临床适用于上呼吸道感染，急性腮腺炎，流行性脑脊髓膜炎等。

风寒感冒冲剂

〔药物组成〕 桂枝 白芷 荆芥穗 羌活 白芍 葛根杏仁

〔功能与主治〕 解表散寒，退热止咳。用于风寒感冒，恶寒发热，头痛颈强，全身酸疼，咳嗽。

〔用法与用量〕 口服，1次1袋，1日3次。

〔剂型与规格〕 冲剂，每袋装12 g

〔附注〕 本品临床适用于风寒型感冒，上呼吸道感染，支气管炎，肺炎。

防 感 片

〔药物组成〕 黄芪 白术等

〔功能与主治〕 益气健脾，扶正固表，止汗。用于体虚感受风邪，头昏乏力，咽喉肿痛，自汗气喘。

〔用法与用量〕 口服，1 次 5～7 片，1 日 2 次。

〔剂型与规格〕 片剂，每片约重 0.32 g

〔附注〕 本品临床适用于老年体虚感冒，上呼吸道感染，支气管哮喘等。

板兰根干糖浆

〔药物组成〕 板兰根 100%

〔功能与主治〕 清热凉血，解毒消肿。用于头面红肿，咽喉肿痛，口渴烦躁，麻疹。

〔用法与用量〕 口服，1 次 5 g，每 4 小时 1 次。

〔剂型与规格〕 颗粒剂，每包装 10 g

〔附注〕 本品具有广谱抗菌和抗病毒作用。临床适用于流行性腮腺炎，流行性脑脊髓膜炎，传染性肝炎，上呼吸道感染等。

复方柴胡注射液

〔药物组成〕 北柴胡 91% 细辛 9%

〔功能与主治〕 和解湿热，发表止痛。用于外感风邪，头痛咳嗽，全身酸痛。

〔用法与用量〕 肌肉注射，1 次 2～4 ml，1 日 1～2 次。

〔剂型与规格〕 注射剂，每支装 2 ml

〔附注〕 本品临床适用于感冒，上呼吸道感染，支气管肺炎，单纯疱疹，病毒性角膜炎等。

芎菊上清丸

〔药物组成〕 大黄 8.6% 栀子 8.6% 川芎 8.6% 防风 8.6% 桔梗 8.6% 菊花 8.6% 黄芩 8.6% 荆芥 4.3% 薄荷 4.3% 滑石 5.6% 甘草 12.8% 黄柏 12.8%

〔功能与主治〕 散风清热。用于上焦风热，头痛头晕，暴发火眼，鼻塞耳鸣。

〔用法与用量〕 口服，1 次 6 g，1 日 2 次。

〔剂型与规格〕 水丸，每 20 粒重 1 g

〔附注〕 处方来源于宋·陈师文《太平惠民和剂局方》。

本品临床适用于上呼吸道感染，神经性头痛，鼻窦炎，鼻炎，眼巩膜炎，高血压症。

清 眩 丸

〔药物组成〕 川芎 28.6% 白芷 28.6% 薄荷 14.3% 荆芥穗 14.3% 石膏 14.2%

〔功能与主治〕 散风清热。用于风热头晕目眩，偏正头痛，鼻塞牙痛。

〔用法与用量〕 口服，1 次 1～2 丸，1 日 2 次。

〔剂型与规格〕 蜜丸，每丸重 6 g

〔附注〕 处方来源于元·罗天盖《卫生宝鉴》。

本品临床适用于感冒头痛，鼻炎，鼻窦炎，三叉神经痛，高血压症等。

抗菌消炎片

〔药物组成〕 金银花 17.8% 大青叶 17.8% 百部 17.8% 金钱草 17.8% 知母 14.6% 黄芩 8.9% 大黄 5.3%

〔功能与主治〕 清热解毒。用于外感风热，咽喉肿痛，疔疖痈肿，下焦湿热。

〔用法与用量〕　口服，1次4～8片，1日3次。

〔剂型与规格〕　片剂，每片重约0.25 g

〔附注〕　本品临床适用于上呼吸道感染，牙周炎，各种皮肤化脓感染症，外伤感染等。

千 里 光 片

〔药物组成〕　千里光100%

〔功能与主治〕　清热解毒。用于内湿外感，咽喉肿痛，湿热泻泄。

〔用法与用量〕　口服，1次3～5片，1日3次。

〔剂型与规格〕　片剂，每片含药2g

〔附注〕　本品临床适用于上呼吸道感染，大叶性肺炎，急性菌痢，急性肠炎，急性阑尾炎，滴虫性阴道炎。

四 季 青 片

〔药物组成〕　四季青叶100%

〔功能与主治〕　清热解毒。用于肺热咳嗽，咽喉肿痛，小便淋沥，涩痛，热疖痈肿，烫伤。

〔用法与用量〕　口服，1次5片，1日3次。

〔剂型与规格〕　片剂，每片含生药4 g

〔附注〕　本品具有广谱抗菌作用。临床适用于急、慢性扁桃体炎，急、慢性菌痢，肠炎，尿路感染，外伤感染等。

金 银 花 露

〔药物组成〕　金银花100%

〔功能与主治〕　清热解毒。用于暑热烦渴，痧痘痈疽，小儿胎毒等。

〔用法与用量〕　口服，1次30～50 ml，1日2～3次。

〔剂型与规格〕　露剂，每瓶装500 ml

〔附注〕 本品临床适用于夏季汗囊炎，皮肤丘疹感染，中暑口干，新生儿皮肤感染等。

一 粒 珠

〔药物组成〕 牛黄 乳香 没药 珍珠 蟾酥 冰片等

〔功能与主治〕 活血，消肿，解毒。用于痈疽疮疖，乳痈乳岩，红肿疼痛，初起末溃或有脓。

〔用法与用量〕 口服，1 次 1.5 g，1 日 1 次。

〔剂型与规格〕 水丸，每 50 粒重 3 g

〔附注〕 处方来源于清·谢元庆《良方集腋》。

本品临床适用于乳腺炎，多发性脓肿，皮肤化脓性感染。

葛根芩连片

〔药物组成〕 葛根 50% 黄芩 18.8% 黄连 18.7% 甘草 12.5%

〔功能与主治〕 解表清里。用于身热，喘而汗出，烦躁口渴，腹痛下痢。

〔用法与用量〕 口服，1 次 3～4 片，1 日 3 次。

〔剂型与规格〕 片剂，每片重 0.3 g

〔附注〕 处方来源于汉·张仲景《伤寒论》。

本品临床适用于急性胃肠炎和细菌性痢疾等。

9　抗风湿药物

冯了性药酒

〔药物组成〕　丁公藤　白芷　五加皮　麻黄　青蒿子　当归尾　桂枝　小茴香　川芎　威灵仙　防己　栀子　羌活　独活

〔功能与主治〕　祛风通络，散寒止痛。用于风寒湿痹，四肢麻木，筋骨酸痛，腰膝乏力。

〔用法与用量〕　口服，1 次 15 ml，1 日 3 次。

〔剂型与规格〕　药酒，每瓶装 500 ml

〔附注〕　本品具有消炎，抗风湿，改善微循环，消肿镇痛作用。临床适用于风湿性、类风湿性关节炎(风寒湿痹)，外伤肿痛。

五加皮药酒

〔药物组成〕　玉竹 23.2%　党参 8.7%　姜黄 8.7%　五加皮 5.8%　陈皮 5.8%　菊花 2.9%　红花 2.9%　牛膝 2.9%　白术 2.2%　白芷 2.2%　当归 1.4%　青风藤 1.4%　川芎 1.4%　威灵仙 1.4%　檀香 1.4%　海风藤 1.4%　豆蔻 1.1%　独活 0.7%　草乌 0.7%　砂仁 0.7%　木香 0.7%　丁香 0.7%　肉桂 0.7%　栀子 16.4%　木瓜 1.4%　川乌 0.7%

〔功能与主治〕　舒筋活血，除湿散风。用于风湿痿痹，手足拘挛，四肢麻木，腰膝疼痛，阴囊湿冷。

〔用法与用量〕　口服，1 次 10~15 ml，1 日 2 次。

〔剂型与规格〕　药酒，每瓶装 500 ml

〔附注〕　本品具有抗炎，镇痛，抗风湿，改善微循环作用。临床适用于风湿性、类风湿性关节炎及老年性肢体麻木等。

本品与冯了性药酒功效相似，但本品的滋补作用较强，对老年及体弱患者具有较好效果。

国 公 酒

〔药物组成〕　玉竹　陈皮　红曲　肉桂　丁香　砂仁　豆蔻　木香　檀香　地黄　老鹳草　当归　牛膝　枳壳　麦门冬　白术　苍术　槟榔　川芎　木瓜　白芷　丹皮　羌活　厚朴　藿香　红花　独活　枸杞子　白芍　补骨脂　佛手　山楂　栀子　香加皮　紫草　防风　蜂蜜

〔功能与主治〕　祛风除湿，养血活络。用于风寒湿痹，四肢麻木，骨节疼痛。

〔用法与用量〕　口服，1次10～15 ml，1日2次。

〔剂型与规格〕　药酒，每瓶装250 ml

〔附注〕　本品具有抗菌，消炎，促进微循环及滋养作用。临床适用于风湿性关节炎，类风湿性关节炎，老年性肢体麻木等。

不可与阿斯匹林、水杨酸钠同服。

风 湿 药 酒

〔药物组成〕　草乌0.9%　红花0.9%　红曲1.3%　老鹳草0.9%　地枫0.4%　薏苡仁0.9%　白术0.4%　麻黄0.9%　生姜0.4%　桂枝0.4%　防己0.4%　黄芪0.4%　马钱子0.4%　赤芍0.4%　肉桂0.4%　草蔻0.4%　香加皮0.4%　威灵仙0.4%　木瓜0.4%　丹参0.4%　穿山龙0.4%　苍术0.4%　橘红0.2%　高良姜0.4%　白酒87.1%

〔功能与主治〕　祛风除湿，通经活络。用于腰腿疼，手足拘挛，半身不遂，风湿痹痛。

〔用法与用量〕　口服，1次15～25 ml，1日2次。

〔剂型与规格〕　药酒，每瓶装250 ml

〔附注〕　本品具有抗风湿，抗炎，镇痛，改善微循环等作用，临床适用于风湿性关节炎，风湿性瘫痪等。

不可与阿斯匹林，水杨酸钠同服。

舒筋活络酒

〔药物组成〕　木瓜 4.1%　桑寄生 6.8%　玉竹 21.6%　续断 2.7%　川牛膝 8.2%　当归 4.1%　川芎 5.4%　红花 4.1%　独活 2.7%　羌活 2.7%　防风 5.4%　白术 8.2%　蚕砂 5.4%　红曲 16.2%　甘草 2.7%

〔功能与主治〕　祛风除湿，舒筋活络。用于风寒湿痹，筋骨疼痛，四肢麻木。

〔用法与用量〕　口服，1 次 20～30 ml，1 日 2 次。

〔剂型与规格〕　酒剂，每瓶装 250 ml

〔附注〕　本品具有抗风湿，抗炎，镇痛，改善微循环等作用。临床适用于风湿性关节炎，肢体麻木，肌肉疼痛等。

孕妇慎用。

狗 皮 膏

〔药物组成〕　枳壳　青皮　大枫子　赤石脂　赤芍　天麻　甘草　乌药　牛膝　羌活　黄柏　补骨脂　威灵仙　生川乌　续断　白蔹　桃仁　生附子　川芎　生草乌　杜仲　远志　香附　白术　川楝子　僵蚕　小茴香　蛇床子　当归　细辛　菟丝子　陈皮　青风藤　木香　肉桂　轻粉　儿茶　丁香　乳香　没药　血竭　樟脑等

〔功能与主治〕　祛风散寒，舒筋活血，止痛。用于风寒湿痹，肩臂腰腿疼痛，肢体麻木，跌打损伤。

〔用法与用量〕　外用，加温软化，贴患处。

〔剂型与规格〕　黑膏药，每张净重 15 g 或 30 g

〔附注〕　本品具有抑菌，消炎，镇痛，改善微循环等作用。临床适用于风湿痛，神经痛，扭伤红肿疼痛。

金不换膏药

〔药物组成〕　当归　独活　秦艽　苍术　白芷　杜仲　羌活　川乌　干姜　高良姜　荆芥　防风　草乌　川芎　地黄　玄参　甘草　麻黄　没药　肉桂　乳香　血竭　龙骨　海螵蛸(去壳)等

〔功能与主治〕　散风活血，消肿止痛。用于风寒湿痹，四肢麻木，腰腿疼痛，跌打损伤，筋骨疼痛。

〔用法与用量〕　外用，加热软化，贴患处。

〔剂型与规格〕　黑膏药，每张净重 10 g

〔附注〕　本品具有抗风湿，消肿镇痛，改善微循环的作用。临床适用于风湿性关节炎，神经痛及扭伤疼痛等。

风湿止痛膏

〔药物组成〕　乳香　没药　冰片　樟脑　薄荷脑　冬青油　丁香　肉桂　红花　生川乌　生草乌　荆芥　防风　干姜　金银花　当归等

〔功能与主治〕　祛风除湿，化瘀止痛。用于风寒湿痹引起的腰肩，四肢，肌肉疼痛。

〔用法与用量〕　外用，将患处洗净擦干，按疼痛大小贴敷。

〔剂型与规格〕　橡胶硬膏剂，每张 5×7 cm

〔附注〕　本品具有抗风湿，消炎镇痛，改善微循环等作用。临床适用于风湿性关节炎，类风湿关节炎，肌纤维炎等引起的腰肩、四肢、关节、肌肉疼痛。

对橡胶膏过敏者慎用。

伤湿祛痛膏

〔药物组成〕　干姜 19.3%　苍术 14.3%　白芷 9.1%　川芎 7.1%　当归 14.3%　麻黄 7.1%　草乌 7.1%　八角茴香 4.6%　山奈 5.8%　樟脑 2%　冬青油 3%　冰片 2%　薄荷脑 4.1%

〔功能与主治〕　祛风除湿，止痛。用于风湿疼痛，肢体麻木，头痛及扭伤肿痛。

〔用法与用量〕　外用，将皮肤洗净擦干，贴于患处。

〔剂型与规格〕　含药橡胶膏，每张 5×6.5 cm

〔附注〕　本品具有抗风湿，抗炎，镇痛，改善微循环等作用。临床适用于风湿性关节炎，肌纤维炎，肌肉拉伤，神经炎等。

凡对橡胶膏药过敏或皮肤有渗出液，外伤出血及化脓者均不宜贴用。

阳和解凝膏

〔药物组成〕　牛蒡草　凤仙透骨草　生川乌　桂枝　大黄　当归　生草乌　生附子　地龙　僵蚕　赤芍　白芷　白蔹　白芨　川芎　续断　防风　荆芥　五灵脂　木香　香木缘　陈皮　肉桂　乳香　没药　苏合香等

〔功能与主治〕　温阳化湿，消肿散结。用于阴疽，瘰疬未溃，寒湿痹痛。

〔用法与用量〕　外用，加温软化，贴患处。

〔剂型与规格〕　黑膏药，每张净重 1.5 g、3 g、6 g

〔附注〕　本品具有抗菌，消炎，抗结核，抗风湿的作用。临床适用于骨结核，腹膜结核，淋巴结核，血栓性脉管炎，慢性风湿性关节炎，肌纤维炎等。

疮疡红肿热痛，或已溃破者禁用。

伤湿宝珍膏

〔药物组成〕 芸香浸膏 薄荷脑 樟脑 冬青油 复方细辛流浸膏等

〔功能与主治〕 除湿祛风，温经行滞。用于跌打损伤，风湿性神经痛、肩背疼痛、腰痛。

〔用法与用量〕 外用，贴敷患处，4～5 天换 1 次。

〔剂型与规格〕 橡皮膏，每袋装 2 张

〔附注〕 本品具有抗炎，抗风湿，改善微循环等作用。临床适用于风湿性关节炎，腰膝疼痛，肌肉拘紧，风湿性神经痛，外伤肿痛。

孕妇忌用。

伤湿止痛膏

〔药物组成〕 伤湿止痛流浸膏 冰片 樟脑 芸香浸膏等

〔功能与主治〕 祛风湿，活血止痛。用于风寒湿痹，筋挛拘急，四肢麻木，肌肉拉伤。

〔用法与用量〕 外用，贴患处，根据疼痛部位及大小决定用量。

〔剂型与规格〕 橡胶膏剂，每袋装 5 张

〔附注〕 本品具有抑菌，消炎，消肿镇痛，改善局部微循环等作用。临床适用于风湿性关节炎，肌纤维炎，肌肉拉伤，肌肉酸痛，扭伤等。

本品作用时间较短，8～12 小时更换 1 次。对橡皮膏过敏及局部有溃破者不宜使用。

镇 江 膏 药

〔药物组成〕 生川乌 生草乌 乌梢蛇 羌活等

〔功能与主治〕 祛风止痛，舒筋活血。用于筋骨疼痛，跌

打损伤，四肢麻木，关节疼痛。

〔用法与用量〕　外用，加温软化，贴于患处。

〔剂型与规格〕　黑膏药，每张重 25 g

〔附注〕　本品具有消炎，镇痛，抗风湿，改善微循环的作用。临床适用于风湿、类风湿性关节炎，神经炎，肌纤维炎，老年性肢体麻木等。

消 络 痛 片

〔药物组成〕　芫花条 99%　绿豆 1%

〔功能与主治〕　散风祛湿，消肿止痛。用于风寒湿痹，关节疼痛。

〔用法与用量〕　口服，1 次 3～4 片，1 日 3 次。

〔剂型与规格〕　糖衣片，每片重约 0.25 g

〔附注〕　本品具有抗菌，消炎，镇痛，消肿，促进关节部位微循环等作用。临床适用于风湿性关节炎，尤其适用于急性期的消肿镇痛。

独活寄生丸

〔药物组成〕　独活 7.4%　秦艽 7.3%　防风 7.3%　细辛 7.3%　杜仲 7.3%　牛膝 7.3%　寄生 7.3%　当归 4.9%　熟地黄 4.9%　白芍 4.9%　川芎 7.3%　党参 7.3%　茯苓 7.3%　甘草 4.9%　肉桂 7.3%

〔功能与主治〕　养血舒筋，祛风逐湿。适用于肝肾不足，风寒湿痹，腰膝疼痛，筋骨拘挛，关节不利。

〔用法与用量〕　口服，1 次 1 丸，1 日 1～2 次。

〔剂型与规格〕　蜜丸，每丸重 9 g

〔附注〕　处方来源于唐·孙思邈《备急千金要方》。

本品临床适用于肝肾两亏，气血不足型慢性关节炎，风湿性坐骨神经痛等。

武力拔寒散

〔药物组成〕 白花菜子等

〔功能与主治〕 祛风散寒，活血止痛。用于风寒湿痹，筋骨麻木，肩背疼痛，胃寒作疼，饮食失调，肾寒精冷，子宫寒冷，行经腹痛，寒湿带下。

〔用法与用量〕 外用，取药适量，用鸡蛋清加温开水少许或用人乳调成糊状，分摊在蜡纸上，贴于穴位或患处。有全身症状者，先贴较重处。

〔剂型与规格〕 散剂，每袋装 16.5 g

〔附注〕 本品具有抑菌消炎，镇痛，改善微循环等作用。临床适用于风湿性关节炎，肌纤维炎，神经炎，疝气，神经性胃痛，痛经等。

忌食生冷食物。肚脐及脚心部位不可贴用。本品有一定刺激性，用时有轻度疼痛为正常现象。每次贴 2～3 小时，揭去。贴之甚痛者可提前揭下。15 岁以下小儿勿用。

豨莶丸

〔药物组成〕 豨莶草 100%

〔功能与主治〕 散风祛湿，强筋健骨。用于风寒湿痹，手足麻木，筋骨萎弱，腰腿酸痛，骨刺疼痛。

〔用法与用量〕 口服，1 次 2 丸，1 日 2 次。

〔剂型与规格〕 蜜丸，每丸重 6 g

〔附注〕 本品具有抗风湿，消炎镇痛，改善微循环作用，临床适用于风湿性关节炎，类风湿性关节炎，肌纤维炎，骨质增生等。

大活络丸

〔药物组成〕 蕲蛇 威灵仙 全蝎 天麻 人参 当归

人工牛黄等

〔功能与主治〕　祛风，舒筋，活络，除湿。用于风寒湿痹引起的肢体疼痛，手足麻木，筋骨拘挛，中风瘫痪，口眼歪斜，半身不遂，言语不清。

〔用法与用量〕　口服，1次2丸，1日2次。

〔剂型与规格〕　蜜丸，每丸重3.6 g

〔附注〕　本品具有消炎，镇痛，抗风湿，促进血液循环等作用。临床适用于风湿性关节炎，风湿性肌纤维炎，神经炎，骨质增生，坐骨神经痛，脑血管意外和脑血管痉挛的恢复期。

孕妇忌服。

天 麻 丸

〔药物组成〕　天麻7.7%　羌活12.8%　独活12.8%　萆薢7.7%　杜仲9%　牛膝7.7%　附子1.3%　地黄20.5%　玄参7.7%　当归12.8%

〔功能与主治〕　散风活血，舒筋止痛。用于风中经络所致筋脉掣痛，手足麻木，腰腿疼痛，行走不便，口眼歪斜，半身不遂。

〔用法与用量〕　口服，1次1丸，1日1～2次。

〔剂型与规格〕　蜜丸，每丸重9 g

〔附注〕　本品具有消炎，镇痛，抗风湿，改善微循环等作用。临床适用于风湿性关节炎，退行性关节病，痛风性关节炎，类风湿性关节炎，脑溢血后遗症，脑血管痉挛，老年性手足挛痛。

小 活 络 丸

〔药物组成〕　胆南星21.2%　川乌21.1%　草乌21.1%　地龙21.2%　乳香7.7%　没药7.7%

〔功能与主治〕　祛风除湿，活血通痹。用于风寒湿痹，肢体疼痛，麻木拘挛。

〔用法与用量〕 口服，1 次 1 丸，1 日 2 次。

〔剂型与规格〕 蜜丸，每丸重 3 g

〔附注〕 本品具有抑菌，消炎，镇痛，抗风湿，改善微循环等作用。临床适用于风湿性关节炎，类风湿性关节炎，肌纤维炎，骨质增生等。

孕妇禁用。不可与阿托品、咖啡因、氨茶碱同服。

九 分 散

〔药物组成〕 马钱子粉 25%　麻黄 25%　乳香 25%　没药 25%

〔功能与主治〕 活血散瘀，消肿止痛。用于跌打损伤，瘀血肿痛。

〔用法与用量〕 饭后服，1 次 0.25 g，1 日 1 次。

〔剂型与规格〕 散剂，每包装 2.7 g

〔附注〕 本品适用于风湿性肌纤维炎，肌无力症，风湿性关节炎。

本品有毒，服用不宜超过 2.7g(1 包)。孕妇及高血压、心肾病患者禁用。小儿及体弱者按医嘱服用。外伤出血者不可外敷。

木 瓜 丸

〔药物组成〕 木瓜 10.8%　牛膝 8.2%　狗脊 5.4%　海风藤 10.8%　威灵仙 10.8%　鸡血藤 5.4%　白芷 10.8%　制川乌 5.4%　制草乌 5.4%　当归 10.8%　川芎 10.8%　人参 5.4%

〔功能与主治〕 散风祛湿，活络止痛。用于风寒湿痹，四肢麻木，遍身疼痛。

〔用法与用量〕 口服，1 次 1 丸，1 日 2 次。

〔剂型与规格〕 蜜丸，每丸重 9 g

〔附注〕 本品具有抗菌消炎，抗风湿，改善微循环作用。

临床适用于风湿性，类风湿性关节炎，病程较长，出现腰膝酸痛，肌肉疼痛无力者，以及老年性四肢麻木，腰膝酸痛。

复方当归注射液

〔药物组成〕　当归 18%　川芎 41%　红花 41%

〔功能与主治〕　活血化瘀。用于各种急慢性劳损，腰腿酸痛，四肢麻木，关节痛，痛经。

〔用法与用量〕　肌肉注射，1 日或隔日 1 次，1 次 2 ml。

〔剂型与规格〕　注射剂，每支装 2 ml

〔附注〕　本品具有改善微循环，抗炎，消肿，镇痛等作用。临床适用于各种急慢性肌纤维劳损，肌纤维炎，神经炎，坐骨神经痛，痛经，关节炎，外伤性截瘫，小儿麻痹症。

有出血倾向者及妇女月经过多者慎用。孕妇禁用。

祛风舒筋丸

〔药物组成〕　防风 5.6%　桂枝 5.6%　麻黄 5.6%　威灵仙 5.6%　川乌 5.6%　草乌 5.6%　苍术 5.6%　茯苓 5.6%　木瓜 5.6%　秦艽 5.6%　骨碎补 5.5%　牛膝 5.5%　甘草 5.5%　海风藤 5.5%　青风藤 5.5%　穿山龙 5.5%　老鹳草 5.5%　茄根 5.5%

〔功能与主治〕　祛风散寒，舒筋活络。用于风寒湿痹，四肢麻木，腰腿疼痛。

〔用法与用量〕　口服，1 次 1 丸，1 日 2 次。

〔剂型与规格〕　蜜丸，每丸重 9 g

〔附注〕　本品具有抗病毒，消炎，抗风湿，改善微循环的作用。临床适用于风湿性关节炎，肌纤维炎，以及感冒引起的发烧，头痛等。

孕妇慎用。

坎 离 砂

〔药物组成〕 麻黄 0.2% 羌活 0.2% 独活 0.2% 防风 0.2% 荆芥 0.2% 透骨草 0.2% 红花 0.2% 白芷 0.2% 当归 0.2% 牛膝 0.2% 生艾绒 0.2% 木瓜 0.2% 桂枝 0.2% 附子 0.2% 干姜 0.2% 铁落花 97.0%

〔功能与主治〕 祛风散寒, 活血止痛。用于腰腿疼痛, 四肢麻木, 筋骨拘挛, 阴寒腹痛, 小肠疝气。

〔用法与用量〕 外用, 1 次 1 袋, 用醋 10~15 g 迅速拌匀, 装入布袋内, 用棉纱盖好, 约 1 小时, 待药物发热后, 熨敷患处。

〔剂型与规格〕 熨剂, 每袋装 30 g

〔附注〕 本品具有抗菌, 消炎, 促进血循环作用, 临床适用于肌纤维炎, 神经炎, 风湿性关节炎等。

注意避风及过热。

伸筋丹胶囊

〔药物组成〕 地龙 25.7% 马钱子 17.9% 红花 17.9% 乳香 7.7% 防己 7.7% 没药 7.7% 香加皮 7.7% 骨碎补 7.7%

〔功能与主治〕 舒筋通络, 活血祛瘀, 消肿止痛。用于风寒湿痹, 腰腿疼痛, 四肢麻木, 筋骨扭伤, 积瘀肿痛。

〔用法与用量〕 口服, 1 次 5 粒, 1 日 3 次。

〔剂型与规格〕 胶囊剂, 每粒装 0.15 g

〔附注〕 本品具有消炎, 镇痛, 促进局部血液循环的作用。临床适用于肩周炎, 坐骨神经痛, 慢性骨性关节炎, 肥大性脊椎炎, 颈椎病, 骨折后遗症等。

孕妇及哺乳期妇女禁用。

10　抗寄生虫病药物

乌　梅　丸

〔药物组成〕　乌梅 19.9%　蜀椒 5%　黄连 20.7%　当归 5%　干姜 12.4%　黄柏 7.4%　桂枝 7.4%　附子 7.4%　人参 7.4%　细辛 7.4%

〔功能与主治〕　补虚温脏，驱蛔止痛。用于蛔厥，肠寒，胃痛吐蛔，或脾虚久痢，手足厥逆。

〔用法与用量〕　口服，1次1丸，1日3次，3岁以下儿童酌减。

〔剂型与规格〕　蜜丸，每丸重 9g

〔附注〕　处方来源于汉·张仲景《伤寒论》。

本品具有杀虫镇痛作用。临床适用于胆道蛔虫，蛔虫性肠梗阻，慢性胆囊炎，也可用于慢性胃肠炎，过敏性结肠炎，菌痢，阿米巴痢，阑尾炎等。

不宜与碳酸氢钠、氢氧化铝、胃舒平、氨茶碱同服。

乌梅安胃丸

〔药物组成〕　乌梅肉 24.0%　黄连 19.0%　附子 7.1%　干姜 11.9%　桂枝 7.1%　党参 7.1%　细辛 7.1%　当归 4.8%　黄柏 7.1%　花椒 4.8%

〔功能与主治〕　安蛔止痛。用于蛔厥，腹部阵痛，手足厥冷，呕恶吐蛔。

〔用法与用量〕　口服，1次9g，1日2次。

〔剂型与规格〕　水丸，每 40 粒重约 2 g。

〔附注〕　处方来源于汉·张仲景《伤寒论》。

本品具有杀虫，镇痛作用。临床适用于胆道蛔虫病。

川 楝 素 片

〔药物组成〕　川楝皮 100%

〔功能与主治〕　杀虫止痒。用于蛔虫，蛲虫，蛲虫腹痛。

〔用法与用量〕　口服，1 次 8～10 片，1 日 1 次，空腹服，小儿每岁以半片计。

〔剂型与规格〕　片剂，每片重 0.3 g

〔附注〕　本品为川楝皮提取物川楝素的制剂，具有抗寄生虫作用。临床适用于蛔虫，蛲虫等消化道寄生虫病。

溃疡病患者不易服用。

驱 虫 片

〔药物组成〕　木香 15.5%　槟榔 15.5%　使君子 15.5%　雷丸 4.5%　白矾 4.5%　芜荑 4.5%　芦荟 4.5%　大黄 15.5%　牵牛子 15.5%　雄黄 4.5%

〔功能与主治〕　杀虫，消积，通便。用于虫积腹痛，不思饮食，面黄肌瘦。

〔用法与用量〕　口服，1 次 8 片，1 日 2 次，小儿酌减。

〔剂型与规格〕　片剂，每片重约 0.3 g。

〔附注〕　本品具有抗寄生虫，缓泻作用。临床适用于蛔虫病，小儿慢性消耗性疾病。

囊 虫 丸

〔药物组成〕　茯苓 16.8%　雷丸 8.4%　生川乌 1.0%　桃仁 12.6%　烫水蛭 2.9%　大黄 4.2%　醋芫花 1.0%　黄连 4.2%　僵蚕 12.6%　橘红 5.0%　干漆炭 2.9%　牡丹皮 8.4%　五灵脂流浸膏 20.0%

〔功能与主治〕　活血化瘀，软坚消囊，镇惊止痛。用于囊肿疮块。

〔用法与用量〕　口服，1次1丸，1日2～3次。

〔剂型与规格〕　蜜丸，每丸重5g

〔附注〕　本品具有杀虫，镇痛作用。临床适用于人体猪囊虫症，脑囊虫及由脑囊虫引起的癫痫症。

使 君 子 丸

〔药物组成〕　使君子50%　天南星25%　槟榔25%

〔功能与主治〕　消积驱虫。用于小儿虫积，腹大胀痛，面黄肌瘦，善食多啼。

〔用法与用量〕　口服，1次9g，1日1次。

〔剂型与规格〕　水丸，每50粒重3g

〔附注〕　处方来源于明·王肯堂《证治准绳》。

本品具有抗寄生虫作用。临床适用于蛔虫病，蛲虫病等。

鳖 甲 煎 丸

〔药物组成〕　鳖甲胶　阿胶　蜂房　鼠妇虫　土鳖虫　蟅螂　硝石　柴胡　黄芩　半夏　党参　干姜　厚朴　桂枝　白芍　射干　桃仁　牡丹皮　大黄　凌霄花　葶苈子　石苇　瞿麦

〔功能与主治〕　活血化瘀，消积化痞。用于疟疾日久，胁肋胀满，心下痞块。

〔用法与用量〕　口服，1次2丸，1日2～3次。

〔剂型与规格〕　蜜丸，每丸重3g

〔附注〕　处方来源于汉·张仲景《金匮要略》。

本品具有抗疟原虫作用。临床适用于疟疾，黑热病，慢性肝炎.血吸虫病。

化 虫 丸

〔药物组成〕　鹤虱20%　槟榔10%　苦楝皮10%　使君

子 10%　雷丸 10%　大黄 10%　牵牛子 10%　玄明粉 20%

〔功能与主治〕　驱虫消积，用于肠道虫积，腹痛肛痒。

〔用法与用量〕　口服，1 次 6~9 g，1 日 1~2 次，3 岁以下小儿酌减。

〔剂型与规格〕　水丸，每 30 粒重 1 g

〔附注〕　处方来源于宋·陈师文《太平惠民和剂局方》。

本品具有杀虫作用。临床适用于肠道蛔虫，钩虫，蛲虫，姜片虫及蛲虫病。

年老体弱，小儿慎用。

霉 滴 净 片

〔药物组成〕　老鹳草　硼酸　雄黄　蛇床子　青黛　玄明粉　樟脑　冰片

〔功能与主治〕　燥湿杀虫。用于湿热下注，阴痒疼痛，赤白带下。

〔用法与用量〕　外用药，1 次 1 片，1 日 1 次，12 天为 1 疗程，每晚清洗阴部后，取药置于阴道深处。

〔剂型与规格〕　片剂，每片重 0.5 g

〔附注〕　本品具有抗菌消炎，杀虫作用。临床适用于霉菌性。滴虫性阴道炎、宫颈炎等。

孕妇慎用，月经期停用。

11 抗肿瘤药物

西 黄 丸

〔药物组成〕 乳香 没药 人工牛黄等

〔功能与主治〕 解毒散结，消肿止痛。用于痈疽疮疡，瘰疬，痰核，流注。

〔用法与用量〕 口服，1次3g，1日2次。

〔剂型与规格〕 水丸，每20粒重1g

〔附注〕 本品临床适用于多种肿瘤，脉管炎初期，多发性脓肿，淋巴结炎，急性蜂窝组织炎，阑尾脓肿，骨髓炎，肺脓肿，肝脓疡等。尤对乳腺癌疗效明显。

孕妇禁用。

片 仔 癀

〔药物组成〕 人工牛黄 蛇胆 三七等

〔功能与主治〕 清热解毒，消肿止痛。用于热毒肿痛，疔疮痈毒，乳蛾。

〔用法与用量〕 口服，1～8岁，1次0.15～0.3g，8岁以上0.6g，1日2～3次；外用，冷开水调敷患处，1日数次。

〔剂型与规格〕 曲剂，每块重3g；胶囊剂，每粒装0.3g

〔附注〕 本品临床适用于急慢性肝炎，耳炎，眼炎，扁桃体炎，牙龈肿痛，口疮，肿瘤及烫伤，灼伤等。

孕妇忌服。

新 癀 片

〔药物组成〕 人工牛黄 三七等

〔功能与主治〕 清热解毒，散瘀消肿。用于热毒肿瘤，疮痈肿毒。

〔用法与用量〕 口服，1次2～4片，1日3次，小儿酌减；外用，水调涂患处。

〔剂型与规格〕 糖衣片，每片重约0.32 g

〔附注〕 本品临床适用于食道癌，贲门癌，急性黄疸性肝炎，胆囊炎，风湿性关节炎，痔疮，外科感染，各种无名肿毒等。

胃与十二指肠溃疡患者，肾功能不全者及孕妇慎用，有消化道出血史忌用。

鸦胆子乳注射液

〔药物组成〕 鸦胆子100%

〔功能与主治〕 清热解毒，散结消肿。用于热毒壅盛，痈疽瘰疬，腹下痞块。

〔用法与用量〕 静脉注射，1日1次，1次5～10 ml，4个月为1疗程。根据病情需要，可以加大剂量至1次10～30 ml。

使用时加5～10%葡萄糖注射液或生理盐水250～500 ml稀释。

〔剂型与规格〕 静脉注射用乳剂，每支装2ml，含本品10%

〔附注〕 本品临床适用于食道癌，胃癌，直肠癌等消化道系统癌症，亦可用于肺癌的治疗。

少数患者用药后有厌油腻、恶心、厌食等消化道反应，经对症治疗可以缓解。

宫 颈 癌 片

〔药物组成〕 掌叶半夏100%

〔功能与主治〕 解毒散结，消肿止痛。用于湿热下注，瘰病，流注。

〔用法与用量〕　口服，1 次 2～3 片，1 日 3 次。

〔剂型与规格〕　糖衣片，每片含醇浸膏 0.3 g

〔附注〕　本品具有抗肿瘤作用。临床适用于子宫颈癌及子宫颈癌前期病变。

核葵注射液

〔药物组成〕　核桃枝 91%　龙葵 9%

〔功能与主治〕　利湿消肿。用于脾肾两虚，湿热壅盛，脘腹胀满。

〔用法与用量〕　肌肉注射，1 次 2～4 ml，1 日 1～2 次，2 个月为 1 疗程；瘤体注射（宫颈癌体注射），1 次 4～8 ml，1 日 1 次。

〔剂型与规格〕　注射剂，每支 2 ml。

〔附注〕　本品具有增强机体免疫功能，抗肿瘤，利尿，镇痛作用。临床适用于多种肿瘤的胸水，腹水，疼痛及宫颈出血。可抑制肺癌，宫颈癌的瘤体生长，对部分宫颈癌患者可缩小肿瘤。

12 外科药物

12.1 伤科用药

跌 打 丸

〔药物组成〕 三七 5.2% 当归 2.6% 白芍 3.9% 赤芍 5.2% 桃仁 2.6% 红花 3.9% 血竭 3.9% 刘寄奴 2.6% 骨碎补 2.6% 续断 25.8% 苏木 3.9% 牡丹皮 2.6% 乳香 3.9% 没药 3.9% 姜黄 1.9% 甜瓜子 2.6% 防风 2.5% 枳实（炒）2.5% 桔梗 2.5% 甘草 3.9% 木通 2.5% 自然铜（煅）2.6% 土鳖虫 2.5% 三棱（醋制）3.9%

〔功能与主治〕 活血散瘀，消肿止痛，祛风活络。用于跌打损伤，瘀血肿痛，闪腰岔气。

〔用法与用量〕 口服，1次1丸，1日2次。

〔剂型与规格〕 蜜丸，每丸重 3 g

〔附注〕 本品具有消炎，镇痛，促进血液循环作用。临床适用于各类骨折，关节，韧带，腰肌损伤等。

孕妇禁用。

中华跌打丸

〔药物组成〕 金不换 半边莲 鹅不食草 杜仲 田基黄 颠茄根等

〔功能与主治〕 消肿止痛，舒筋活络，止血生肌。用于筋骨挫伤，创伤，风湿痹痛。

〔用法与用量〕 口服，1次1丸，1日2～3次；外用，白酒调，搽患处。

〔剂型与规格〕　蜜丸，每丸重 6 g

〔附注〕　本品临床适用于各种外伤，扭伤，跌伤，刀伤，风湿性关节炎等。

内服药丸后，如有喉干或口苦现象，可饮一些清凉剂。如患外感发烧，咳嗽痰稠，应停服。

七　厘　散

〔药物组成〕　血竭　乳香　没药　红花　儿茶　冰片　朱砂等

〔功能与主治〕　化瘀消肿，止痛止血。用于跌扑损伤，血瘀疼痛，外伤出血。

〔用法与用量〕　口服，1 次 1～1.5 g，1 日 1～3 次

〔剂型与规格〕　散剂，每瓶装 1.5 g

〔附注〕　本品具有抗炎镇痛，止血，促进局部血液循环作用。临床适用于各种扑伤出血，扭挫伤，骨折，软组织损伤，韧带劳损等，可试用于中毒性心肌炎，冠心病心绞痛。亦可用于一切无名肿毒，烧伤，烫伤及带状疱疹。

不宜与溴化钾，溴化钠，碘化钠同服。

骨折挫伤散

〔药物组成〕　乳香　没药　大黄　红花　鳖虫等

〔功能与主治〕　舒筋活血，接骨止痛，消肿散瘀。用于跌打损伤，瘀血肿痛，风湿痹痛。

〔用法与用量〕　口服，1 次 9 粒，1 日 3 次。

〔剂型与规格〕　胶囊剂，每粒重约 0.4 g

〔附注〕　本品具有抗炎，促进局部血液循环，骨折愈合的作用。临床适用于各种挫伤，韧带拉伤，风湿性关节炎等。

三七伤药片

〔药物组成〕 三七 3.1% 草乌（蒸）3.1% 冰片 0.06% 雪上一枝蒿 3.1% 骨碎补 29.2% 接骨木 46.84% 红花 9.4% 赤芍 5.2%

〔功能与主治〕 舒筋活血，散瘀止痛。用于挫伤，扭伤，跌打损伤。

〔用法与用量〕 口服，1 次 3 片，1 日 3 次。

〔剂型与规格〕 糖衣片，每片重约 0.33 g

〔附注〕 本品具有消炎，镇痛作用。临床适用于各种外伤，关节痛，神经痛及软组织损伤等。临床 305 例伤科患者用本品治疗，总有效率达 91.8%。

跌 打 药 精

〔药物组成〕 红花 儿茶 归尾 安息香 乳香 没药等

〔功能与主治〕 散瘀消肿，活络止痛。用于跌伤，筋骨扭伤，积瘀肿痛。

〔用法与用量〕 口服，每次 5～10 ml；外用涂搽患处。

〔剂型与规格〕酒剂，每瓶装 50 g

〔附注〕 本品具有消炎，镇痛，促进局部血液流动作用。临床适用于伤科各种肿痛。

一粒止痛丹

〔药物组成〕 （略）

〔功能与主治〕 活血散瘀，消肿止痛。用于跌打损伤，瘀血肿痛，月经痛。

〔用法与用量〕 口服，1 次 1 丸，1 日 2～3 次。

〔剂型与规格〕 微丸，每 10 粒重 1 g

〔附注〕 本品具有显著的镇痛作用，并可抗炎消肿。临床适用于刀伤，跌打损伤，痛经等局部疼痛，对部分晚期恶性肿瘤疼痛也有较好疗效。

接 骨 散

〔药物组成〕 麻黄 16.7% 土鳖虫 16.7% 乳香 16.7% 没药 16.7% 地龙 16.6% 自然铜 16.6%

〔功能与主治〕 活血止痛，续筋接骨。用于伤筋动骨，瘀血肿痛。

〔用法与用量〕 口服，1次 1/3～1袋，1日1～2次；外用，白酒调敷患处。

〔剂型与规格〕 散剂，每袋重 9 g

〔附注〕 本品具有镇痛，促进肉芽组织生长的作用。临床适用于伤科各种肿胀疼痛。

五 虎 散

〔药物组成〕 当归 21.3% 红花 21.3% 防风 21.3% 天南星 21.3% 白芷 14.8%

〔功能与主治〕 活血散瘀，消肿止痛。用于跌打损伤，瘀血不散，红肿疼痛或皮肉青紫。

〔用法与用量〕 口服，1次 6 g，1日2次；外用，适量，白酒调敷患处。

〔剂型与规格〕 散剂，每包重 6 g

〔附注〕 本品具有促进血液循环及镇痛作用。临床适用于跌伤，扭伤，风湿性关节炎等。

孕妇忌服。

正 骨 水

〔药物组成〕 大力王 丢了棒 薄荷脑 碎骨木等

〔功能与主治〕 舒筋活络，活血止痛。用于跌打损伤，筋骨疼痛。

〔用法与用量〕 搽患处，重症者用药液湿透药棉敷患处，上肢敷 1 小时，下肢敷 1 小时半。1 日 2～3 次

〔剂型与规格〕 酊水剂，每瓶装 15 ml

〔附注〕 本品具有促进局部血液流动、镇痛作用。临床适用于各种骨折，挫伤，脱臼肿胀。

孕妇禁用。不可内服。患处肤破出血，应先止血，忌搽伤口。

红 药 片

〔药物组成〕 三七 46.0% 土鳖虫 10.8% 当归 10.8% 白芷 10.8% 川芎 10.8% 红花 10.8%

〔功能与主治〕 活血止痛，祛瘀生新。用于跌打损伤，筋骨肿痛，风湿麻木。

〔用法与用量〕 口服，1 次 2 片，1 日 2 次。

〔剂型与规格〕 糖衣片，每片（基片）重 0.25 g

〔附注〕 本品具有消炎、镇痛，促进血液循环作用。临床适用于各种骨折及软组织损伤。

跌打损伤丸

〔药物组成〕 麻黄 20% 马钱子适量（相当于含土的 0.228%） 土鳖虫 30% 当归 20% 红花 20% 自然铜（醋煅）10%

〔功能与主治〕 活血祛瘀，消肿止痛。用于跌打损伤，闪腰岔气，伤筋动骨，瘀血肿痛。

〔用法与用量〕 口服，首服半丸，1 日 2 次，如无唇麻等反应，可继服每次 1 丸，1 日 2 次，服后应轻微发汗。

〔剂型与规格〕 蜜丸，每丸重 3 g

〔附注〕 本品具有消炎、镇痛，促进血液循环作用。临床

适用于一切外科损伤，肿胀疼痛。

心脏病患者，孕妇及儿童忌服。

跌打活血散

〔药物组成〕 红花 2.6% 当归 12.8% 血竭 3.0% 三七 4.3% 骨碎补 12.8% 续断 12.8% 乳香 12.8% 没药 12.8% 儿茶 8.4% 大黄 8.4% 冰片 0.9% 大鳖虫 8.4%

〔功能与主治〕 舒筋活血，散瘀止痛。用于跌打损伤，瘀血肿痛，闪腰岔气。

〔用法与用量〕 口服，1 次 3 g，1 日 2 次；外用，黄酒或醋调敷患处。

〔剂型与规格〕 散剂，每包重 3 g

〔附注〕 本品具有改善微循环，消肿，镇痛作用。临床适用于各种跌伤，扭伤肿痛。

孕妇忌用。

腰 痛 丸

〔药物组成〕 吉祥草 15% 山药 30% 补骨脂 30% 怀牛膝 7.5% 续断 10%

〔功能与主治〕 行气活血，散瘀止痛。用于闪跌扭伤，瘀血肿痛。

〔用法与用量〕 口服，1 次 1～2 丸，1 日 2 次。

〔剂型与规格〕 蜜丸，每丸重 9 g

〔附注〕 本品具有消炎，镇痛作用。临床适用于伤科各种肿痛，腰痛及急性腰肌劳损等。

药 艾 条

〔药物组成〕 艾叶 74.0% 桂枝 3.9% 降香 5.4% 高良姜 3.9% 广藿香 1.6% 香附 1.6% 白芷 3.1% 陈皮 1.6%

丹参 1.6%　　生川乌 2.3%　　雄黄 0.4%

〔功能与主治〕　　行气血，逐寒湿。用于风寒湿痹，肌肉酸麻，关节四肢疼痛，腹冷痛。

〔用法与用量〕　　外用，点燃灸烤，至皮肤红晕为度，1 日 2 次。

〔剂型与规格〕　　灸熨剂，每支重 29.6 g

〔附注〕　　本品具有抗炎，镇痛作用。临床适用于慢性风湿性关节炎所致肌肉酸麻疼痛。

12.2　外科用药

梅花点舌丹

〔药物组成〕　　珍珠　蟾酥　雄黄　朱砂　硼砂　葶苈子　乳香　没药　血竭　沉香　冰片等

〔功能与主治〕　　清热解毒，消肿止痛。用于疔疮痈肿初起，咽喉牙龈肿痛，口舌生疮。

〔用法与用量〕　　口服，1 次 3 粒，1 日 1～2 次；外用，醋调敷患处。

〔剂型与规格〕　　水丸，每 10 粒重 1 g

〔附注〕　　本品具有抗菌，消炎，镇痛作用。临床适用于腮腺炎，乳腺炎，急性淋巴结炎，脓毒败血症，扁桃体炎，牙周炎，咽炎，无名肿毒等。

紫　金　锭

〔药物组成〕　　山慈姑　红大戟　千金子霜　五倍子等

〔功能与主治〕　　辟秽化浊，清热解毒，活血消肿，用于中暑，腹胀痛，恶心呕吐，泄泻，外治痈疽，疔疮，痄腮，丹毒，喉风。

〔用法与用量〕　　口服，1 次 0.6～1.5 g，1 日 2 次；外用，

醋调敷患处。

〔剂型与规格〕　锭剂，每支 0.3 g

〔附注〕　本品临床适用于暑夏肠胃型感冒，急性胆囊炎，腮腺炎，淋巴结炎，虫蛇咬伤，无名肿毒等。

小 金 丸

〔药物组成〕　木鳖子　草乌　枫香脂　乳香　没药　五灵脂　当归　地龙　香墨等

〔功能与主治〕　散瘀消肿，活血止痛。用于阴疽初起，肿硬作痛，疮疡瘰疬，痰核瘿瘤。

〔用法与用量〕　打碎后口服，1 次 1.5 g，1 日 2 次，小儿酌减。

〔剂型与规格〕　糊丸，每丸重 0.6 g，水丸，每 50 粒重 3 g

〔附注〕　本品具有消炎，抗菌，镇痛，抗结核作用。临床适用于多发性脓肿，骨结核，肠系膜淋巴结核，甲状腺瘤，淋巴结炎，乳腺炎，乳腺癌等。

孕妇忌服。

如意金黄散

〔药物组成〕　姜黄 12.5%　大黄 12.5%　黄柏 12.5%　苍术 5%　厚朴 5%　陈皮 5%　甘草 5%　生天南星 5%　白芷 12.5%　天花粉 25%

〔功能与主治〕　解毒消肿，止痛。用于痈疽肿毒初起，肿未形成，局部红肿坚硬，灼热疼痛。

〔用法与用量〕　外用，调敷，1 日数次。

〔剂型与规格〕　散剂，每包重 15 g

〔附注〕　处方来源于明·陈实功《外科正宗》。

本品具有抗菌消炎作用。临床适用于外科急性化脓性感染，急性蜂窝组织炎，溶血性链球菌感染引起的急性体表炎症，急性淋巴结炎，腮腺炎，乳腺炎，毛囊炎，湿疹，丹毒以及外伤肿胀疼痛。

醒 消 丸

〔药物组成〕　雄黄　乳香　没药等

〔功能与主治〕　活血散瘀，消肿止痛。用于痈疽肿毒，红肿热痛。

〔用法与用量〕　口服，1 次 1.5～3 g，1 日 2 次。

〔剂型与规格〕　水丸，每 20 粒重 1 g

〔附注〕　本品具有抗菌消炎，消肿作用。临床适用于丹毒，脓毒败血症，淋巴结核，乳腺炎，硬节性红斑，肿瘤等。

孕妇禁用。

阳 和 丸

〔药物组成〕　熟地黄 55.6%　鹿角胶 16.7%　肉桂 5.6%　炮姜 2.8%　麻黄 2.8%　白芥子 11.1%　甘草 5.6%

〔功能与主治〕　温阳补血，散寒消痰。用于一切阴疽，附骨疽，流注，鹤膝风等局部漫肿无头，皮色不变症。

〔用法与用量〕　口服，1 次 3 g，1 日 2 次。

〔剂型与规格〕　水丸，每 30 粒重 1 g

〔附注〕　处方来源于清。王洪绪《外科证治全生集》。

本品具有抗菌、消炎，抗结核作用。临床适用于骨结核，腹膜结核，淋巴结核，血栓闭塞性脉管炎，骨髓炎，慢性深部脓肿，慢性支气管炎，妇女痛经，慢性关节炎，腰椎间盘突出，腰椎肥大等。

疡疮肿疽已溃者禁用。

拔 毒 膏

〔药物组成〕　蜜陀僧 0.97%　木鳖子 0.97%　白芨 0.5%　白蔹 0.5%　夏枯草 1.9%　苍耳子 0.97%　猪牙皂 0.97%　紫草 0.5%　地丁 0.5%　山慈姑 0.5%　大枫子 0.5%　蛇床子 0.5%　益母草 0.96%　连翘 0.96%　血竭 0.5%　没药 0.5%　乳香 0.5%　儿茶 0.5%　冰片 0.5%　白矾 0.5%　黄蜡 3.9%　植物油 62.5%　黄丹 19.4%

〔功能与主治〕　拔毒止痛，化腐生肌。用于皮肤诸疮，脓溃肿痛，蝎鳖虫咬，无名肿毒。

〔用法与用量〕　外用，贴患处。

〔剂型与规格〕　膏药，每张净重 0.125 g

〔附注〕　本品具有抗菌消炎，促进创伤组织愈合的作用。临床适用于疖肿，化脓性感染，蜂窝组织炎，蝎毒感染等。

蟾 酥 丸

〔药物组成〕　蟾酥　雄黄　轻粉　枯矾　寒水石　铜绿　乳香　没药　胆矾　蜗牛等

〔功能与主治〕　清热解毒，消肿止痛。用于疔疮，发背，乳痈等恶疮。

〔用法与用量〕　口服，1 次 5～15 粒，1 日 1～2 次；外用，醋调敷患处。

〔剂型与规格〕　水丸，每 30 粒重 1 g

〔附注〕　本品具有抗菌消炎，镇痛作用。临床适用于各种化脓性感染，蜂窝组织炎，化脓性淋巴结炎等。

孕妇忌服，已溃烂者不宜外敷。

紫 草 膏

〔药物组成〕　紫草 35.8%　白芷 10.7%　防风 10.7%　乳

香 10.7%　　没药 10.7%　　当归 10.7%　　地黄 10.7%

〔功能与主治〕　　化腐生肌，消肿止痛。用于疮疡已溃，疼痛不止，久不收口。

〔用法与用量〕　　外用，涂患处，每 2～3 日换药 1 次。

〔剂型与规格〕　　软膏剂，每盒装 15 g

〔附注〕　　处方来源于清·顾世澄《疡医大全》。

本品具有消炎，镇痛，促进创口愈合的作用。临床适用于各种化脓性感染，溃破流脓血，水痘溃烂，冻伤，烫伤，烧伤等。

内消瘰疬片

〔药物组成〕　　夏枯草 26.18%　　浙贝母 3.2%　　海藻 3.2%　　白蔹 3.2%　　天花粉 3.2%　　连翘 3.2%　　熟大黄 3.2%　　玄明粉 3.2%　　蛤壳 3.2%　　大青盐 16.1%　　枳壳 3.2%　　桔梗 3.2%　　薄荷冰 0.02%　　地黄 3.2%　　当归 3.2%　　玄参 16.1%　　甘草 3.2%

〔功能与主治〕　　软坚散结，解毒消肿。用于痰凝气滞引起的瘰疬痰核，颈项瘿瘤。

〔用法与用量〕　　口服，1 次 4～8 片，1 日 1～2 次。

〔剂型与规格〕　　片剂，每片重 0.6 g

〔附注〕　　处方来源于清·顾世澄《疡医大全》。

本品具有抗菌，抗结核，镇痛作用。临床适用于慢性淋巴结炎，淋巴结核，甲状腺肿大等。

栀子金花丸

〔药物组成〕　　栀子　黄连　黄芩　黄柏　大黄　金银花　知母　天花粉

〔功能与主治〕　　清热泻火，凉血解毒。用于肺胃热盛，口舌生疮，牙龈肿痛，目赤眩晕，咽喉肿痛，大便燥结。

〔用法与用量〕　　口服，1 次 9 g，1 日 1 次。

〔剂型与规格〕 水丸，每 50 粒重 3 g；蜜丸，每丸重 9 g

〔附注〕 处方来源于金·刘宏素《宣明论方》。

本品具有抗菌消炎作用；临床适用于慢性咽炎，牙周炎，口疮，丹毒，蜂窝组织炎，肛门直肠周围感染，鼻出血等。

孕妇忌服

荆防败毒丸

〔药物组成〕 荆芥 11.4% 防风 11.4% 茯苓 11.3% 前胡 11.3% 桔梗 11.3% 羌活 7.5% 独活 7.5% 柴胡 7.5% 川芎 7.5% 枳壳 7.5% 甘草 3.9% 薄荷 1.9%

〔功能与主治〕 清热解毒，疏风散结。用于疮疡初起，发热肿痛，以及外感风寒。

〔用法与用量〕 口服，1 次 6 g，1 日 3 次。

〔剂型与规格〕 水丸，每 20 粒重 1 g

〔附注〕 处方来源于《摄生众妙方》。

本品具有抗菌消炎，抗病毒作用。临床适用于疥癣，湿疹，荨麻疹等皮肤病及疔疖，乳腺炎，流行性感冒，流行性腮腺炎。

阑尾消炎片

〔药物组成〕 金银花 14.3% 大青叶 14.3% 败酱草 14.3% 蒲公英 14.3% 红藤 14.3% 川楝子 2.9% 大黄 4.3% 木香 4.3% 冬瓜子 4.3% 桃仁 2.9% 赤芍 5.5% 黄芩 4.3%

〔功能与主治〕 活血散瘀，消肿止痛。用于肠痈脓肿，脘腹胀满，腹痛拒按。

〔用法与用量〕 口服，1 次 10～15 片，1 日 3 次。

〔剂型与规格〕 糖衣片，每片（基片）重约 0.25 g

〔附注〕 本品具有抗菌消炎作用，临床适用于急、慢性阑尾炎。

腮 腺 炎 片

〔药物组成〕 蓼大青叶 21.4% 板兰根 21.4% 连翘 21.4% 蒲公英 21.4% 夏枯草 14.26% 人工牛黄 0.14%

〔功能与主治〕 清热解毒, 消肿散结。用于散结, 痈疽肿痛。

〔用法与用量〕 口服, 1 次 6 片, 1 日 3 次。

〔剂型与规格〕 片剂, 每片重 0.3 g

〔附注〕 本品具有抗病毒, 消炎作用。临床适用于流行性腮腺炎。

12.3 抗骨质增生药

骨 刺 片

〔药物组成〕 地黄 20% 鸡血藤 15% 威灵仙 12.5% 淫羊藿 12.5% 肉苁蓉 7.5% 鹿衔草 12.5% 骨碎补 12.5% 莱菔子 7.5%

〔功能与主治〕 补肾活血, 祛风软坚。用于颈项强直, 沉酸胀痛, 胳臂麻木, 腰腿疼痛。

〔用法与用量〕 口服, 1 次 5 片, 1 日 3 次。

〔剂型与规格〕 糖衣片, 每片 (基片) 重约 0.3 g

〔附注〕 本品具有改善血液微循环, 消炎镇痛作用。临床适用于骨质增生引起的颈椎肥大, 腰椎肥大, 胸椎肥大以及四肢关节增生等。

服药后部分病人出现轻度消化道反应, 可自行消失。

骨质增生丸

〔药物组成〕 熟地 21.4% 肉苁蓉 14.3% 骨碎补 14.3% 淫羊藿 14.3% 鸡血藤 14.3% 莱菔子 7.1% 鹿衔草

14.3%

〔功能与主治〕 补腰肾，强筋骨，活血利气止痛。用于腰膝酸软，颈背强直，四肢疼痛，活动不利。

〔用法与用量〕 口服，蜜丸，1 次 1 丸，浓缩丸 1 次 10～15 粒，1 日 2～3 次。

〔剂型与规格〕 蜜丸，每丸重 3 g，浓缩丸，每 8 粒重 1 g

〔附注〕 本品具有改善血液微循环，消炎镇痛作用。临床适用于肥大性脊椎炎，颈椎病，腰椎、胸椎肥大，跟骨刺，大骨节病以及增生性关节炎等。

骨 刺 丸

〔药物组成〕 穿山龙 徐长卿 制马钱子 鸡血藤等

〔功能与主治〕 通经活络，祛湿止痛，软坚散结。用于风寒湿痹，颈项强直，沉酸胀痛，腰腿疼痛。

〔用法与用量〕 口服，1 次 1 丸，1 日 2～3 次。

〔剂型与规格〕 蜜丸，每丸重 6 g

〔附注〕 本品具有改善血液微循环，消炎镇痛作用。临床适用于骨质增生，风湿性关节炎，类风湿性关节炎，风湿病等。

骨 仙 片

〔药物组成〕 骨碎补 广防己 熟地黄 黑豆 菟丝子等

〔功能与主治〕 填精益髓，壮腰健肾，舒筋活络。用于四肢麻木，腰腿酸痛，颈项强直。

〔用法与用量〕 口服，1 次 4～6 片，1 日 3 次，30～50 天为 1 疗程。

〔剂型与规格〕 糖衣片，每片重 0.5 g

〔附注〕 本品具有改善血液微循环，消炎镇痛作用。临床适用于骨质增生症，足跟骨骨质增生，膝关节骨质增生，腰椎，胸椎，颈椎等诸骨关节增生。

感冒发烧者勿用

骨刺消痛液

〔药物组成〕　川乌　木瓜　威灵仙　乌梅　怀牛膝　桂枝等

〔功能与主治〕　活血，利湿，止痛。用于风寒湿痹，湿热蕴结引起颈项强直，沉酸胀痛，四肢麻木，腰腿疼痛。

〔用法与用量〕　口服，1 次 10～15 ml，1 日 2 次。

〔剂型与规格〕　酒剂，每瓶装 30 ml

〔附注〕　本品具有改善血液微循环，消炎镇痛作用。临床适用于腰椎，胸椎肥大，颈椎病，风湿性，类风湿性关节炎。

不宜和阿斯匹林，水杨酸钠同服。

12.4　痔瘘用药

痔　瘘　丸

〔药物组成〕　大黄　胡黄连　芒硝　郁李仁　槐花　地榆　桃仁　乳香　没药　象牙屑　滑石　雄黄　荆芥穗　石决明　当归

〔功能与主治〕　清热解毒，消肿通便，化痔散结。用于湿热下注，血热所致痔疮肿痛，痔瘘下血。

〔用法与用量〕　口服，1 次 9 g，1 日 2 次。

〔剂型与规格〕　蜜丸，每丸重 9 g

〔附注〕　本品具有消炎，止血作用。临床适用于内、外痔，混合痔出血，肛裂，脱肛等。

槐　角　丸

〔药物组成〕　槐角 28.5%　地榆 14.3%　黄芩 14.3%　枳壳 14.3%　当归 14.3%　防风 14.3%

〔功能与主治〕　清肠疏风，凉血止血。用于大肠热盛，痔瘘肿痛，大便出血。

〔用法与用量〕　口服，1次1丸，1日2次。

〔剂型与规格〕　蜜丸，每丸重9g

〔附注〕　处方来源于《沈氏尊生书》。本品具有消炎，止血作用。临床适用于内、外痔，混合痔，肛裂出血，便血等。

消 痔 灵 片

〔药物组成〕　五倍子4.8%　白蔹23.5%　卷柏23.5%　地榆23.5%　槐花23.5%　牛羊胆膏1.2%

〔功能与主治〕　清热凉血，消肿解毒。用于痔瘘肿痛，大便下血。

〔用法与用量〕　口服，1次3～5片，1日3次。

〔剂型与规格〕　糖衣片，每片（基片）重约0.3g

〔附注〕　本品具有消炎，止血，促进创面愈合作用。临床适用于内外痔疮，混合痔，肛裂出血等。

化 痔 灵 片

〔药物组成〕　黄连1.5%　琥珀1.5%　三七3.8%　五倍子30%　石榴皮30%　枯矾17.4%　雄黄6.3%　槐花3.2%　乌梅3.1%　诃子（去核）3.2%

〔功能与主治〕　清热，凉血，收剑。用于痔瘘肿毒，大便下血。

〔用法与用量〕　口服，1次4～6片，1日3次。

〔剂型与规格〕　糖衣片，每片重约0.3g

〔附注〕　本品具有抗菌消炎，促进创面愈合作用。临床适用于内、外痔疮，混合痔，肛裂出血等。

12.5 烧伤、烫伤用药

京万红烫伤药膏

〔药物组成〕 地榆 栀子 大黄 冰片等

〔功能与主治〕 消肿止痛,化腐生肌。用于各种烧烫伤,脓疡溃烂。

〔用法与用量〕 外用,涂敷患处。

〔剂型与规格〕 油膏剂,每瓶装 30 g

〔附注〕 本品具有抗菌消炎,镇痛,促进创面愈合作用。临床适用于Ⅰ~Ⅱ度烧伤,烫伤,内外痔疮、褥疮等。

獾 油

〔药物组成〕 獾油 97% 冰片 3%

〔功能与主治〕 润肤生肌,消肿止痛。用于水火烫伤,皮肤红肿,起泡溃烂。

〔用法与用量〕 外用,涂敷患处。

〔剂型与规格〕 油膏剂,每瓶装 15 g

〔附注〕 本品具有消炎、镇痛,护肤作用。临床适用于轻度烧伤,烫伤所致皮肤起泡,溃烂以及痔疮,疮癣等。

烧伤气雾剂

〔药物组成〕 五倍子 诃子等

〔功能与主治〕 清热解毒,利湿收敛。用于烧烫伤,肿痛溃烂。

〔用法与用量〕 外用,喷患处,1 日 3~4 次。

〔剂型与规格〕 气雾剂,每瓶装 20 ml

〔附注〕 本品具有抑菌,促进创面愈合作用。临床适用于烫伤,火焰烧伤,化学烧伤,电击伤,复合烧伤等。

12.6　蛇伤用药

云 南 蛇 药

〔药物组成〕　（略）

〔功能与主治〕　解热消肿，止血止痛。用于毒蛇咬伤。

〔用法与用量〕　外用，涂搽患处。

〔剂型与规格〕　酊水剂，每瓶装 200 ml。

〔附注〕　本品具有消炎解毒，止血作用。临床适用于各种毒蛇咬伤。

季德胜蛇药片

〔药物组成〕　（略）

〔功能与主治〕　解热消肿，止血止痛。用于毒蛇、毒虫咬伤。

〔用法与用量〕　口服，1 次 1 片，1 日 3 次。

〔剂型与规格〕　片剂，每片重 0.3 g

〔附注〕　本品具有解毒，镇痛作用。主要用于毒蛇、毒虫咬伤。

13　妇产科药物

13.1　月经失调用药

艾附暖宫丸

〔药物组成〕　艾叶 13.2%　肉桂 2.2%　香附 26.0%　当归 13.0%　吴茱萸 8.7%　川芎 8.7%　白芍 8.7%　地黄 4.3%　黄芪 8.7%　续断 6.5%

〔功能与主治〕　理气补气，暖宫调经。用于妇女子宫虚寒，月经不调，经来腹痛，腰酸带下。

〔用法与用量〕　口服，1 次 1 丸，1 日 2 次。

〔剂型与规格〕　蜜丸，每丸重 9 g

〔附注〕　处方来源于明·龚廷贤《寿世保元》。

本品具有镇痛，调整子宫功能，滋养，强壮作用。临床适用于不孕症，月经失调，痛经，白带。

乌鸡白凤丸

〔药物组成〕　乌鸡 25.1%　鹿角胶 5.0%　鳖甲 2.5%　桑螵蛸 1.9%　牡蛎 1.9%　人参 5.0%　黄芪 1.3%　当归 5.6%　香附 5.0%　白芍 5.0%　天冬 2.5%　甘草 1.3%　熟地黄 10.0%　地黄 10.0%　银柴胡 1.0%　川芎 2.5%　芡实 2.5%　丹参 5.0%　鹿角霜 1.9%　山药 5.0%

〔功能与主治〕　补气养血，调经止带。用于气血两虚，身体瘦弱，腰膝酸软，经血不调，崩漏带下。

〔用法与用量〕　口服，1 次 1 丸，1 日 2 次。

〔剂型与规格〕　蜜丸，每丸重 9 g

〔附注〕　本品具有滋养，强壮，调整子宫功能及收敛作用。临床适用于月经失调，功能性子宫出血，女性生殖器炎症，白带。

女 金 丹

〔药物组成〕 当归 7.0% 白芍 3.5% 熟地黄 3.5% 川芎 3.5% 党参 2.5% 白术 3.5% 益母草 10.0% 茯苓 3.5% 牡丹皮 3.5% 甘草 3.5% 没药 3.5% 肉桂 3.5% 延胡索 3.5% 藁本 3.5% 白芷 3.5% 黄芩 3.5% 香附 7.5% 白薇 3.5% 赤石脂 3.5% 砂仁 2.5% 鹿角霜 7.5% 陈皮 7.0% 阿胶 3.5%

〔功能与主治〕 养血调经，理气止痛。用于气滞血瘀，经血不调，痛经，腰腿酸痛，四肢无力。

〔用法与用量〕 口服，1 次 1 丸，1 日 2 次。

〔剂型与规格〕 蜜丸，每丸重 9 g

〔附注〕 处方来源于明·韩懋胜，金丹方。

本品具有滋养，强壮，调整子宫功能，镇痛作用。临床适用于月经失调，痛经，功能性子宫出血，女性生殖器炎症，白带。

孕妇慎用。

妇科调经片

〔药物组成〕 香附 51.4% 当归 18.5% 大枣 10.3% 赤芍 1.5% 熟地黄 6.2% 白术 3.0% 延胡索 4.1% 川芎 2.1% 白芍 1.5% 甘草 1.4%

〔功能与主治〕 补血，益气，调经。用于月经不调，经来腹痛，月经量少色淡，质清稀，头晕眼花，面色苍白，小腹绵绵作痛，按之痛减。

〔用法与用量〕 口服，1 次 4 片，1 日 3 次。

〔剂型与规格〕 片剂，每片重约 0.3 g

〔附注〕 本品具有滋养，强壮，调整子宫功能，镇痛作用。临床适用于月经失调，经期腹痛。

妇科十味片

〔药物组成〕 香附 76.8% 党参 2.2% 白术 2.2% 茯苓 2.2% 甘草 1.1% 大枣 7.7% 熟地黄 3.1% 当归 3.1% 白芍 0.8% 川芎 0.8%

〔功能与主治〕 补气养血，调经止痛。用于月经不调，经来腹痛。

〔用法与用量〕 口服，1 次 4 片，1 日 3 次。

〔剂型与规格〕 片剂，每片重 0.25 g

〔附注〕 本品具有滋养，强壮，镇痛，调整子宫功能作用。临床适用于月经失调，经期腹痛。

妇科通经丸

〔药物组成〕 巴豆 红花 干漆 沉香 香附 木香 大黄 郁金 莪术 黄芩 三棱 艾叶 鳖甲 硇砂等

〔功能与主治〕 破瘀通经，解郁止痛。用于经行腹痛，经闭，胸膈痞闷，腰腹胀痛。

〔用法与用量〕 每早空腹，小米汤或黄酒送服，1 次 30 粒，1 日 1 次。

〔剂型与规格〕 水丸，每 10 粒重 1 g，每袋装 3 g

〔附注〕 本品具有扩张血管，改善血液循环，解除郁血，调整子宫功能作用。临床适用于痛经，闭经。

腹泻及孕妇忌服。服药期间，忌食生冷，辛辣，荞麦面等。

逍 遥 丸

〔药物组成〕 柴胡 16.7% 当归 16.7% 白芍 16.7% 白术 16.7% 茯苓 16.7% 甘草 13.4% 薄荷 3.1%

〔功能与主治〕 疏肝和中，养血调经。用于肝郁血虚，胸胁胀痛，月经不调，乳房作胀。

〔用法与用量〕　口服，1次6～9g，1日1～2次。

〔剂型与规格〕　水丸，每20粒重1g

〔附注〕　处方来源于宋，陈师文《太平惠民和剂局方》。

本品具有消炎，镇痛，调节子宫活动机能的作用。临床适用于妇女月经失调，慢性肝炎，慢性胃炎，神经衰弱，胸膜炎等。

八宝坤顺丸

〔药物组成〕　熟地黄7.9%　地黄7.9%　白芍7.9%　当归7.9%　川芎7.9%　人参3.9%　白术7.9%　茯苓7.9%　甘草3.9%　黄芩7.9%　益母草3.9%　牛膝3.9%　橘红7.9%　沉香3.9%　木香1.6%　砂仁3.9%　琥珀3.9%

〔功能与主治〕　养血调经。用于气血两虚，月经不调，经行腹痛，腰腿酸痛，足跗浮肿。

〔用法与用量〕　口服，1次1丸，1日2次。

〔剂型与规格〕　蜜丸，每丸重9g

〔附注〕　本品具有滋养，强壮，镇痛，调整子宫功能作用。临床适用于月经失调，痛经。

血府逐瘀丸

〔药物组成〕　桃仁16.8%　红花12.0%　川芎6.0%　当归12.0%　牛膝12.0%　赤芍8.0%　枳壳8.0%　桔梗6.0%　生地黄12.0%　柴胡4.0%　甘草4.0%

〔功能与主治〕　活血祛瘀，理气止痛。用于胸中血瘀，血行不畅所致头痛，胸痛日久不愈，痛如针刺而有定处，或呃逆日久，或内热烦闷，心悸失眠，入暮渐热及血瘀闭经，痛经。

〔用法与用量〕　口服，1次1丸，1日2次。

〔剂型与规格〕　蜜丸，每丸重9g

〔附注〕　处方来源于清·王清任《医林改错》。

本品临床适用于冠心病心绞痛，风湿性心脏病，胸部挫伤与肋软骨炎之胸痛，脑震荡后遗症之头痛头晕，精神抑郁，失眠健忘，闭经、痛经。

孕妇忌服。

温 经 丸

〔药物组成〕　党参 18.5%　茯苓 11.1%　白术 18.5%　黄芪 7.4%　附子 3.7%　肉桂 11.2%　吴茱萸 7.4%　干姜 7.4%　厚朴 3.7%　沉香 3.7%　郁金 7.4%

〔功能与主治〕　温经散寒，健脾理气。用于妇女脾虚血寒之痛经，经血不调，寒湿带下，腰膝酸软，手足不温，食少乏力。

〔用法与用量〕　口服，1 次 1 丸，1 日 2 次。

〔剂型与规格〕　蜜丸，每丸重 9 g

〔附注〕　本品临床适用于妇女痛经，月经失调，白带，亦可用于中上腹疼痛。

痛 经 丸

〔药物组成〕　当归 7.6%　白芍 5.1%　熟地黄 10.0%　川芎 3.8%　香附 7.6%　木香 1.3%　山楂 7.6%　青皮 1.3%　延胡索 5.1%　炮姜 1.3%　茺蔚子 2.5%　肉桂 1.3%　益母草 30.4%　丹参 7.6%　五灵脂 5.0%　红花 2.5%

〔功能与主治〕　活血散寒，调经止痛。用于寒凝血滞，经来少腹冷痛，得热痛减，经血量少，色黑有块。

〔用法与用量〕　口服，1 次 6～9 g，1 日 1～2 次，临经前服。

〔制剂与规格〕　水丸，每袋装 6 g

〔附注〕　本品具有扩张血管，调整子宫功能，镇痛作用。临床适用于痛经。

妇 康 宁 片

〔药物组成〕 白芍 39.3% 当归 4.9% 麦门冬 9.8% 党参 5.9% 香附 5.9% 三七 3.9% 益母草 29.5% 艾叶炭 0.8%

〔功能与主治〕 养血调经，理气止痛。用于妇女气血两亏，经血不调，经行腹痛，面色苍白，头晕眼花，气短懒言，乏力，唇甲色淡。

〔用法与用量〕 口服，1 次 4 片，1 日 2~3 次，或经前 4~5 天服用。

〔剂型与规格〕 片剂，每片重 0.5 g

〔附注〕 本品具有滋养，强壮，镇痛，调整子宫功能作用。临床适用于月经失调，痛经。

当归养血丸

〔药物组成〕 益母草 18.0% 川芎 4.5% 泽兰 9.0% 肉桂 1.8% 当归 18.1% 厚朴 9.0% 木香 4.5% 香附 9.0% 赤芍 9.0% 枳实 7.2% 三棱 1.8% 红花 2.7% 茴香 2.7% 莪术 2.7%

〔功能与主治〕 温经活血。用于妇女受寒月经不调，瘀血腹痛，产后血寒腹痛。

〔用法与用量〕 1 次 60 丸，睡前温开水送服。

〔剂型与规格〕 水丸，每 20 粒重约 1 g

〔附注〕 本品具有扩张血管，解除郁血，调整子宫功能作用。临床适用于妇女月经失调，闭经，经期腹痛，产后下腹部疼痛。

孕妇及阴虚有热者忌服。

当归浸膏片

〔药物组成〕　当归 100%

〔功能与主治〕　活血调经。用于月经不调，痛经。

〔用法与用量〕　口服，1 次 4～6 片，1 日 3 次。

〔剂型与规格〕　片剂，每片重 0.5 g

〔附注〕　本品具有镇痛，调整子宫功能作用。临床适用于月经失调，痛经。

七制香附丸

〔药物制成〕　香附 25.0%　当归 7.1%　三棱 3.6%　赤芍 7.1%　莪术 3.6%　川芎 7.1%　延胡索 3.6%　地黄 7.1%　青皮 3.6%　乌药 3.6%　益母草 14.2%　桃仁 2.7%　地骨皮 2.7%　蒲黄 3.6%　红花 3.6%　木香 1.8%

〔功能与主治〕　理气解郁，活血止痛。用于气滞血瘀，两胁胀痛，月经不调，行经腹痛。

〔用法与用量〕　口服，1 次 6 g，1 日 2～3 次。

〔剂型与规格〕　水丸，每 20 粒重约 1 g

〔附注〕　本品具有扩张血管，镇痛，调整子宫功能作用。临床适用于月经失调，痛经.

益 母 丸

〔药物组成〕　益母草 54.2%　当归 27.1%　川芎 13.6%　木香 5.1%

〔功能与主治〕　活血调经，行气止痛。用于气滞血瘀，月经不调，痛经，产后瘀血腹痛。

〔用法与用量〕　口服，1 次 1 丸，1 日 2 次。

〔剂型与规格〕　蜜丸，每丸重 9 g

〔附注〕　本品具有扩张血管，改善血循环，镇痛，调整子宫功能作用。临床适用于月经失调，痛经，产后下腹部疼痛等。

孕妇及月经过多者忌服。

益 母 草 膏

〔药物组成〕　益母草 100%

〔功能与主治〕　活血调经。用于闭经，痛经及产后血瘀腹痛。

〔用法及用量〕　口服，1 次 10 g，1 日 1～2 次。

〔剂型与规格〕　煎膏剂，每瓶装 100 g

〔附注〕　本品具有显著增强子宫肌肉的收缩力和紧张性作用。临床适用于闭经，痛经，产后下腹部疼痛。

孕妇忌用。

13.2　白带用药

固 经 丸

〔药物组成〕　黄柏 20%　白芍 20%　黄芩 13%　椿皮 10%　香附 10%　龟板 27%

〔功能与主治〕　滋阴清热，固精止带。用于阴虚血热，月经先期，量多，色紫黑，赤白带下。

〔用法与用量〕　口服，1 次 6 g，1 日 2 次。

〔剂型与规格〕　水丸，每 20 粒重 1 g

〔附注〕　处方来源于宋·陈自明《妇人良方大全》。

本品具有调整子宫功能，利尿作用。临床适用于妇女月经周期缩短，白带，亦可用于男性神经衰弱，遗精，遗尿，失眠等症。

千 金 止 带 丸

〔药物组成〕　白术 3.6%　党参 3.6%　香附 14.2%　当归

7.1%　小茴香 3.6%　白芍 3.6%　延胡索 3.6%　川芎 7.1%
杜仲 3.6%　木香 3.6%　补骨脂 3.6%　砂仁 3.6%　椿皮
14.2%　续断 3.6%　牡蛎 3.6%　青黛 3.6%　鸡冠花 14.2%

〔功能与主治〕　补虚止带，和血调经。用于赤白带下，月经不调，腰酸腹痛。

〔用法与用量〕　口服，1 次 6~9 g，1 日 2~3 次。

〔剂型与规格〕　水丸，每袋装 18 g

〔附注〕　本品具有滋养，强壮，利尿，调整子宫功能作用。临床适用于白带，月经失调。

白　带　丸

〔药物组成〕　黄柏 21.4%　椿皮 42.9%　香附 7.1%　白芍 14.3%　当归 14.3%

〔功能与主治〕　清湿热，止带下。用于湿热下注，赤白带下，症见带下量多，色黄绿如脓，或挟血液，或浑浊如米泔，有秽臭气，阴中瘙痒，小便短赤。

〔用法与用量〕　口服，1 次 6 g，1 日 2 次。

〔剂型与规格〕　水丸，每袋装 18 g

〔附注〕　本品临床适用于白带。

13.3　妊娠病用药

保　胎　丸

〔药物组成〕　黄芪 9.3%　茯苓 9.3%　白术 9.3%　当归 9.3%　艾叶 9.3%　白芍 9.3%　熟地黄 9.3%　川芎 4.7%　菟丝子 9.3%　川贝母 2.3%　枳壳 4.7%　党参 2.3%　厚朴 2.3%　羌活 1.2%　桑寄生 4.7%　荆芥穗 2.3%　甘草 1.1%

〔功能与主治〕　补气，养血，安胎。用于气血两亏，胎元不固，胎动不安，腰酸腹痛，胎漏滑胎。

〔用法与用量〕 口服，1 次 1 丸，1 日 3 次。

〔剂型与规格〕 蜜丸，每丸重 6 g

〔附注〕 本品临床适用于先兆流产，习惯流产。

安 胎 丸

〔药物组成〕 当归 12% 川芎 12% 白芍 12% 黄芩 12% 白术 6% 续断 12% 艾叶 12% 桑寄生 6% 菟丝子 12% 阿胶 4%

〔功能与主治〕 养血安胎。用于胎动不安，滑胎。

〔用法与用量〕 口服，1 次 1 丸，早晚各 1 次。

〔剂型与规格〕 蜜丸，每丸重 6 g

鹿 胎 膏

〔药物组成〕 茯苓 鹿角胶 白术 熟地黄 当归 人参 白芍 川芎 甘草 阿胶

〔功能与主治〕 养血益气，温肾调经。用于肾虚，妇女气血两亏，经血不调，经行腹痛。

〔用法与用量〕 开水化服，1 次 3 g，1 日 2 次。

〔剂型与规格〕 煎膏剂，每瓶装 50 g

〔附注〕 本品临床适应于妇女月经失调，经期腹痛，不孕症，亦可用于神经衰弱，性神经衰弱，糖尿病，慢性肾炎。

实热火盛者勿服。

13.4 产后病用药

生 化 汤 丸

〔药物组成〕 当归 25.8% 川芎 12.9% 红花 1.6% 桃仁 3.2% 干姜 1.6% 甘草 3.2% 益母草 51.7%

〔功能与主治〕 祛瘀活血，温经止痛。用于产后血瘀腹痛，恶露不尽。

〔用法与用量〕　口服，1 次 1～2 丸，1 日 2 次。

〔剂型与规格〕　蜜丸，每丸重 9 g

〔附注〕　本品具有扩张血管，解除郁血，镇痛，调整子宫功能作用。临床适用于产后下腹部疼痛，恶露过多，产后胎盘残留，产后大出血。

服用期间宜忌食生冷之物。

八珍益母丸

〔药物组成〕　益母草 29.7%　党参 7.4%　熟地黄 14.8%　当归 14.8%　白术 7.4%　茯苓 7.4%　白芍 7.4%　川芎 7.4%　甘草 3.7%

〔功能与主治〕　补气养血，调经。用于妇女气血两虚，体弱无力，精血不调，经行腹痛，色淡经少，食欲不振。

〔用法与用量〕　口服，1 次 1 丸，1 日 2 次。

〔剂型与规格〕　蜜丸，每丸重 9 g

〔附注〕　处方来源于明·张介宾《景岳全书》。

本品具有调整子宫功能，镇痛作用。临床适用于妇女月经失调，痛经，产褥热及其它产后发热性疾患，亦可用于贫血。

失 笑 散

〔药物组成〕　蒲黄 50%　五灵脂 50%

〔功能与主治〕　活血祛瘀，止痛。用于瘀血阻滞，胸脘疼痛，或产后恶露不行，或月经不调，小腹急痛。

〔用法与用量〕　口服，1 次 6～9 g，1 日 1～2 次。

〔剂型与规格〕　散剂，每袋装 18 g

〔附注〕　处方来源于宋·陈师文《太平惠民和剂局方》。

本品临床适用于月经失调、痛经，闭经，宫外孕，产后恶露滞留，冠心病心绞痛，急、慢性胃炎，胃、十二指肠溃疡（血瘀型），病毒性肝炎，血尿。

孕妇忌服。

下乳涌泉散

〔药物组成〕　当归 5.1%　白芍 5.1%　桔梗 5.1%　川芎 5.1%　地黄 5.1%　白芷 5.1%　天花粉 2.6%　甘草 2.6%　柴胡 2.6%　通草 15.4%　漏芦 15.4%　王不留行 18.0%　麦芽 12.8%

〔功能与主治〕　养血催乳。用于产后少乳。

〔用法与用量〕　1 次 1 袋，水煎 2 次，煎液混合后分 2 次服。

〔剂型与规格〕　散剂，每袋重 30 g

〔附注〕　服用期间忌食辛辣之物。

产后身痛片

〔药物组成〕　照山白 100%

〔功能与主治〕　祛风散寒，活血通络。用于妇女产后因受风寒引起的腰痛，四肢关节麻木疼痛，月经不调，痛经，经闭。

〔用法与用量〕　口服，1 次 2 片，1 日 2 次。

〔剂型与规格〕　片剂，每片重约 0.25 g

〔附注〕　本品临床适用于产后腰痛，产后关节痛，月经失调，痛经，闭经。

孕妇忌服。服药期间忌食生冷之物。

13.5　杂病用药

大黄䗪虫丸

〔药物组成〕　土鳖虫 2.3%　熟大黄 22.7%　水蛭 4.5%　桃仁 9.1%　虻虫 3.4%　黄芩 4.5%　蛴螬 3.4%　地黄

22.7%　干漆 2.3%　白芍 9.1%　苦杏仁 9.1%　甘草 6.9%

〔功能与主治〕　活血破瘀，通经消癥。用于瘀血内停，腹部肿块，肌肤甲错，目眶黯黑，潮热羸瘦，经闭不行，癥瘕积聚。

〔用法与用量〕　口服，1 次 1～2 丸，1 日 1～2 次。

〔剂型与规格〕　蜜丸，每丸重 3 g

〔附注〕　处方来源于汉·张仲景《金匮要略》。

本品具有扩张血管，祛除瘀血，促进吸收，调整子宫功能作用。临床适用于腹部肿块，肝脾肿大，闭经等。

孕妇禁用。若出现皮肤过敏者停服。

少腹逐瘀丸

〔药物组成〕　盐茴香 6.6%　当归 19.7%　炮干姜 1.4%　川芎 6.6%　醋延胡索 6.6%　官桂 6.6%　炒没药 6.6%　赤芍 13.1%　醋五灵脂 13.1%　蒲黄 19.7%

〔功能与主治〕　活血逐瘀，祛寒止痛。用于寒凝瘀滞引起的少腹硬痛，以及产后恶露不下，瘀血上攻，痛不可忍，或经期腰酸腹胀，月经不调，其色黑紫有瘀块等。

〔用法与用量〕　口服，1 次 1 丸，1 日 1～2 次。

〔剂型与规格〕　蜜丸，每丸重 6 g

〔附注〕　处方来源于清·王清任《医林改错》。

本品具有扩张血管，消除瘀血，促进吸收，调整子宫功能，镇痛作用。临床适用于腹部肿块，产后恶露滞留，痛经，月经失调。

孕妇忌服。

化症回生丸

〔药物组成〕　益母草　红花　花椒　当归　水蛭　苏木　三棱　川芎　竹节香附　降香　香附　人参　没药　高良姜　苦

杏仁　姜黄　小茴香　大黄　五灵脂　延胡索　桃仁　蒲黄　虻虫　乳香　鳖甲胶　干漆　丁香　吴茱萸　白芍　艾叶　阿魏　熟地黄　肉桂　紫苏子

〔功能与主治〕　消癥化瘀。用于癥积血痹，妇女干血痨，产后血瘀，少腹疼痛拒按。

〔用法与用量〕　口服，1次1丸，1日2次。

〔剂型与规格〕　蜜丸，每丸重6g

〔附注〕　本品具有扩张血管，解除郁血，促进吸收作用。临床适用于腹部肿块，产后瘀血，肝脾肿大，子宫肌瘤，外伤（血瘀型）。

孕妇禁用。

调经至宝丸

〔药物组成〕　大黄72.0%　木香4.0%　牵牛子2.0%　陈皮2.0%　枳实2.0%　黄芩2.0%　苍术2.0%　山楂3.2%　五灵脂2.0%　当归1.0%　香附2.8%　槟榔2.0%　三棱1.0%　莪术1.0%　鳖甲1.0%

〔功能与主治〕　破瘀，通经。用于妇女血瘀积聚，月经闭止，行经腹痛。

〔用法与用量〕　口服，1次6g，1日2次。

〔剂型与规格〕　水丸，每20粒重1g

〔附注〕　本品具有扩张血管，改善血循环，消除瘀血，镇痛，调整子宫功能作用。临床适用于妇女腹部肿块，闭经，痛经。

体质衰弱及孕妇忌服。

金鸡冲剂

〔药物组成〕　金樱根18.0%　鸡血藤33.7%　功劳木18.0%　两面针6.7%　千斤拔18.0%　穿心莲5.6%

〔功能与主治〕 清热解毒，活血通络。用于尿频，带下量多，臭秽，月经不调，经来腹痛。

〔用法与用量〕 口服，1次1包，1日2次，十日为1疗程，必要时可连服2～3个疗程。

〔剂型与规格〕 冲剂，每袋装6 g

〔附注〕 本品临床适用于子宫附件炎，子宫内膜炎，盆腔炎，月经失调，痛经，白带，阴囊湿疹。也用于放节育环，人工流产后预防感染。

孕妇慎服。

妇科分清丸

〔药物组成〕 当归16.3% 白芍8.2% 川芎12.2% 地黄16.3% 栀子8.2% 黄连4.1% 石苇4.1% 海金砂2.0% 甘草8.2% 关木通8.2% 滑石12.2%

〔功能与主治〕 清热利湿，活血止痛。用于湿热下注膀胱，小便频数，尿道刺痛，短赤浑浊。

〔用法与用量〕 口服，1次9 g，1日2次。

〔剂型与规格〕 水丸，每丸50粒重3 g

〔附注〕 本品临床适用于膀胱炎，尿道炎，急性前列腺炎，泌尿系结石及急性肾炎，急性肾盂炎。

孕妇慎用。

14 儿科药物

小儿至宝丸

〔药物组成〕 紫苏叶 广藿香 薄荷 羌活 白附子 陈皮 白芥子 胆南星 山楂 川贝母 六神曲 槟榔 麦芽 茯苓 琥珀 冰片 天麻 钩藤 僵蚕 蝉蜕 全蝎 人工牛黄 雄黄 滑石

〔功能与主治〕 疏风镇惊,化痰导滞。用于小儿感受风寒,发热鼻塞,咳嗽痰多,停食停乳,呕吐泄泻,惊惕抽搐。

〔用法与用量〕 口服,1次1丸,1日2~3次。

〔剂型与规格〕 蜜丸,每丸重1.5 g

〔附注〕 本品临床适用于小儿胃肠型感冒,急性感染性疾病引起的惊厥。

妙 灵 丹

〔药物组成〕 薄荷 葛根 羌活 川贝母 化桔红 前胡 桔梗 法半夏 天南星 赤芍 钩藤 朱砂 冰片 木通 玄参 地黄 天麻 水牛角浓缩粉

〔功能与主治〕 清热宣肺,化痰镇惊。用于小儿感冒,症见发烧,头痛眩晕,内热咳嗽,呕吐痰涎,鼻干口燥,咽喉肿痛,小便不利,惊惕啼叫,睡卧不宁。

〔用法与用量〕 口服,周岁以上1次1丸,周岁以下1次1／2丸,1日2次。

〔剂型与规格〕 蜜丸,每丸重1.5 g

〔附注〕 本品临床适用于小儿上呼吸道感染。

解肌宁嗽丸

〔药物组成〕 紫苏叶 4.8% 前胡 8.0% 葛根 8.0% 苦杏仁 8.0% 桔梗 8.0% 陈皮 8.0% 半夏 8.0% 浙贝母 8.0% 天花粉 8.0% 枳壳 8.0% 茯苓 6.4% 木香 2.4% 玄参 8.0% 甘草 6.4%

〔功能与主治〕 解表宣肺，止咳化痰。用于小儿伤风感冒，身热头痛，咳嗽痰多，口渴咽干，鼻流清涕，呕吐痰涎。

〔用法与用量〕 口服，小儿周岁 1 次半丸，2 至 3 岁 1 次 1 丸；1 日 2 次。

〔剂型与规格〕 蜜丸，每丸重 3 g

〔附注〕 本品具有解热，镇咳，祛痰作用。临床适用于小儿上呼吸道感染，急性支气管炎。

小儿金丹片

〔药物组成〕 西河柳 荆芥穗 前胡 薄荷 牛蒡子 防风 羌活 大青叶 朱砂 天麻 水牛角浓缩粉 川贝母 半夏（制） 橘红 枳壳 胆南星 桔梗 玄参 木通 赤芍 甘草 冰片 葛根 地黄

〔功能与主治〕 祛风清热，镇惊化痰。用于小儿伤风感冒，发热头痛，鼻流清涕，咳嗽气促，咽喉肿痛，高热惊风，疹出迟缓。

〔用法与用量〕 口服，1 次 3 片，1 日 2 次，周岁以内酌减。

〔剂型与规格〕 片剂，每片重 0.2 g

〔附注〕 本品临床适用于小儿上呼吸道感染，急性感染性疾病引起的惊厥及发疹性传染病初期。

小儿止嗽丸

〔药物组成〕 玄参 8.7% 麦冬 8.7% 苦杏仁 8.7% 胆南星 8.7% 紫苏子 4.4% 槟榔 6.5% 天花粉 6.5% 紫苏叶 4.4% 川贝母 6.5% 知母 4.4% 栝蒌子 6.5% 甘草 6.5% 桔梗 6.5% 竹茹 6.5% 桑白皮 6.5%

〔功能与主治〕 清热化痰，润肺止咳。用于小儿内热发烧，咳嗽痰黄，口干舌燥，腹胀便秘，久嗽痰盛。

〔用法与用量〕 口服，1 次 1 丸，1 日 2 次，周岁以下小儿酌减。

〔剂型与规格〕 蜜丸，每丸重 3 g

〔附注〕 本品具有解热，祛痰，镇咳作用。临床适用于小儿上呼吸道感染，发热，咳嗽，便秘。

小儿止咳糖浆

〔药物组成〕 桔梗流浸膏 14.3% 甘草流浸膏 71.4% 橙皮酊 9.5% 氯化铵 4.8%

〔功能与主治〕 化痰止咳。用于小儿感冒，咳嗽。

〔用法与用量〕 口服，2～5 岁，1 次 5 ml，1 日 3 次；5 岁以上，1 次 5～10 ml，一日 3 次；2 岁以下，酌情递减。

〔剂型与规格〕 糖浆剂，每瓶装 100 ml

〔附注〕 本品具有祛痰、镇咳作用。临床适用于小儿上呼吸道感染，急慢性支气管炎引起的咳嗽。

小儿牛黄清心散

〔药物组成〕 天麻 8.5% 胆南星 6.8% 黄连 12.8% 赤芍 6.8% 大黄 12.8% 全蝎 6.8% 水牛角浓缩粉 8.5% 人工牛黄 0.85% 僵蚕（麸炒）8.5% 琥珀 2.1% 雄黄 6.4% 冰片 2.15% 金礞石（煅）8.5% 朱砂 8.5%

〔功能与主治〕 清热化痰，镇惊止痉。用于小儿内热，急惊痰喘，四肢抽搐，神志昏迷。

〔用法与用量〕 日服，周岁以内 1 次 1／2 袋，1 岁至 3 岁 1 次 1 袋，3 岁以上酌增，1 日 1～2 次。

〔剂型与规格〕 散剂，每袋重 0.6 g

〔附注〕 本品临床适用于小儿高热，急性感染性疾病引起的惊厥。

风寒感冒，痘疹期间引起的内热发烧忌服。

保婴镇惊丸

〔药物组成〕 大黄 53.6% 朱砂 10.7% 甘草 35.7%

〔功能与主治〕 泻热，导滞，镇惊。用于小儿实热便秘，腹胀呕吐，惊风，目赤口疮。

〔用法与用量〕 口服，6 岁以下 1 次 1 丸，1 日 1 次，周岁小儿减半服用。

〔剂型与规格〕 蜜丸，每丸重 1.5 g

〔附注〕 本品临床适用于小儿便秘，惊厥，抽搐，手足搐搦。

小儿惊风丸

〔药物组成〕 麻黄 苍术 丁香 细辛 栀子 天麻 甘草 僵蚕 猪牙皂 全蝎 蜈蚣 胆南星 钩藤 冰片 朱砂

〔功能与主治〕 祛风散寒，开窍镇惊。用于小儿急惊风，四时感冒，发冷发热。

〔用法与用量〕 口服，初生小儿，1 次 5 粒；半岁至 1 岁，1 次 10 粒；1 至 2 岁，1 次 15 粒；2 岁以上，1 次 20 粒；1 日 3 次。

〔剂型与规格〕 水丸，每 100 粒重 0.6 g

〔附注〕 本品临床适用于小儿急性感染性疾病引起的惊

厥，上呼吸道感染。

婴儿安片

〔药物组成〕 鸡内金（醋炒）15% 清半夏10% 川贝母10% 天竺黄10% 陈皮10% 钩藤10% 天麻10% 朱砂10% 琥珀15%

〔功能与主治〕 祛风镇惊，消食，化痰，退热。用于小儿发热，咳嗽，食水不化，痰热惊风。

〔用法与用量〕 口服，不满1岁1次1/2片，1岁至3岁1次1片，4岁至7岁1次2片，8岁至12岁1次3片，每晚服1次。

〔剂型与规格〕 片剂，每片重约0.32g

〔附注〕 本品临床适用于小儿发热，咳嗽，消化不良，惊厥，抽搐，手足搐搦。

忌食生冷、油腻之物。

小儿健脾丸

〔药物组成〕 人参4.6% 白术1.3% 甘草4.6% 茯苓1.3% 法半夏4.6% 陈皮9.3% 白扁豆9.3% 山药9.3% 莲子9.3% 砂仁4.6% 六神曲9.3% 桔梗4.6% 麦芽9.3% 玉竹9.3% 南山楂9.3%

〔功能与主治〕 健脾，和胃，化滞。用于小儿脾胃虚弱，不思饮食，大便溏泻，体弱无力。

〔用法与用量〕 口服，1次2丸，1日3次。

〔剂型与规格〕 蜜丸，每丸重3g

〔附注〕 本品具有健胃，助消化作用。临床适用于小儿消化不良，厌食，营养不良。

小儿消食片

〔药物组成〕 鸡内金　山楂　六神曲　槟榔　麦芽　陈皮

〔功能与主治〕 消食化滞，健脾和胃。用于脾胃不和，消化不良，食欲不振，腹胀便秘，食滞，疳积。

〔用法与用量〕 口服，1 岁至 3 岁 1 次 2～4 片，3 岁至 7 岁 1 次 4～6 片，1 日 3 次。

〔剂型与规格〕 片剂，每片重约 0.3 g

〔附注〕 本品具有健胃，助消化作用。临床适用于小儿消化不良，厌食，便秘，营养不良。

小儿消积丸

〔药物组成〕 枳壳 4.1%　黄芩 2.5%　三棱 4.1%　槟榔 16.4%　莪术 4.1%　陈皮 4.1%　厚朴 4.1%　大黄 8.2%　青皮 4.1%　木香 4.1%　牵牛子 16.4%　巴豆霜 8.2%　香附 16.4%　朱砂 3.2%

〔功能与主治〕 消食导滞，理气和胃。用于小儿乳积，食滞，腹胀腹痛。

〔用法与用量〕 口服，1～3 个月 1 次 5 粒，4～6 个月 1 次 10 粒，1～2 岁 1 次 30 粒，3～6 岁 1 次 50 粒，7～12 岁 1 次 80 粒。

〔剂型与规格〕 水丸，每 320 粒重 1 g

〔附注〕 本品临床适用于小儿消化不良，便秘。体质弱，腹泻者忌服。

香苏正胃丸

〔药物组成〕 广藿香 11.8%　紫苏叶 23.6%　厚朴 11.8%　香薷 11.8%　枳壳 2.9%　陈皮 5.9%　白扁豆 5.9%　砂仁 2.9%　山楂 2.9%　茯苓 2.9%　六神曲 2.9%　甘草

1.6%　麦芽 2.9%　滑石 9.7%　朱砂 0.5%

〔功能与主治〕　解表和中，消食行滞。用于小儿暑湿感冒，停食停乳，头痛发热，呕吐泄泻，腹痛胀满，小便不利。

〔用法与用量〕　口服，1次1丸，1日1～2次，周岁以内小儿酌减。

〔剂型与规格〕　蜜丸，每丸重3g

〔附注〕　本品临床适用于胃肠型感冒，急性胃肠炎。

香　橘　丸

〔药物组成〕　茯苓 7.8%　白术 7.8%　苍术 7.8%　陈皮 7.8%　香附 7.8%　山药 5.2%　白扁豆 5.2%　法半夏 5.2%　薏苡仁 5.2%　莲子 5.2%　山楂 5.2%　泽泻 2.6%　枳实 5.2%　木香 1.2%　麦芽 5.2%　砂仁 2.6%　厚朴 5.2%　甘草 2.6%　六神曲 5.2%

〔功能与主治〕　健脾开胃，燥湿止泻。用于小儿脾胃虚弱，脘腹胀满，呕吐泄泻，不思饮食。

〔用法与用量〕　口服，1次1丸，1日3次，3岁以下小儿酌减。

〔剂型与规格〕　蜜丸，每丸重3g

〔附注〕　本品具有健胃，助消化作用。临床适用于小儿寄生虫病，小儿单纯性消化不良等慢性消耗性疾病。

婴　儿　散

〔药物组成〕　白扁豆（炒）4.5%　川贝母 0.97%　鸡内金（炒）13.5%　木香 13.5%　山药（炒）13.5%　人工牛黄 0.03%　白术（炒）13.5%

〔功能与主治〕　健脾，消食，止泻。用于消化不良，乳食不进，腹痛腹泻。

〔用法与用量〕　口服，不满周岁1次0.25 g，1至3岁1次

0.5~1g，1 日 2 次。

〔剂型与规格〕　散剂，每包重 0.5 g

〔附注〕　本品具有健胃，助消化，止泻作用。临床适用于小儿消化不良，厌食，腹泻。

小儿止泻片

〔药物组成〕　山药　白术　白矾　车前子　枣树皮等

〔功能与主治〕　健脾利水，涩肠止泻。用于小儿脾胃虚弱，腹泻腹痛，消化不良，不思饮食，面黄肌瘦。

〔用法与用量〕　口服，周岁以内 1 次 2 片；1~2 岁 1 次 3 片；3~4 岁 1 次 4 片，1 日 3 次。

〔剂型与规格〕　片剂，每片重 0.25 g

〔附注〕　本品临床适用于小儿腹泻。
痢疾初起禁用，腹胀者慎用。

牛黄抱龙片

〔药物组成〕　人工牛黄　朱砂　腰黄　琥珀　胆南星　全蝎　茯苓　人工竺黄　僵蛹

〔功能与主治〕　清热化痰，祛风镇惊。用于小儿急惊，身热昏睡，牙关紧闭，手足抽搐，痰喘平壅，两目上视。

〔用法与用量〕　口服，1 次 2 片，1 日 1~2 次，周岁以内酌减。

〔剂型与规格〕　片剂，每袋装 4 片。

〔附注〕　本品临床适用于小儿高热，咳嗽，急性感染性疾病引起的惊厥。

七 珍 丸

〔药物组成〕　僵蚕（炒）　全蝎　朱砂　雄黄　胆南星　天竺黄　巴豆霜　寒食曲

〔功能与主治〕 定惊豁痰，消积通便。用于小儿急惊风，身热，昏睡，气粗，烦躁，痰涎壅盛，停食停乳，大便秘结。

〔用法与用量〕 口服，小儿3至4个月，1次3粒；5至7个月，1次4～5粒；周岁，1次6～7粒；1日1～2次。周岁以上及体实者酌加用量。

〔剂型与规格〕 水丸，每200粒重约3g

〔附注〕 本品临床适用于小儿急性感染性疾病引起的惊厥，发热，厌食，便秘。

本品含巴豆霜，应注意控制剂量，不可久服。

牛黄镇惊丸

〔药物组成〕 胆南星 人工牛黄 川贝母 竹黄 雄黄 大黄 钩藤 天麻 全蝎 禹白附 地龙（肉） 冰片 郁金 石菖蒲 沉香 羌活 薄荷 川乌 川芎 茯苓 珍珠 琥珀 朱砂

〔功能与主治〕 清热镇惊，驱风化痰。用于小儿急热惊风，发烧气促，痰涎壅盛，惊痫抽搐，牙关紧闭，神志不清。

〔用法与用量〕 口服，1次1丸，1日2次，周岁以内酌减。

〔剂型与规格〕 蜜丸，每丸重1.5g

〔附注〕 本品临床适用于小儿癫痫，急性感染性疾病引起的惊厥。

导 赤 丸

〔药物组成〕 连翘12.5% 黄连6.3% 栀子12.5% 木通6.2% 玄参12.5% 赤芍6.2% 天花粉12.5% 大黄6.3% 黄芩12.5% 滑石12.5%

〔功能与主治〕 清热泻火，利尿通便。用于口舌生疮，咽喉疼痛，心胸烦热，小便短赤，大便秘结。

〔用法与用量〕 口服，1次1丸，1日2次，周岁以内小儿酌减。

〔剂型与规格〕 蜜丸，每丸重3g

〔附注〕 本品临床适用于口腔溃疡，急性咽炎，喉炎，扁桃体炎，急性膀胱炎，急性尿道炎，急性肾盂肾炎。

腹泻及体弱者忌服。

保 赤 散

〔药物组成〕 六神曲（炒）23.8%　巴豆霜14.3%　天南星（制）38.1%　朱砂23.8%

〔功能与主治〕 消食导滞，化痰镇惊。用于小儿冷积，停乳停食，大便秘结，腹部胀满，痰涎壅盛，惊悸不安。

〔用法与用量〕 口服，小儿6个月至1岁1次0.09g；2至4岁1次0.18g，1日1~2次，6个月以内小儿酌减。

〔剂型与规格〕 散剂，每瓶装0.09g

〔附注〕 本品临床适用于小儿厌食，消化不良，便秘，腹胀及因惊吓引起的精神神经症状。

本品含巴豆，不可服用过量。腹泻者忌服。

小儿升血灵冲剂

〔药物组成〕 大枣　皂矾　山楂等

〔功能与主治〕 补气养血，消积理脾。用于小儿血虚，虚劳。

〔用法与用量〕 开水冲服，1岁以下1次5g；1岁至3岁1次10g；3岁至7岁1次15g，1日3次。

〔剂型与规格〕 冲剂，每袋装10g。

〔附注〕 本品具有增加红细胞及提高血红蛋白作用。临床适用于小儿缺铁性贫血。

据临床报道，本品治疗小儿缺铁性贫血300例，经治疗10

天后治愈率 67.0%，治疗 20 天后治愈率 79.0%，治疗 30 天后治愈率 91.7%。

禁用茶水冲服。

稚儿灵冲剂

〔药物组成〕　党参　孩儿参　南沙参　地黄　首乌　当归白术　黑大豆　白芍　木香　白扁豆　山药　仙鹤草　茯苓五味子　石菖蒲　浮小麦　甘草　牡蛎　陈皮　远志　大枣

〔功能与主治〕　益气，健脾，补脑，强身。用于小儿食欲不振，大便溏泄，面黄体弱，夜寝不宁，睡后盗汗等症。

〔用法与用量〕　开水冲服，1 次 9～15 g，1 日 2 次。

〔剂型与规格〕　冲剂，每瓶装 400 g

〔附注〕　本品具有滋养，强壮，健胃作用。临床适用于小儿厌食，营养不良，消化不良及发育迟缓。

五粒回春丹

〔药物组成〕　西河柳　金银花　牛蒡子　连翘　蝉蜕　薄荷　桑叶　防风　麻黄　羌活　僵蚕　橘红　胆南星　川贝母苦杏仁　茯苓　赤芍　淡竹叶　甘草　羚羊角粉　冰片　人工牛黄

〔功能与主治〕　宣肺透表，清热解毒。用于小儿瘟毒引起头痛高烧，流涕多泪，咳嗽气促，烦躁口渴，麻疹初期，疹出不透。

〔用法与用量〕　口服，1 次 5 粒，1 日 2 次。

〔剂型与规格〕　糊丸，每 100 粒重 3 g

〔附注〕　本品临床适用于小儿急性感染性疾病，颜面丹毒，猩红热，白喉，流行性腮腺炎及麻疹初期。

忌食生冷油腻厚味。

清 疹 散

〔药物组成〕　石膏　水牛角浓缩粉　知母　蝉蜕　重楼　薄荷叶　金银花　连翘　僵蚕　芦根

〔功能与主治〕　清热解毒，解表透疹。用于疹毒不透，咽肿音哑，呼吸急促，腹痛便溏，神昏谵语，抽搐。

〔用法与用量〕　口服，小儿1岁以上1次1／2袋，3岁以上1次1袋，5岁以上1次$1\frac{1}{2}$袋。

〔剂型与规格〕　散剂，每袋装 0.625 g

〔附注〕　本品具有解热，抗菌作用。临床适用于小儿麻疹、风疹、猩红热等急性发疹性疾病，白喉等症。

牛黄至宝丸

〔药物组成〕　野山人参　朱砂　人工牛黄　天南星　冰片　人工天竺黄　琥珀　水牛角浓缩粉　玳瑁　腰黄

〔功能与主治〕　清热解毒，镇惊开窍。用于温邪内陷，热入心包，神昏谵语，斑疹隐现，小儿急热惊风。

〔用法与用量〕　口服，1次1丸，用温开水化服。

〔剂型与规格〕　蜜丸，每丸重 3 g

〔附注〕　本品临床适用于流行性乙型脑炎，流行性脑脊髓膜炎，败血症，中毒性肺炎，中毒性菌痢引起的昏迷，小儿急性感染性疾病引起的惊厥。

孕妇慎用。

小儿退热冲剂

〔药物组成〕　大青叶 14.9%　板兰根 9.0%　金银花 9.0%　连翘 9.0%　栀子 9.0%　牡丹皮 9.0%　黄芩 9.0%　淡竹叶 5.9%　地龙 5.9%　重楼 4.4%　柴胡 9.0%　白薇 5.9%

〔功能与主治〕 清热解表。用于小儿感冒发烧。

〔用法与用量〕 口服，5岁以下1次5g，5岁至10岁1次15g，1日3次。

〔剂型与规格〕 冲剂，每袋重5g

〔附注〕 本品临床适用于小儿上呼吸道感染，流行性感冒，发烧。

小儿奇应丸

〔药物组成〕 沉香 雄黄 水牛角浓缩粉 法半夏 朱砂 党参 桔梗 白附子 盐酸奎宁 樟脑 人工牛黄 冰片 牛胆汁浸膏

〔功能与主治〕 清热，镇惊，熄风。用于小儿急慢惊风，高热，感冒咳嗽，麻疹未透，疳疾。

〔用法与用量〕 口服，1岁以下，1次6～8丸；1～3岁，1次12丸；4～6岁，1次15丸；7～10岁，1次20丸，1日2次，重症1日3次。

〔剂型与规格〕 水丸，每10粒重0.05g

〔附注〕 本品临床适用于小儿急性感染性疾病引起的惊厥，慢性疾病引起的抽搐，高热，麻疹初期等症。

小儿解热栓

〔药物组成〕 金银花22.3% 羌活11.1% 大青叶44.4% 拳参11.1% 大黄11.1%

〔功能与主治〕 清热解毒，疏风解表，化瘀消肿。用于伤风感冒，痄腮，高热。

〔用法与用量〕 先将肛门周围洗净，然后把药栓送入距肛门口约2cm处，1次1粒，1日2～3次。

〔剂型与规格〕 栓剂，每枚1g

〔附注〕 本品临床适用于小儿高热，上呼吸道感染，流行性感冒，流行性腮腺炎。

疳 积 散

〔药物组成〕　石燕 18.2%　茯苓 18.2%　石决明 18.2%
谷精草 9.0%　使君子仁 18.2%　威灵仙 9.1%　鸡内金 9.1%

〔功能与主治〕　消积治疳。用于小儿疳积，面黄肌瘦，腹
部膨胀，消化不良，目翳夜盲。

〔用法与用量〕　1 次 9 g，用热米汤加糖少许调服，1 日 2
次，3 岁以内小儿酌减。

〔剂型与规格〕　散剂，每瓶装 3 g

〔附注〕　本品具有助消化，杀虫作用。临床适用于小儿营
养不良，消化不良，寄生虫病等引起的形体干瘦，结核病等慢性
消耗性疾病。

肥 儿 丸

〔药物组成〕　肉豆蔻 10.6%　木香 4.3%　麦芽 10.6%
胡黄连 21.3%　六神曲 21.3%　槟榔 10.6%　使君子仁 21.3%

〔功能与主治〕　健胃，消积，杀虫。用于小儿消化不良，
虫积腹痛，面黄肌瘦，食少腹胀泄泻。

〔用法与用量〕　口服，1 次 1～2 丸，1 日 1～2 次，3 岁以
内小儿酌减。

〔剂型与规格〕　蜜丸，每丸重 3 g

〔附注〕　处方来源于宋·陈师文《太平惠民和剂局方》。

本品具有健胃，助消化，驱虫作用。临床适用于小儿蛔虫
病，消化不良，营养不良。

服本品后泻下酸粘腐臭或蛔虫等即可停药，一般服药不过三
日。

小儿肝炎冲剂

〔药物组成〕 茵陈 24.2% 黄芩 12.1% 栀子（姜制）6.1% 黄柏 12.1% 山楂 18.2% 郁金 3.0% 大豆黄卷 18.2% 通草 6.1%

〔功能与主治〕 清利湿热，退黄。用于小儿湿热黄疸，目黄身黄，腹胀恶心，身热体倦，食欲不振，肝区疼痛。

〔用法与用量〕 口服，1岁至3岁1次0.5～1块，3岁至7岁1次2块，7岁以上酌增，1日3次。

〔剂型与规格〕 冲剂，每块重7.5g

〔附注〕 本品临床适用于小儿急性黄疸型肝炎。

万 应 锭

〔药物组成〕 胡黄连 黄连 儿茶 冰片 香墨 牛胆汁等

〔功能与主治〕 清热镇惊，解毒祛暑，凉血消肿。用于小儿高热，惊风，中暑，口舌生疮，牙齿疼痛，牙龈，咽喉肿痛，痈肿。

〔用法与用量〕 口服，1次2～4粒，1日1～2次，3岁以内小儿酌减。

〔剂型与规格〕 水丸，每10粒重1.5g

〔附注〕 本品临床适用于小儿高热、感染、中毒、营养和代谢障碍、癫痫、中暑等所致惊厥，疖，疔，有头疽，急性咽炎，急性扁桃体炎，阿弗他口炎，急性根尖脓肿。

五福化毒丸

〔药物组成〕 水牛角浓缩粉 4.7% 连翘 14.0% 青黛 4.7% 黄连 1.2% 牛蒡子 11.6% 玄参 14.0% 地黄 11.5% 桔梗 11.5% 芒硝 1.2% 赤芍 11.6% 甘草 14.0%

〔功能与主治〕 清热解毒，凉血消肿。用于小儿热毒实火所致疮疖，痱毒，咽喉肿痛，口舌生疮，牙龈出血，痄腮。

〔用法与用量〕 口服，1次1丸，1日2～3次。

〔剂型与规格〕 蜜丸，每丸重3 g

〔附注〕 处方来源于明·龚廷贤《寿世保元》。

本品临床适用于小儿疖，疔，有头疽，汗腺炎，急性咽炎，急性扁桃体炎，阿弗他口炎，流行性腮腺炎及传染病出疹后期的治疗。

百 日 咳 片

〔药物组成〕 禽胆膏100%

〔功能与主治〕 止咳，化痰，定喘。用于小儿顿咳。

〔用法与用量〕 口服，每岁1次1片，1日3次。

〔剂型与规格〕 片剂，每片重50 mg

〔附注〕 本品为家禽新鲜胆汁浓缩制成的稠膏，临床适用于小儿百日咳。

15   五官科药物

15.1   眼科用药

杞菊地黄丸

〔药物组成〕   枸杞子 6.9%   菊花 6.9%   山茱萸 13.8%
山药 13.8%   牡丹皮 10.3%   泽泻 10.3%   熟地黄 27.7%   茯
苓 10.3%

〔功能与主治〕   滋肾养肝。用于肝肾阴亏，眩晕耳鸣，羞
明畏光，迎风流泪，视物昏花。

〔用法与用量〕   口服，1 次 1 丸，1 日 2 次。

〔剂型与规格〕   蜜丸，每丸重 9 g

〔附注〕   处方来源于《医级》。

本品具有滋养，保护肝脏，消炎作用。临床适用于流泪症，
青光眼，畏光，老年性白内障，玻璃体混浊，急性视神经炎，中
心性视网膜炎，视网膜脱离，视神经萎缩，单纯性疱疹性角膜
炎，沙眼性角膜炎，病毒性角膜炎，耳鸣，耳源性眩晕。

石斛夜光丸

〔药物组成〕   人参   茯苓   天门冬   山药   麦门冬   地黄
熟地黄   枸杞子   决明子   牛膝   菟丝子   菊花   苦杏仁   石
斛   肉苁蓉   甘草   五味子   防风   白蒺藜   黄连   枳壳   川芎
青箱子   水牛角浓缩粉   羚羊角

〔功能与主治〕   滋阴降火，养阴明目。用于肝肾不足，阴
虚火旺所致内障目疾，视物昏花，瞳仁散大或变色，羞明怕光
等。

〔用法与用量〕   口服，1 次 1 丸，1 日 2 次。

〔剂型与规格〕 蜜丸，每丸重 9 g

〔附注〕 处方来源于明·傅仁宇《审视瑶函》。

本品具有滋养，保护肝脏，消炎，泻下作用。临床适用于白内障，青光眼，视网膜炎，脉络膜炎，视神经炎，神经性头痛，玻璃体混浊，畏光。

明目地黄丸

〔药物组成〕 熟地黄 18.6% 山药 9.2% 山茱萸 9.2% 茯苓 7.0% 牡丹皮 7.0% 泽泻 7.0% 枸杞子 7.0% 菊花 7.0% 白蒺藜 7.0% 当归 7.0% 石决明 7.0% 白芍 7.0%

〔功能与主治〕 滋养肝肾，明目。用于肝肾阴虚，虚火上炎所致目涩羞明，视物昏花，迎风流泪，雀目。

〔用法与用量〕 口服，1 次 1 丸，1 日 2 次。

〔剂型与规格〕 蜜丸，每丸重 9 g

〔附注〕 本品具有滋养，保护肝脏，消炎作用。临床适用于中心性视网膜炎，视网膜脱离，视神经炎，视神经萎缩，玻璃体混浊，流泪症，畏光，夜盲（肝肾阴虚型）。

黄连羊肝丸

〔药物组成〕 黄连 密蒙花 决明子（炒） 龙胆 石决明（煅） 黄柏 芜蔚子 黄芩 夜明砂 柴胡 胡黄连 木贼 青皮（醋炒） 鲜羊肝

〔功能与主治〕 泻火，明目。用于肝火内盛，目暗羞明，胬肉攀睛。

〔用法与用量〕 口服，1 次 1 丸，1 日 1～2 次。

〔剂型与规格〕 蜜丸，每丸重 9 g

〔附注〕 本品具有解热、抗菌、消炎作用。临床适用于翼状胬肉，畏光，夜盲，青光眼，白内障（肝火内盛型）。

明目羊肝丸

〔药物组成〕 鲜羊肝 20.8%　木贼 6.9%　枸杞子 3.6%　地黄 6.9%　决明子（炒）6.9%　当归 6.9%　夜明砂 6.9%　蝉蜕 6.9%　沙苑子（盐炒）6.9%　黄连 6.9%　蒺藜（盐炒）6.9%　菊花 6.9%　荆芥穗 1.0%　防风 3.6%　羌活 1.0%　川芎 1.0%

〔功能与主治〕 滋补肝肾，祛风明目。用于雀目流泪，视物昏花。

〔用法与用量〕 口服，1 次 1 丸，1 日 2 次。

〔剂型与规格〕 蜜丸，每丸重 9 g

〔附注〕 本品具有滋养，保护肝脏，消炎作用。临床适用于夜盲，流泪症，玻璃体混浊（肝肾阴虚型）。

障 眼 明 片

〔药物组成〕 山萸肉 8%　蕤仁肉 10%　枸杞子 12%　肉苁蓉 12%　防党参 12%　绵黄芪 15%　密蒙花 8%　升麻 2%　蔓荆子 6%　川芎 3%　石菖蒲 2%　菊花 10%

〔功能与主治〕 补益肝肾，健脾调中，退翳明目。用于圆翳内障，视瞻昏渺，云雾移睛，高风内障，青盲及视力疲劳，精神困倦，头晕眼花，腰酸健忘等症。

〔用法与用量〕 口服，1 次 4 片，1 日 3 次。（每个疗程用药 3～6 个月）。

〔剂型与规格〕 片剂，每瓶装 100 片。

〔附注〕 本品具有增强眼的新陈代谢，促进角膜上皮组织再生作用。临床适用于初期及中期老年性白内障，视网膜中央血管阻塞，视网膜静脉周围炎，视网膜脱离，急性视神经炎，中心性视网膜脉络膜炎，玻璃体混浊，视网膜色素变性，视神经萎缩等陈旧性眼底病及视力疲劳。

光 明 眼 膏

〔药物组成〕　炉甘石（煅）72.5%　冰片 20.3%　硼砂 3.4%　硫酸铜 2.4%　重硫酸黄连素 1.4%

〔功能与主治〕　清热解毒，燥湿止痛。用于风热眼，鱼子石榴，砂眼。

〔用法与用量〕　涂于眼皮内，1 日 3～4 次，用后休息片刻。

〔剂型与规格〕　软膏剂，每支装 2 g

〔附注〕　本品具有消炎，收敛作用。临床适用于眼结膜炎，结膜溃疡，翼状胬肉，砂眼。

15.2　耳鼻喉科用药

耳聋左慈丸

〔药物组成〕　磁石（煅）3.7%　熟地黄 29.6%　山茱萸（制）14.7%　山药 14.7%　牡丹皮 11.2%　茯苓 11.2%　竹叶柴胡 3.7%　泽泻 11.2%

〔功能与主治〕　滋肾平肝。用于肝肾阴虚，耳鸣耳聋，头晕目眩。

〔用法与用量〕　口服，1 次 1 丸，1 日 2 次。

〔剂型与规格〕　蜜丸，每丸重 9 g

〔附注〕　本品具有滋养，保护肝脏作用。临床适用于耳鸣，耳聋，急性、慢性非化脓性中耳炎，美尼尔氏病（肝肾阴虚型）。

藿 胆 丸

〔药物组成〕　广藿香 90%　猪胆膏 10%

〔功能与主治〕　清风热，通鼻窍。用于风热上扰引起的鼻塞不通，时流浊涕。

〔用法与用量〕 口服，1 次 3～6 g，1 日 2 次。

〔剂型与规格〕 水丸，每瓶丸重 36 g

〔附注〕 处方来源于清·吴谦《医宗金鉴》。

本品具有抗炎，消肿，解热作用。临床适用于慢性鼻炎，慢性副鼻窦炎，鼻窦炎。

鼻 炎 片

〔药物组成〕 苍耳子 辛夷 白芷 防风 荆芥 连翘 黄柏 知母 野菊花 麻黄 细辛 桔梗 五味子 甘草

〔功能与主治〕 清热，散风，消肿，通窍。用于伤风鼻塞，鼻窒。

〔用法与用量〕 口服，1 次 3～4 片，1 日 3 次，小儿酌减。

〔剂型与规格〕 片剂，每片重 0.3 g

〔附注〕 本品具有抗菌、消炎作用。临床适用于急、慢性鼻炎、副鼻窦炎。

鼻 炎 糖 浆

〔药物组成〕 黄芩 16.8% 白芷 16.8% 苍耳子 16.8% 辛夷 16.8% 鹅不食草 16.8% 麻黄 7.9% 薄荷 8.1%

〔功能与主治〕 清热解毒，消肿通窍。用于伤风鼻塞，鼻窒。

〔用法与用量〕 口服，1 次 20 ml，1 日 3 次。

〔剂型与规格〕 糖浆剂，每瓶装 200 ml

〔附注〕 本品具有解热，抗菌，消肿作用。临床适用于急、慢性鼻炎。

鼻 渊 丸

〔药物组成〕　金银花　野菊花　辛夷　苍耳子等

〔功能与主治〕　清热毒，通鼻窍。用于鼻窒，鼻渊。

〔用法与用量〕　口服，1次5粒，1日3次。

〔剂型与规格〕　浓缩丸，每10粒重1g

〔附注〕　本品具有抗菌，消炎作用。临床适用于急、慢性鼻炎，急、慢性鼻窦炎。

六 神 丸

〔药物组成〕　（略）

〔功能与主治〕　清热解毒，消肿止痛。用于瘟疫白喉，咽喉肿痛，单双乳蛾，喉风，喉烂丹痧等症。

〔用法与用量〕　含服，1次10粒，1日1～2次，小儿1岁服1粒，4～8岁服5～6粒，9～15岁服8粒；外用，取10粒用开水或米醋少许溶成糊状，每日数次敷搽。

〔剂型与规格〕　微丸，每330粒重1g

〔附注〕　本品具有抗炎，镇痛，抗病毒，强心作用。临床适用于白喉，急性咽炎，急性喉炎，扁桃体炎，口腔炎，齿冠周炎，急性根尖脓肿，腮腺炎，猩红热及一般疮疖。

据报道，本品可作为强心药使用。可用于肺源性心脏病合并心衰，慢性肝炎的肝区痛。

孕妇忌服。疖肿破溃后不可局部外涂。

喉 症 丸

〔药物组成〕　板兰根 41.3%　冰片 1.4%　人工牛黄 2.9%　青黛 1.2%　猪胆汁 39.3%　雄黄 4.5%　玄明粉 2.0%　硼砂 2.0%　蟾酥（酒制）3.9%　百草霜 1.5%

〔功能与主治〕　清热解毒，消肿止痛。用于咽喉肿痛，单双乳蛾及一般疮疡肿毒。

〔用法与用量〕 含化，3 岁至 10 岁 1 次 3～5 粒，成人每次 5～10 粒，1 日 2 次。外用疮疖初起，红肿热痛未破者，将丸用凉开水化开，涂于红肿处，日涂数次。

〔剂型与规格〕 微丸，每 224 粒重 1 g

〔附注〕 本品临床适用于咽炎、喉炎、扁桃体炎及一般疮疖等症。

孕妇忌服。疮已溃破者不可外敷。

清 音 丸

〔药物组成〕 桔梗 15.2%　寒水石 15.2%　薄荷 15.1%　诃子 15.2%　甘草 15.1%　乌梅 15.2%　硼砂 3.0%　青黛 3.0%　冰片 3.0%

〔功能与主治〕 清音，利膈。用于肺热，胃热所致急喉喑，口干舌燥，声音不扬，嘶哑失音。

〔用法与用量〕 口服或含化，1 次 1 丸，1 日 2 次。

〔剂型与规格〕 蜜丸，每丸重 6 g

〔附注〕 本品具有抗菌，消炎作用。临床适用于急性喉炎。

炎得平胶囊

〔药物组成〕 穿心莲 100%

〔功能与主治〕 清热，解毒，凉血消肿。用于肺热咳嗽，咽喉肿痛，口舌生疮，泄泻痢疾。

〔用法与用量〕 口服，1 次 2 粒，1 日 3 次。

〔剂型与规格〕 胶囊剂，每粒装量 0.3 g

〔附注〕 本品具有抗菌消炎作用，临床适用于急性扁桃体炎、咽喉炎、流行性腮腺炎、支气管炎、肺炎、细菌性痢疾、急性胃肠炎、外伤感染等。

15.3 口腔科用药

冰 硼 散

〔药物组成〕 硼砂（炒）45.0% 冰片 4.5% 朱砂 5.5% 玄明粉45.0%

〔功能与主治〕 清热解毒，消肿止痛。用于咽喉、牙龈肿痛，口舌生疮。

〔用法与用量〕 取少许涂抹患处吹入咽喉。

〔剂型与规格〕 散剂，每瓶装 3 g

〔附注〕 处方来源于明·陈实功《外科正宗》。

本品具有抗菌，镇静作用。临床适用于急性咽炎，急性喉炎，急性喉阻塞，咽部神经官能症，急性扁桃体炎，口腔炎，舌炎，舌溃疡，牙周炎，急性根尖脓肿，化脓性中耳炎，鼻炎，急性结膜炎，阴道白色念珠菌感染（热毒型）。

锡 类 散

〔药物组成〕 青黛 41.6% 人工牛黄 3.8% 壁钱（炭）7.0% 冰片 2.1% 象牙屑 21.0% 珍珠 21.0% 人指甲（烫）3.5%

〔功能与主治〕 清热解毒，化腐。用于咽喉红肿，糜烂，唇舌肿痛。

〔用法与用量〕 取少许，吹入患处，内服遵医嘱。

〔剂型与规格〕 散剂，每瓶装 0.3 g

〔附注〕 处方来源于清·尤在泽《金匮翼》。

本品具有解热，消炎，镇痛作用。临床适用于口腔粘膜溃疡，口腔炎，鹅口疮，急性咽炎，急性喉炎，扁桃体炎，咽后壁脓肿，急性会厌炎（外服治疗）及慢性菌痢，慢性结肠炎，胃、十二指肠溃疡（内服治疗）。

双料喉风散

〔药物组成〕 珍珠 人工牛黄 冰片 青黛 黄连 甘草等。

〔功能与主治〕 清热解毒，消肿止痛。用于咽喉肿痛，口腔糜烂，牙龈疼痛，鼻渊，失荣等症。

〔用法与用量〕 取少许，吹入患处，或遵医嘱。

〔剂型与规格〕 散剂，每瓶装 1.25 g

〔附注〕 本品具有抗菌，消炎，镇静作用。临床适用于咽炎，喉炎，扁桃体炎，口腔炎，齿冠周炎，鼻窦脓肿，鼻咽癌患部发炎，化脓性中耳炎及皮肤溃疡。

牛黄益金片

〔药物组成〕 黄柏 人工牛黄等

〔功能与主治〕 清热利咽，消肿止痛。用于咽喉肿痛，口舌生疮；梅核气及大便秘结。

〔用法与用量〕 含化或吞服，含化 1 次 1~2 片，1 日 3 次；吞服 1 次 4~6 片，1 日 3 次，或遵医嘱。

〔剂型与规格〕 片剂，每片重约 0.5 g

〔附注〕 本品具有解热，镇静，消炎作用。临床适用于急、慢性咽炎，咽部神经官能症，口腔溃疡及便秘。

牙痛一粒丸

〔药物组成〕 蟾酥 41.0% 朱砂 8.0% 雄黄 10.0% 甘草 41.0%

〔功能与主治〕 止痛消肿。用于各种风火牙痛，牙龈肿痛。

〔用法与用量〕 每次取 1~2 粒，填入龋齿洞内或肿痛的齿缝处，外塞 1 块消毒棉花，防止药丸滑脱，并注意将含药后渗出的唾液吐出，不可咽下。

〔剂型与规格〕 微丸，每 125 粒重 0.3 g

〔附注〕 本品具有消炎，镇静作用。临床适用于各种牙痛，龋齿，牙周炎。

16　皮肤科药物

肤螨灵软膏

〔药物组成〕　大枫子仁　苦杏仁　等

〔功能与主治〕　杀虫，止痒，止痛。用于酒渣鼻。

〔用法与用量〕　外用，每晚用温水和药皂洗去面部油腻，搓擦药膏于患部。

〔剂型与规格〕　软膏，每盒装 5 g

〔附注〕　本品对蠕形螨有明显的杀虫作用。临床适用于蠕形螨性酒渣鼻。

用药期间勿用化妆品。过敏者勿用，患光感性皮炎或过敏性皮炎，面部有湿疹者不宜用；孕妇忌用。用药后，如发生红肿、痒、脱屑时，可暂时停药，待症状消失后再用。

养容祛斑药膏

〔药物组成〕　硬脂酸　羊毛脂　柿叶提取液　珍珠粉等

〔功能与主治〕　消斑润肤。用于面部黎黑斑，轻度雀斑。

〔用法与用量〕　先将面部用温水洗净擦干后搽，1 日 1~2 次。

〔剂型与规格〕　霜膏，每管装 30g

〔附注〕　本品具有改善微循环，促进表皮色素细胞的代谢，保护皮肤作用。临床适用于面部黄褐斑、雀斑及过敏性剌痒的辅助治疗。

外用药切勿入口。

白 癜 风 丸

〔药物组成〕 补骨脂 3.7% 黄芪 3.7% 红花 3.7% 川芎 3.7% 当归 3.7% 香附 3.7% 桃仁 3.7% 丹参 3.7% 乌梢蛇 3.7% 紫草 3.7% 白藓皮 3.7% 山药 3.7% 白蒺藜 48.1% 干姜 3.7% 硫酸铜 0.1% 龙胆 3.7%

〔功能与主治〕 活血通络，解毒利湿，驱风止痒，补气祛斑。用于白癜风。

〔用法与用量〕 口服，蜜丸 1 次 1 丸；浓缩丸 1 次 6 粒，1 日 2 次。

〔剂型与规格〕 蜜丸，每丸重 6 g；浓缩丸，每 10 粒重 2 g

〔附注〕 本品具有改善微循环，增加皮肤黑色素作用。临床适用于白癜风。

紫归治裂膏

〔药物组成〕 紫草 11.1% 当归 11.1% 白蔹 5.6% 甘草 5.6% 羊毛脂 3.9% 冰片 2.2% 氧化锌 21.1% 松香 16.7% 液状石蜡 1.7% 橡胶 17.8% 二甲基亚砜 1.1% 凡士林 2.1%

〔功能与主治〕 活血，生肌，止痛。用于手足皲裂。

〔用法与用量〕 洗净患处后，用热水稍加浸泡，揩干，将药膏贴于患处，2~3 天换药 1 次。

〔剂型与规格〕 膏药剂，每张 5×7 cm

〔附注〕 本品具有扩张血管，镇痛，促用伤口愈合作用。临床适用于手足皮肤皲裂症。

冻 疮 水

〔药物组成〕 辣椒 樟脑

〔功能与主治〕　温通血脉、消肿。用于冻疮未溃。

〔用法与用量〕　取药适量，擦患处，1日3～5次。

〔剂型与规格〕　酊剂，每瓶装10 ml

〔附注〕　本品具有改善微循环，促进表皮细胞新生作用。临床适用于冻疮未破溃者。

鹅掌风药水

〔药物组成〕　土荆皮20%　蛇床子10%　大风子仁10%　百部10%　防风4%　当归8%　凤仙透骨草10%　侧柏叶8%　吴茱萸3.8%　花椒10%　蝉蜕6%　斑蝥0.2%

〔功能与主治〕　祛风除湿，止痒杀虫。用于鹅掌风、灰指甲、湿癣、脚癣。

〔用法与用量〕　外用，将患处洗净，1日擦3～4次。灰指甲应先除去空松部分，使药易渗入。

〔剂型与规格〕　酊水剂，每瓶装20 ml

〔附注〕　本品具有杀虫、止痒、抗霉菌作用。临床适用于寄生虫性、霉菌性湿癣、脚癣、手癣等。

17 滋养、强壮药物

17.1 调节机体功能、抗衰老药

青 春 宝

〔药物组成〕　人参　天门冬　地黄等

〔功能与主治〕　益气补血，养阴生津。用于气虚血亏，未老先衰，心肾不交，健忘失眠，腰膝酸软，食欲不振等。

〔用法与用量〕　口服，1次3~5片，1日2次。

〔剂型与规格〕　片剂

〔附注〕

本品具有健脑安神，抗疲劳，提高人体免疫力等作用。临床适用于未老先衰，须发早白，贫血，神经衰弱，心脏病，各种疾病恢复治疗。

实验证明，本品可延长老龄小鼠生存期，能促进巨噬细胞吞噬功能，增强机体免疫功能，可减轻因辐射所致器官的损伤，无毒副作用。

服药期间忌食生萝卜

补中益气丸

〔药物组成〕　黄芪 30.3%　党参 9.1%　甘草 15.1%　白术 9.1%　当归 9.1%　升麻 9.1%　柴胡 9.1%　陈皮 9.1%

〔功能与主治〕　补中益气，升阳举陷。用于脾胃虚弱，中气下陷，体倦乏力，食少腹胀，久泻，脱肛，子宫脱垂。

〔用法与用量〕　口服，1次1丸，1日2~3次。

〔剂型与规格〕　蜜丸，每丸重 9 g

〔附注〕　处方来源于金·李杲《脾胃论》。

本品具有增强机体抵抗力，调节胃肠功能等作用。临床适用于各种营养不良性贫血，神经衰弱，单纯性体位性低血压，子宫脱垂，胃下垂，慢性胃肠炎，慢性肝炎，各种出血疾患等。

十全大补丸

〔药物组成〕　党参 10.8%　白术 10.8%　茯苓 10.8%　甘草 5.4%　当归 16.2%　川芎 5.4%　白芍 10.8%　肉桂 2.8%　熟地黄 16.2%　黄芪 10.8%

〔功能与主治〕　温补气血。用于气血两亏，面色苍白，气短心悸，头晕自汗，体倦乏力，四肢不温。

〔用法与用量〕　口服，1 次 1 丸，1 日 2～3 次。

〔剂型与规格〕　蜜丸，每丸重 9 g

〔附注〕　处方来源于宋·陈师文《太平惠民和剂局方》。

本品具有调节胃肠功能，增强肾上腺皮质功能，改善微循环、抗胃溃疡、抗贫血、提高机体免疫力等作用。临床适用于各种妇科病的治疗，各种贫血，胃下垂，糖尿病，肝硬化，肺气肿等慢性病的辅助治疗。

人　参　精

〔药物组成〕　人参 100%

〔功能与主治〕　补气、生津止渴，安神益智。用于气虚心悸，津亏口渴，自汗虚脱，健忘失眠，肾虚阳痿等。

〔用法与用量〕　口服，1 次 2～3 ml，1 日 3 次。

〔剂型与规格〕　口服液，每瓶 10 ml

〔附注〕　本品具有调节机体功能、抗衰老等作用。临床适用于神经衰弱，精神病，心血管系统疾患，贫血，性功能减退，糖尿病，出血性休克等。

双 宝 素

〔药物组成〕　人参　蜂王浆

〔功能与主治〕　滋补强壮，益气健脾。用于病后体虚，疲乏无力，食欲减退，健忘失眠等。

〔用法与用量〕　口服，胶囊 1 次 1～2 粒，1 日 3 次；口服液 1 次 10 ml，1 日 2 次。

〔剂型与规格〕　口服液，每支装 10 ml；胶囊，每瓶装 30 粒。

〔附注〕　本品具有促进新陈代谢，改善大脑功能，提高机体免疫力等作用。临床适用于心脏病，肝炎，胃溃疡，贫血，未老先衰，风湿性关节炎，神经衰弱等。

王 浆 片

〔药物组成〕　王浆　100%

〔功能与主治〕　滋补强身。用于脾胃气虚，食欲不振，头晕耳鸣，健忘失眠，心悸等。

〔用法与用量〕　口服，1 次 2～3 片，1 日 2～3 次。

〔剂型与规格〕　片剂，每片重 0.25 g

〔附注〕　本品临床适用于神经官能症，神经炎，营养不良，风湿性关节炎，风湿热，肝炎，对高血压、十二指肠溃疡、心血管疾病、结核病、糖尿病可作为辅助治疗。

五加参冲剂

〔药物组成〕　刺五加

〔功能与主治〕　安神益智，补肾健脾，强筋壮骨。用于体虚衰弱，全身无力，食欲不振，失眠健忘，心悸气短等。

〔用法与用量〕　口服，1 次 1 块，1 日 2～3 次。

〔剂型与规格〕　冲剂，每块重 12.25 g

〔附注〕 本品具有提高机体功能，抗过敏，抗疲劳，抗辐射，调节血压，增加冠脉血流量等作用。临床适用于慢性气管炎，神经官能症，原发性高血压，性机能减退，风湿性关节炎，各种贫血等。

六味地黄丸

〔药物组成〕 熟地 32.0%　山茱萸 16.0%　丹皮 12.0%　山药 16.0%　茯苓 12.0%　泽泻 12.8%

〔功能与主治〕 滋阴补肾。用于肾阴亏损，头晕耳鸣，腰膝酸软，骨蒸潮热，盗汗遗精，消渴。

〔用法与用量〕 口服，1 次 1 丸，1 日 2 次。

〔剂型与规格〕 蜜丸，每丸重 9 g

〔附注〕 处方来源于宋·钱乙《小儿药证直诀》。

本品具有改善肾功能，降压，利尿，抗炎，抗肿瘤作用。临床适用于先天性小儿发育迟缓，慢性肾炎，高血压，糖尿病，类风湿性关节炎，脊椎肥大症，肺结核，甲状腺机能亢进，视神经炎，青光眼，牙周脓肿等。

灵 芝 片

〔药物组成〕 灵芝

〔功能与主治〕 强壮安神。用于健忘失眠，多梦，食欲不振等。

〔用法与用量〕 口服，1 日 3 次，1 次 3 片。

〔剂型与规格〕 片剂，每片含药 1 g

〔附注〕 本品具有增强机体免疫力，强心，降低血脂，调节血压，调节中枢神经功能，镇咳，祛痰作用。临床适用于喘息性气管炎，支气管哮喘，传染性肝炎，慢性肠炎，菌痢，血小板减少性紫癜，风湿性关节炎，冠心病，胃及十二指肠溃疡等。

八 珍 丸

〔药物组成〕 党参 12.1% 白术 12.1% 茯苓 12.1% 当归 18.2% 甘草 6.1% 白芍 12.1% 川芎 9.1% 熟地黄 18.2%

〔功能与主治〕 补气益血。用于气血两虚，面色萎黄，食欲不振，四肢乏力，月经不调等。

〔用法与用量〕 口服，1 次 1 丸，1 日 2 次。

〔剂型与规格〕 蜜丸，每丸重 9 g

〔附注〕 处方来源于《瑞竹堂经验方》。

本品具有调节胃肠功能，促进红细胞再生等作用。临床适用于各种贫血，慢性胃炎，胃及十二指肠溃疡，视神经萎缩，月经失调等。

大 补 阴 丸

〔药物组成〕 熟地黄 21.4% 知母 14.4% 黄柏 14.4% 龟板 21.4% 猪骨髓 28.4%

〔功能与主治〕 滋阴降火。用于阴虚火旺，潮热盗汗，咳嗽咯血，耳鸣遗精。

〔用法与用量〕 口服，1 次 6 g，1 日 2～3 次。

〔剂型与规格〕 蜜丸，每丸重 3 g

〔附注〕 处方来源于元·朱震亨《丹溪心法》。

本品具有改善肾功能，降压，利尿，抗炎等作用。临床适用于甲状腺机能亢进，肾结核，骨结核，糖尿病等。

参苓白术丸

〔药物组成〕 人参 13.8% 茯苓 13.8% 白术 13.8% 山药 13.8% 白扁豆 10.3% 砂仁 6.9% 薏苡仁 6.9% 桔梗 6.9% 甘草 13.8%

〔功能与主治〕 补脾胃，益肺气。用于脾胃虚弱，食少便溏，气短咳嗽，肢倦乏力。

〔用法与用量〕 口服，1 次 6～9 g，1 日 2～3 次。

〔剂型与规格〕 水丸，每 20 粒重 1 g

〔附注〕 处方来源于宋·陈师文《太平惠民和剂局方》。

本品具有调节胃肠功能，抗炎，助消化，增强机体免疫力作用。临床适用于慢性胃肠炎，贫血，肺结核，慢性肾炎，消化不良等。

康宝口服液

〔药物组成〕 蜂王浆 刺五加 黄精 党参 桑椹 砂仁 黄芪 山楂 枸杞子 淫羊藿等

〔功能与主治〕 益气补肾，健脾和胃，养心安神。用于健忘失眠，头晕耳鸣，视减听衰，食欲不振，腰膝酸软，心慌气短，中风后遗症等。

〔用法与用量〕 口服，1 次 10～20 ml，1 日 2 次。

〔剂型与规格〕 口服液，每支装 10 ml

〔附注〕 本品具有改善大脑功能，促进新陈代谢等作用。临床适用于神经衰弱，冠心病，脱发，慢性肾炎，脑血管栓塞，妇女更年期综合症等。

人参蜂王浆

〔药物组成〕 人参 王浆 蜂蜜

〔功能与主治〕 滋补强壮，益气健脾。用于食欲不振，病后体虚，疲乏无力等。

〔用法与用量〕 口服，1 次 10 ml，1 日 1 次，早或晚空腹时服。

〔剂型与规格〕 口服液，每支装 10 ml

〔附注〕 本品具有改善大脑功能，促进新陈代谢、滋养强壮等作用。临床适用于各种贫血、神经衰弱、神经官能症、慢性肝炎、肺心病、慢性气管炎、风湿性关节炎、慢性肾炎、肺结核等。

参杞冲剂

〔药物组成〕　党参　枸杞子

〔功能与主治〕　补气血，健脾胃，养肝肾。用于脾胃虚弱，头晕眼花，体倦乏力。

〔用法与用量〕　口服，1 次 1 袋，1 日 2 次。

〔剂型与规格〕　冲剂，每袋装 10 g

〔附注〕　本品具有改善机体功能，降血脂等作用。临床适用于慢性肝炎、动脉硬化症、高血脂症，贫血，神经官能症等。

泰山灵芝精

〔药物组成〕　灵芝 38.2%　人参 0.5%　丹参 1.5%　杜仲 1.5%　枸杞子 1.5%　何首乌 1.5%　酸枣仁 1.5%　五味子 1.5%　熟地黄 1.5%　当归 1.2%　蜂蜜 49.6%

〔功能与主治〕　补益气血，养心安神。用于气血两虚，心肾不交，惊悸怔忡，健忘失眠，腰膝酸软，食欲不振等。

〔用法与用量〕　口服，1 次 10 ml，1 日 2 次，早饭或临睡前服用。

〔制剂与规格〕　口服液，每瓶装 10 ml

〔附注〕　本品具有调节机体功能，促进血液循环，祛痰等作用。临床适用于神经衰弱、冠心病、慢性肝炎、十二指肠及胃溃疡、神经官能症、脱发、贫血等。

当归补血精

〔药物组成〕　当归 76.2%　熟地黄 4.8%　白芍 4.8%　川芎 2.3%　党参 4.8%　黄芪 4.8%　甘草 2.3%

〔功能与主治〕 滋补气血。用于贫血、头晕、心悸健忘、妇女月经不调，产后血虚、体弱。

〔用法与用量〕 口服，1次5 ml，1日2次。

〔剂型与规格〕 糖浆剂，每瓶150 ml，（每1ml含生药0.19 g）

〔附注〕 本品具有滋养、镇静、增强机体免疫力等作用。临床适用于各种贫血、功能性子宫出血，月经不调、神经衰弱、过敏性紫癜等。

首 乌 丸

〔药物组成〕 何首乌42.7% 地黄2.4% 牛膝4.7% 桑椹膏8.3% 女贞子4.7% 桑叶4.7% 黑芝麻1.9% 墨旱莲膏5.7% 补骨脂4.7% 豨莶草9.5% 金银花2.4% 金樱子膏8.3%

〔功能与主治〕 补肝肾；强筋骨，乌须发。用于肝肾两虚，头晕耳鸣，腰膝酸软，须发早白等。

〔用法与用量〕 口服，1次6 g，1日2次。

〔剂型与规格〕 水丸，每20粒重1 g

〔附注〕 本品具有抗炎，降血脂，降低胆固醇等作用。临床适用于风湿性关节炎，须发早白症，动脉硬化，冠心病，荨麻疹，神经衰弱，精神病等。

玉 屏 风 丸

〔药物组成〕 黄芪50% 防风16.7% 白术33.3%

〔功能与主治〕 益气，固表，止汗。用于气虚自汗，表虚易感风寒等症。

〔用法与用量〕 口服，1次6 g，1日2次。

〔剂型与规格〕 水丸，每瓶装125 g

〔附注〕 处方来源于明·张介宾《景岳全书》。

本品具有增强机体免疫功能作用。临床适用于慢性气管炎，体虚感冒，慢性鼻炎，荨麻疹，预防感冒等。

青娥丸

〔药物组成〕　杜仲 48.5%　补骨脂 24.2%　核桃仁 15.2%　大蒜 12.1%

〔功能与主治〕　补肾强腰。用于肾虚腰痛，起坐不利，膝软乏力。

〔用法与用量〕　口服，1 次 1 丸，1 日 2～3 次。

〔剂型与规格〕　蜜丸，每丸重 9 g

〔附注〕　处方来源于宋·陈师文《太平惠民和剂局方》。
本品具有改善肾功能、降压、利尿作用。临床适用于慢性肾炎，肾结核，腰椎结核，骨结核等。

人参养荣丸

〔药物组成〕　党参 8.3%　黄芪 8.3%　陈皮 8.3%　甘草 8.3%　白芍 12.4%　茯苓 5.8%　生姜 4.1%　肉桂 8.3%　熟地黄 5.7%　当归 8.3%　远志 4.1%　白术 8.3%　五味子 5.7%　大枣 4.1%

〔功能与主治〕　补气养血，健脾安神。用于脾肺虚损，气血不足，食欲不振，惊悸盗汗，健忘。

〔用法与用量〕　口服，1 次 9 g，1 日 2 次。

〔剂型与规格〕　水蜜丸，每 10 粒重 1 g

〔附注〕　本品具有调节胃肠功能，镇静等作用。临床适用于血栓闭塞性脉管炎，各种肿瘤，慢性胃肠炎，传染病后期及手术后恢复性辅助治疗。

生发丸

〔药物组成〕　当归 12.3%　侧柏叶 12.3%　地黄 12.3%

女贞子 12.3%　柏子仁 12.4%　枸杞子 3.7%　桑椹子 12.4%
黄柏 3.7%　菟丝子 12.4%　白鲜皮 6.2%

〔功能与主治〕　滋补肝肾，养血生发。用于脱发、斑秃。

〔用法与用量〕　口服，1 次 1 丸，1 日 2 次，重者酌加。

〔剂型与规格〕　大蜜丸，每丸重 9 g

〔附注〕　本品具有生发作用。临床适用于脂溢性皮炎，神经衰弱，代谢障碍引起的脱发等。

忌食动物脂肪，避免精神过度紧张。

乌 发 丸

〔药 物 组 成〕　地黄 25.0%　旱莲草 12.5%　何首乌 25.0%　黑豆 12.5%　女贞子 12.5%　黑芝麻 12.5%

〔功能与主治〕　滋肾补脑，养血乌发。用于青少年白发症。

〔用法与用量〕，口服，1 次 1 丸，1 日 2～3 次。

〔剂型与规格〕　蜜丸，每丸重 9 g

〔附注〕　本品具有增强机体免疫力等作用。临床适用于各种原因引起的白发症。

防止精神过度紧张，忌食辛辣食物。

七宝美髯丸

〔药 物 组 成〕　何首乌 42.2%　菟丝子 10.5%　牛膝 10.5%　补骨脂 5.3%　当归 10.5%　枸杞子 10.5%　茯苓 10.5%

〔功能与主治〕　滋补肝肾，填精养血。用于精血不足，须发早白等。

〔用法与用量〕　口服，1 次 1 丸，1 日 2 次。

〔剂型与规格〕　大蜜丸，每丸重 9 g

〔附注〕　处方来源于唐·邵元节《经验方》

本品具有调节机体机能，促进新陈代谢等作用。临床适用于未老先衰，须发早白等。

17.2　性神经衰弱用药、强壮用药

至宝三鞭丸

〔药物组成〕　蜂蜜　黄芪　人参　当归　鹿茸　梅花鹿鞭　大蛤蚧　菟丝子　地黄　枸杞　蜂乳　小茴香　川椒　甘松　沉香　海狗鞭　广狗鞭　大海马　飞阳起石　五花龙骨　净萸肉　补骨脂　牛夕　淫羊藿　云苓　桑螵蛸　山药　巴戟天　杜仲　肉桂　覆盆子　何首乌　粉丹皮　川黄柏　杭白芍　白术　肉苁蓉　泽泻　苇菖蒲　远志

〔功能与主治〕　补血生精，健脑补肾。用于体质虚弱，腰背酸痛，肾亏遗精，健忘失眠，气虚食减，贫血头晕，妇女血亏，年老气喘等。

〔用法与用量〕　口服，浓缩丸，1次8粒；大蜜丸，1次1丸，1日1次。

〔剂型与规格〕　大蜜丸，每丸重 6.25 g；浓缩丸，每粒重 0.2 g

〔附注〕　本品具有改善大脑功能，促进性腺机能等作用。临床适用于各种机体功能低下症，性神经衰弱，各种贫血，慢性胃肠炎，胃及十二指肠溃疡，神经衰弱等。

龟　龄　集

〔药物组成〕　人参　鹿茸　海马　莲子　茯苓　天冬　麦冬　穿山甲　肉苁蓉　锁阳　补骨脂　淫羊藿　葫芦巴　菟丝子　沙菀子　杜仲　附子　紫梢花　怀牛膝　细辛　地黄　石斛　当归　砂仁　母丁香　菊花　车前子　莱服子　石燕　食盐　贯众　阿胶　朱砂　甘草

〔功能与主治〕 补肾壮阳。用于肾阳虚弱，阳痿遗精，气虚咳嗽，腰膝冷痛，小腹拘急，头晕耳鸣，记忆减退，妇女崩漏，赤白带下，五更泄泻等症。

〔用法与用量〕 口服，1次1.5g，1日1～2次。

〔剂型与规格〕 散剂，每瓶装3 g

〔附注〕 本品具有调节肾上腺皮质功能，促进生长发育，增强机体抵抗力等作用。临床适应于身体虚弱症，性神经衰弱，慢性肾炎，妇女月经不调，更年期综合症，不孕症等。

孕妇忌服，忌生冷食物。

海龙蛤蚧精

〔药物组成〕 海龙 蛤蚧 人参 羊鞭 鹿茸 地黄 肉苁蓉 陈皮 沉香 枸杞子 黄芪 肉桂 当归 川芎 白叩甘草 等

〔功能与主治〕 补肝肾，益精血。用于气血两亏，健忘失眠，头晕耳鸣，腰膝酸软，阳痿遗精，妇女血崩等。

〔用法与用量〕 口服，1次10 ml，1日2次。

〔剂型与规格〕 口服液，每支装10 ml

〔附注〕 本品具有改善大脑功能，促进能量代谢，增强性腺机能等作用。临床适用于神经衰弱，神经官能症，性神经衰弱，各种贫血，肺气肿，慢性胃肠炎，支气管哮喘，男性不育症，前列腺炎，妇女更年期综合症等。

还 少 丹

〔药物组成〕 巴戟天 小茴香 肉苁蓉 人参 山药 枸杞 山茱萸 牛膝 杜仲 五味子 茯苓 地黄 当归 肉桂黄芪 阿胶等

〔功能与主治〕 滋补强身，安神。用于肾气不足，下腹寒冷，梦遗滑精，气虚血亏，头晕眼花，脾胃虚弱，腰膝乏困，妇女赤白带下。

〔用法与用量〕　口服，1次1丸，1日2次。

〔剂型与规格〕　蜜丸，每丸重10 g

〔附注〕　处方来源于元·朱震亨《丹溪心法》。

本品具有强壮、兴奋肾上腺皮质和增强免疫机能作用。临床适用于年老体衰，性机能衰退，各种造血机能障碍等疾患。

孕妇及高血压患者忌服。

全　鹿　丸

〔药物组成〕　鲜鹿肉 39.2%　鹿角胶 0.9%　鹿茸 0.5%　鹿肾 0.4%　鹿尾 0.2%　人参 2.0%　黄芪 2.0%　白术 2.0%　茯苓 2.0%　甘草 1.9%　山药 1.9%　熟地黄 1.9%　生地黄 1.9%　当归 1.9%　川芎 1.9%　枸杞子 1.9%　菟丝子 1.9%　楮实子 2.0%　覆盆子 2.0%　胡芦巴 2.0%　杜仲 2.0%　续断 2.0%　牛膝 2.0%　补骨脂 2.0%　巴戟天 2.0%　肉苁蓉 2.0%　锁阳 2.0%　大青盐 0.9%　秋石 2.0%　天万冬 2.0%　麦门冬 2.0%　茴香 0.9%　花椒 0.9%　沉香 0.9%　陈皮 2.0%　芡实 2.0%　五味子 2.0%

〔功能与主治〕　补阳填精，补气养血。用于阴阳两虚，身体虚弱，头晕耳鸣，梦遗滑精，腰膝酸痛，食少乏力，自汗盗汗，妇女崩漏带下。

〔用法与用量〕　口服，1次1丸，1日2次。

〔剂型与规格〕　蜜丸，每丸重9 g

〔附注〕　处方来源于明·张介宾《景岳全书》。

本品临床适用于性神经衰弱，神经官能症，糠尿病，前列腺炎，慢性肾炎，慢性胃肠炎，肺结核，神经衰弱等。

男　　宝

〔药物组成〕　驴肾　狗肾　人参　当归　杜仲　鹿茸　海

马　阿胶　丹皮　黄芪　熟地黄　茯苓　白术　山茱萸　淫羊藿　补骨脂　枸杞子　菟丝子　附子　巴戟天　肉苁蓉　覆盆子　葫芦巴　麦门冬　锁阳　仙茅　续断　牛膝　玄参　甘草

〔功能与主治〕　补肾壮阳。用于肾阳不足，阳痿滑泄，腰腿酸痛，肾囊湿冷，精神萎靡，食欲不振等症。

〔用法与用量〕　口服，1 次 2～3 粒，1 日 2 次，早晚分服。

〔剂型与规格〕　胶囊，每粒重 0.3 g

〔附注〕　本品具有强壮、调节肾上腺皮质功能，促进性腺机能作用。临床适用于性功能减退症，慢性肾炎，前列腺炎，神经衰弱，胃肠神经官能症，造血功能障碍等。

三　肾　丸

〔药物组成〕　鹿肾　狗肾　驴肾　黄芪　龟板　人参　山茱萸　当归　附子　熟地黄　淫羊藿　茯苓　补骨脂　枸杞子　沙蒺藜　白术　鱼鳔　阿胶　杜仲　菟丝子　鹿茸　肉桂

〔功能与主治〕　滋阴益气，补肾壮阳。用于阳痿不举，腰腿酸痛，精神疲倦，食欲不振。

〔用法与用量〕　口服，1 次 1 丸，1 日 1～2 次。

〔剂型与规格〕　蜜丸，每丸重 6 g

〔附注〕　本品具有强壮，安神，增强性腺机能，提高机体免疫力等作用。临床适用于性功能减退症，神经衰弱，各种贫血，慢性肾炎，前列腺炎，不孕症等。

五子衍宗丸

〔药物组成〕　枸杞子 34.8%　菟丝子 34.8%　覆盆子 17.4%　五味子 4.3%　车前子 8.7%

〔功能与主治〕　补肾益精。用于肾虚腰痛，尿后余沥，遗精早泄，阳痿不育。

〔用法与用量〕　口服，1次1丸，1日2次。

〔剂型与规格〕　蜜丸，每丸重9 g

〔附注〕　处方来源于元·朱震亨《丹溪心法》。

本品具有促进性腺机能，镇静，利尿，强壮等作用。临床适用于性神经衰弱，精子缺乏症，慢性膀胱炎，慢性肾炎，慢性前列腺炎等。

海马补肾丸

〔药物组成〕　大海马　人参　鹿茸　鹿筋　虎骨　龙骨　枸杞子　当归　熟地黄　蛤蚧　黄芪　茯苓　鲜对虾　山萸肉　母丁香　核桃仁

〔功能与主治〕　滋阴补肾，强腰健脑。用于气血两虚，肾气不足，头晕耳鸣，腰膝酸痛，体倦乏力，心悸气短，梦遗滑精等。

〔用法与用量〕　口服，1日2次，1次10粒。

〔剂型与规格〕　浓缩丸，每瓶装120粒

〔附注〕　本品具有促进新陈代谢、增强机体抵抗力等作用。临床适用于神经衰弱，风湿性关节炎，慢性肾炎，慢性气管炎，性神经衰弱症等。

雏　凤　精

〔药物组成〕　鸡胎　狗鞭　羊鞭　羊外肾　人参　鹿茸　山药　杜仲　枸杞子　熟地黄　砂仁　肉桂　沉香　补骨脂　覆盆子　当归等

〔功能与主治〕　温肾壮阳，补气养血。用于气血两虚，腰酸背痛，头晕耳鸣，健忘失眠，心悸不宁，肾亏滑泄，妇女子宫虚冷，月经不调等。

〔用法与用量〕　口服，1次10 ml，1日2次。

〔剂型与规格〕　口服液，每瓶装10 ml

〔附注〕　本品具有强壮，促进血液循环，促进新陈代谢等作用。临床适用于各种贫血症，妇女月经不调，功能性子宫出血，不孕症，神经衰弱，慢性肾炎，慢性胃肠炎，性神经衰弱，神经官能症，妇女更年期综合症等。

补肾宁片

〔药物组成〕　羊外肾　人参等

〔功能与主治〕　温肾助阳，益气固本。用于肾阳虚弱，阳痿遗精，腰膝酸软，健忘失眠，妇女宫冷带下，血崩等。

〔用法与用量〕　口服，1次3～5片，1日3次。

〔剂型与规格〕　片剂，每片重约0.2 g

〔附注〕　本品具有调节肾上腺皮质功能，促进性腺机能等作用。临床适用于性神经衰弱症，前列腺炎，慢性肾炎，妇女更年期综合症等。

二　仙　膏

〔药物组成〕　人参　鹿角胶　鹿茸等

〔功能与主治〕　滋阴助阳，益气养血。用于气血两虚，神疲体倦，阳痿遗精，心悸气短，腰膝酸软。

〔用法与用量〕　口服，1次20 g，1日2次。

〔剂型与规格〕　煎膏剂，每瓶装250 g

〔附注〕　本品具有改善大脑功能，促进性腺机能，增强机体抵抗力等作用。临床适用于性神经衰弱，慢性肾炎，前列腺炎，各种贫血症，各种妇女产后虚弱症。

锁阳固精丸

〔药物组成〕　锁阳 3.8%　肉苁蓉 4.7%　巴戟天 5.7%　补骨脂 4.7%　菟丝子 3.8%　杜仲 4.7%　大茴香 4.7%　韭菜子 3.8%　芡实 3.8%　莲子 3.8%　莲须 4.7%　牡蛎 3.8%　龙

骨 3.8%　鹿角霜 3.8%　熟地黄 10.6%　山茱萸 3.2%　丹皮 2.1%　山药 10.6%　茯苓 2.1%　泽泻 2.1%　知母 0.7%　黄柏 0.7%　牛膝 3.8%　大青盐 4.5%

〔功能与主治〕　温肾固精。用于肾虚滑精，腰膝酸软，眩晕耳鸣，四肢无力。

〔用法与用量〕　口服，1 次 1 丸，1 日 2 次。

〔剂型与规格〕　蜜丸，每丸重 9 g

〔附注〕　本品具有调节肾上腺皮质功能，促进新陈代谢等作用。临床适用于性神经衰弱，慢性肾炎，神经官能症，慢性胃肠炎等。

补肾强身片

〔药物组成〕　淫羊藿 29.4%　菟丝子 17.6%　金樱子 17.6%　狗脊 17.7%　女贞子 17.7%

〔功能与主治〕　补肾强身。用于腰酸足软，头晕耳鸣，眼花心悸，阳痿遗精。

〔用法与用量〕　口服，1 次 3 片，1 日 3 次。

〔剂型与规格〕　片剂，每片重约 0.25 g

〔附注〕　本品具有促进性腺机能，镇静等作用。临床适用于神经衰弱，慢性肾炎，性功能减退症，慢性气管炎，神经官能症等。

鹿 角 胶

〔药物组成〕　鹿角 100%

〔功能与主治〕　温肾助阳，添精补髓。用于肾虚，阳痿，子宫寒冷，崩漏带下。

〔用法与用量〕　口服，1 次 3～6 g，1 日 1～2 次，溶化兑服。

〔剂型与规格〕　胶剂，每块重约 4.5 g

〔附注〕　本品具有促进生长发育，改善造血功能等作用。临床适用于性神经衰弱，小儿发育不良，各种贫血，风湿性心脏病，功能性子宫出血等。

海 龙 胶

〔药物组成〕　海龙 53.3%　黄明胶 40%　当归 0.8%　川芎 0.5%　肉苁蓉 0.5%　黄芪 0.5%　白芍 0.3%　肉桂 0.8%　枸杞子 0.3%　陈皮 0.3%　甘草 2.7%

〔功能与主治〕　温肾养血，填精补髓。用于阳痿，血虚痛经，腰膝酸软，头晕耳鸣。

〔用法与用量〕　烊化兑服，1 次 6～9 g，1 日 1～2 次。

〔剂型与规格〕　胶剂，每块重 15 g

〔附注〕　本品具有强壮作用。临床适用于性神经衰弱，月经不调，妇女更年期综合症，各种贫血等。

18 其他药物

藿香正气水

〔药物组成〕 苍术 11.6% 陈皮 11.6% 厚朴 11.6% 白芷 17.4% 茯苓 17.4% 大腹皮 17.4% 生半夏 11.6% 甘草浸膏 1.2% 广藿香油 0.1% 紫苏叶油 0.1%

〔功能与主治〕 解表化湿，理气和中。用于外感风寒，内伤湿滞，头痛昏重，脘腹胀痛，呕吐泄泻。

〔用法与用量〕 口服，1 次 5～10 ml，1 日 2 次。用时摇匀。

〔制剂与规格〕 酊剂，每瓶 10 ml

〔附注〕 处方来源于宋·陈师文《太平惠民和剂局方》。

本品具有解热、健胃、止呕作用。临床适用于夏季中暑引起的头晕、呕吐、腹痛、腹泻，胃肠型流感，急性胃肠炎等。

祛 暑 丸

〔药物组成〕 藿香 18.8% 紫苏叶 18.8% 香薷 7.5% 木瓜 5.8% 茯苓 29.3% 檀香 2.8% 丁香 2.8% 甘草 14.2%

〔功能与主治〕 清暑祛湿，和胃止泻。用于中暑外感，恶寒发热，头痛身倦，腹胀吐泻。

〔用法与用量〕 口服，1 次 1 丸，1 日 1～2 次。

〔制剂与规格〕 蜜丸，每丸重 9 g

〔附注〕 处方来源于宋·陈师文《太平惠民和剂局方》。

本品具有解热、健胃、镇静、止呕作用。临床适用于夏季中暑感冒，急性胃肠炎等。

清暑益气丸

〔药物组成〕 黄芪 9.6%　苍术 9.6%　黄柏 2.9%　青皮 3.8%　当归 5.8%　党参 9.6%　麦门冬 5.8%　白术 11.5%　六神曲 9.6%　橘皮 9.6%　葛根 3.9%　泽泻 9.6%　五味子 2.9%　甘草 3.9%　升麻 1.9%

〔功能与主治〕 清暑祛湿，益气生津。用于体虚感受暑邪引起的头痛发热，四肢倦怠，口渴心烦，自汗尿赤。

〔用法与用量〕 口服，1 次 1～2 丸，1 日 2 次。

〔制剂与规格〕 蜜丸，每丸重 9 g

〔附注〕 处方来源于金·李杲《脾胃论》。

本品具有增强机体免疫力，解热、镇痛等作用。临床适用于体弱者夏季中暑引起的发烧、咽干、头痛、小便不利等症。

六 一 散

〔药物组成〕 滑石粉 85.7%　甘草 14.3%

〔功能与主治〕 清暑利湿。用于暑热身倦，口渴泄泻，小便黄少。外治痱子刺痒。

〔用法与用量〕 调服或包煎服汤，1 次 6～9 g，1 日 1～2 次；外用扑撒患处。

〔剂型与规格〕 散剂，每袋重 18 g

〔附注〕 处方来源于金·刘河间《伤寒标本》。

本品具有抗炎、利尿、解热作用。临床适用于夏季胃肠型流感，急性肾炎，急性膀胱炎等。

痧 药

〔药物组成〕 丁香　苍术　天麻　麻黄　大黄　甘草　冰片　蟾酥　雄黄　朱砂

〔功能与主治〕 祛暑解毒，辟秽开窍。用于夏令贪凉饮冷，猝然闷乱烦躁，腹痛吐泻，牙关紧闭，四肢厥冷。

〔用法与用量〕 口服，1 次 10～15 粒，1 日 1 次。外用，研细吹鼻取嚏。

〔剂型与规格〕 水丸，每 33 粒重 1 g

〔附注〕 处方来源于《济世养生集》。

本品具有发汗、抗菌消炎、强心等作用。临床适用于夏季急性胃肠炎，食物中毒等。

孕妇忌服。

暑 症 片

〔药物组成〕 猪牙皂 10.3% 细辛 10.3% 薄荷 8.8% 广藿香 8.9% 白芷 2.9% 防风 5.9% 陈皮 5.9% 桔梗 5.9% 白矾 2.9% 木香 5.9% 朱砂 7.3% 雄黄 7.3% 贯众 5.9% 半夏 5.9% 甘草 5.9%

〔功能与主治〕 祛暑开窍，辟温解毒。用于中暑昏厥，牙关紧闭，腹痛吐泻，四肢发麻。

〔用法与用量〕 口服，1 次 2 片，1 日 2～3 次。

〔剂型与规格〕 片剂，每片含药 0.8 g

〔附注〕 本品具有解热、健胃、止呕、强心等作用。临床适用于夏季中暑性休克，急性胃肠炎等。

暑湿正气丸

〔药物组成〕 广藿香 半夏 青木香 陈皮 丁香 肉桂 苍术 白术 茯苓 朱砂 硝石 硼砂 雄黄 金礞石 (煅) 冰片

〔功能与主治〕 祛暑散寒，止痛止泻。用于暑天受寒，腹痛吐泻，头痛恶寒，肢体酸重。

〔用法与用量〕 口服，1 次 1.5～3 g，1 日 1～2 次。

〔剂型与规格〕 水丸，每 200 粒重 3 g，每瓶装 3 g

〔附注〕 本品具有解热、健胃、止呕、镇静作用。临床适用于急性胃肠炎，食物中毒，消化不良等。

益 元 散

〔药物组成〕 滑石 82.2% 甘草 13.7% 朱砂 4.1%

〔功能与主治〕 清暑利湿，镇心安神。用于暑热身倦，心烦口渴，小便黄少。

〔用法与用量〕 包煎服，每次 3～6 g，每日 1～2 次。

〔剂型与规格〕 散剂，每袋重 30 g

〔附注〕 处方来源于金·刘河间《河间六书》。

本品具有抗炎、利尿、镇静作用。临床适用于泌尿系统感染，口腔炎，急性胃肠炎等。

行 军 散

〔药物组成〕 珍珠 人工牛黄 冰片 硝石 硼砂 姜粉雄黄等

〔功能与主治〕 辟瘟、解毒、开窍。用于夏伤暑热，头目眩晕，腹痛吐泻。

〔用法与用量〕 口服，1 次 0.3～0.9 g，1 日 1～2 次。

〔剂型与规格〕 散剂，每瓶重 0.9 g

〔附注〕 本品具有解热、抗菌消炎作用。临床适用于夏季中暑感冒伴有胃肠道症状者，急性胃肠炎等。

孕妇忌服

仁 丹

〔药物组成〕 薄荷脑 草豆蔻 冰片 干姜 肉桂 丁香木香 甘草等

〔功能与主治〕 祛风舒气，生津健胃。用于晕船、晕车及高温闷热所引起的消化呆滞。

〔用法与用量〕　口服或含服，每次 4～8 粒。

〔剂型与规格〕　水丸，每 75 粒重 3 g

〔附注〕　本品具有解热、健胃、止呕、促进消化等作用。临床适用于夏季中毒引起的头痛头晕、消化不良等症。

不宜同溴化钾、溴化钠、碘化钠同服。

清　凉　丹

〔药物组成〕　薄荷脑　薄荷油　樟脑　肉豆蔻　生姜　丁香　儿茶　甘草　肉桂　胡椒　冰片

〔功能与主治〕　祛风健胃，凉喉止渴。用于中暑头昏，喉干舌燥，晕车晕船，闷热不适。

〔用法与用量〕　含化，每次 1～2 格。

〔剂型与规格〕　块剂，每块重 5 g（划分为 25 小格）。

〔附注〕　本品具有解热、健胃等作用。临床适用于夏季中暑引起的口干、头晕、消化不良等症。

清　凉　油

〔药物组成〕　薄荷脑　樟脑　薄荷油　桉叶油　樟脑油桂皮油　丁香油

〔功能与主治〕　局部刺激药。具有清凉作用。用于头疼，皮肤瘙痒，蚊叮虫咬，较轻灼伤等。

〔用法与用量〕　外用。擦于太阳穴或患处。

〔剂型与规格〕　软膏剂，每盒重 3 g

〔附注〕　本品具有局部消炎、镇痛、止痒等作用。临床适用于感冒头痛，蚊叮虫咬等。

风　油　精

〔药物组成〕　薄荷油　桉叶油　樟脑　丁香油　香精油叶绿素　等

〔功能与主治〕 局部刺激药。具有清凉作用。用于伤风感冒引起的头痛头晕，牙痛，蚊叮虫咬。

〔用法与用量〕 外用，涂搽患处；口服，每次 4～6 滴。

〔剂型与规格〕 油剂，每瓶 10 ml

〔附注〕 本品具有局部消炎、镇痛、止痒、驱风作用。临床适用于感冒头痛，蚊叮虫咬引起的皮肤病症。

十 滴 水

〔药物组成〕 樟脑粉 桂皮 大黄 干姜 辣椒 大茴香 桉叶油

〔功能与主治〕 用于中暑而引起的头晕恶心、腹痛 肠胃不适等症。

〔用法与用量〕 口服，1 次 0.5～1 ml。

〔剂型与规格〕 酊剂，每瓶 10 ml

〔附注〕 本品具有镇静止痛、健胃止呕等作用。临床适用于夏季中暑引起的头晕、呕吐、腹痛、消化不良等症。

孕妇忌服。

冰霜梅苏丸

〔药物组成〕 薄荷 紫苏叶 乌梅 葛根 白糖

〔功能与主治〕 清解暑热，生津止渴。用于感受暑热引起的口渴咽干，胸中满闷，头目眩晕。

〔用法与用量〕 含化，每次 1～2 丸，每日数次。

〔剂型与规格〕 水丸，每袋重 30 g

〔附注〕 处方来源于清·汪昂《汤头歌诀》。

本品具有解表、健胃、止呕等作用。临床适用于夏季中暑引起的口干、消化不良等症。

痱 子 粉

〔药物组成〕 滑石粉 冰片

〔功能与主治〕 清凉舒爽，除湿止痒。用于夏令痱子刺痒难忍。

〔用法与用量〕 外用，扑撒患处，每日 4～6 次。

〔剂型与规格〕 散剂，每盒装 100 g

〔附注〕 本品具有局部消炎作用。临床适用于夏季汗囊炎。

附录 1

中医门类药名索引

内科

风　痰　门

人参再造丸	伤湿止痛膏
大活络丸	局方牛黄清心丸
小活络丸	医痫丸
万氏牛黄清心丸	苏冰滴丸
牛黄至宝丹	伸筋丹胶囊
牛黄降压片	杜仲降压片
木瓜丸	鸡血藤浸膏片
心可舒片	坎离砂
天麻丸	环心丹
风湿止痛膏	罗布麻降压片
五加皮药酒	降压平片
风湿药酒	降脂灵胶丸
白金丸	金不换膏药
冯了性药酒	狗皮膏
再造丸	国公酒
羊痫疯丸	武力拔寒散
伤湿宝珍膏	骨刺丸
伤湿祛痛膏	独活寄生丸
红花注射液	活心丸

冠心苏合丸   益心丸

祛风舒筋丸   速效救心丸

复方丹参片   消络痛片

复方罗布麻片   消栓通络片

脉络通片   舒心降压片

冠心通脉灵片   舒筋活络酒

骨刺消痛液   愈心宁心片

复方丹参注射液 解心痛片

复方当归注射液 豨莶丸

脉安冲剂   镇江膏药

消栓再造丸   保心丸

脑立清丸

补 益 门

十全大补丸   双宝素

七宝美髯丸   王浆片

八珍丸   五味子冲剂

人参归脾丸   五加参冲剂

人参养荣丸   生发丸

人参健脾丸   玉泉丸

二仙膏   玉屏风丸

人参精   四君子丸

人参蜂王浆   生脉饮口服液

三肾片   至宝三鞭丸

大补阴丸   朱砂安神丸

山东阿胶膏   全鹿丸

乌发丸   安神补心丸

六味地黄丸   当归补血精

六君子丸   当归养血片

还少丹

补中益气丸

男宝

龟龄集

补肾强力丸

灵芝片

阿胶

金匮肾气丸

青娥丸

枕中丹

参苓白术丸

青春宝

参杞冲剂

柏子养心丸

骨质增生丸

首乌丸

骨仙片

骨刺片

健脑丸

健脑补肾丸

消渴丸

脑灵素片

海龙胶

海龙蛤蚧精

黄明胶

鹿角胶

康宝口服液

锁阳固精丸

腰痛丸

新阿胶

雏风精

痰 嗽 门

二母宁嗽丸

二陈丸

二冬膏

川贝止咳糖浆

小青龙合剂

小半夏合剂

止嗽青果丸

止嗽定喘丸

止咳喘热参片

川贝枇杷止咳冲剂

半夏露

艾叶油气雾剂

百合固金丸

百花定喘丸

苏子降气丸

杏仁止咳糖浆

牡荆油胶丸

芸香油滴丸

定喘丸

炙甘草合剂

罗汉果冲剂

养阴清肺膏

茯苓丸 控涎丸

复方喘贝精片 蛇胆川贝末

复方百部止咳糖浆 蛇胆陈皮末

通宣理肺丸 蛤蚧定喘丸

消咳喘糖浆 紫花杜鹃片

桃花散 喘舒片

润肺补膏 痰喘丸

莱阳梨止咳糖浆 痰咳净

清肺抑火丸 鲜竹沥口服液

麻杏止咳糖浆 橘红丸

清气化痰丸 礞石滚痰丸

气滞积聚门

九气拈痛丸 香砂六君丸

元胡止痛片 香砂枳术丸

开胸顺气丸 烂积丸

木香顺气丸 复肝宁片

木香槟榔丸 逍遥丸

平胃丸 益肝灵片

肚痛丸 健肝片

沉香化气丸 舒肝丸

沉香化滞丸 舒肝和胃丸

良附丸 越鞠丸

时感瘟疫门

九味羌活丸 牛黄清脑片

万氏牛黄清心丸 安宫牛黄丸

川芎茶调丸 防风通圣丸

小青龙合剂 防感片

局方至宝丹　　　　　　银翘解毒片

复方柴胡注射液　　　　西羚感冒片

桑菊感冒片　　　　　　西羚解毒片

银翘解毒丸　　　　　　紫雪丹

羚翘解毒丸　　　　　　腮腺炎片

银黄片　　　　　　　　感冒冲剂

清瘟解毒丸　　　　　　感冒清热冲剂

暑 湿 门

十枣水　　　　　　　　利胆排石片

十滴丸　　　　　　　　肾炎四味丸

八正合剂　　　　　　　金银花露

三金片　　　　　　　　祛暑丸

三仁合剂　　　　　　　茵陈五苓丸

仁丹　　　　　　　　　消炎利胆片

分清正淋丸　　　　　　益元散

五苓散　　　　　　　　清暑益气丸

六一散　　　　　　　　清凉油

玉枢丹　　　　　　　　清凉丹

风油精　　　　　　　　排石冲剂

石淋通片　　　　　　　暑湿正气丸

舟车丸　　　　　　　　痧药

冰霜梅苏丸　　　　　　暑症片

行军散　　　　　　　　痱子粉

利胆片　　　　　　　　藿香正气水

燥 火 门

千里光片　　　　　　　牛黄解毒丸

牛黄上清丸　　　　　　牛黄消炎丸

五仁醇胶囊	复方大青叶注射液
云芝肝太冲剂	复肝宁片
左金丸	栀子金花丸
龙胆泻肝丸	益肝灵片
戊己丸	银黄片
四季青片	黄芩素铝胶囊
连翘败毒丸	清宁丸
鸡骨草丸	黄连上清丸
抗菌消炎片	清脑丸
炎得平胶囊	舒肝和胃丸
板兰根干粉浆	犀羚解毒片

血 疟 门

十灰散	化症回生丸
三七片	荷叶丸

脾 胃 门

大山楂丸	枳实导滞丸
小建中合剂	保和丸
五仁润肠丸	麻仁丸
四神丸	清宁丸
四消丸	清胃保安片
安胃片	强肝丸
附子理中丸	槟榔四消丸

泻 痢 门

香连丸	痢必灵片
消炎抗菌丸	

外科

疮 疡 门

一粒珠
小金丹
内消瘰疬片
化痔灵片
牛黄消炎片
风湿止痛膏
阳和丸
如意金黄散
阳和解凝膏
沈阳红膏
冻疮水
拔毒膏
栀子金花丸
荆防败毒丸
宫颈癌片
脏连丸

海藻丸
桃花散
夏枯草膏
核葵注射液
消痔灵片
梅花点舌丹
鹅掌风药水
紫归治裂膏
猴菇菌片
阑尾消炎片
西黄丸
槐角丸
新癀片
鳖甲煎丸
醒消丸
蟾酥丸

外 伤 门

一粒止痛丹
七厘散
三七伤药片
九分散
万应散
片仔癀
五虎散
云南蛇药

云南白药
中华跌打丸
正骨水
京万红烫伤药膏
季德胜蛇药片
骨折挫伤散
烧伤气雾剂
接骨散

跌打药酒	跌打损伤丸
紫草膏	跌打丸
跌打活血散	玀油

妇科

经 带 门

八珍益母丸	妇科十味片
七制香附丸	妇科五淋丸
大黄䗪虫丸	妇科通经丸
女金丹	妇科调经片
千金止带丸	坤顺丸
少腹逐瘀丸	固经丸
乌鸡白凤丸	金鸡冲剂
艾附暖宫丸	益母丸
白带丸	调经至宝丸
当归补血精	益母草膏
当归养血丸	鹿胎膏
当归浸膏丸	痛经丸
血府逐瘀丸	温经丸

胎 前 门

安胎丸	鹿胎膏
保胎丸	

产 后 门

下乳通泉散	产后身痛片
生化汤丸	益母草膏
失笑散	益母丸

儿科

惊 风 门

七珍丹
小儿奇应丸
小儿惊风丸
小儿牛黄清心散
牛黄至宝丹

牛黄镇惊丸
牛黄抱龙片
五粒回春丹
保婴镇惊丸
婴儿安片

疳 积 门

小儿健脾丸
小儿消积丸
小儿奇应丸
小儿消食片
乌梅丸
乌梅安胃丸

肥儿丸
保赤丸
香桔丸
香苏正胃丸
婴儿散

儿科其他门

小儿止嗽丸
小儿至宝丸
万应锭
小儿止咳糖浆
小儿肝炎冲剂
小儿退热冲剂
小儿解热栓
小儿升血灵

小儿止泻片
五粒回春丹
五福化毒丹
导赤丸
百日咳片
妙灵丹
清疹散
稚儿灵冲剂

五官科

眼 目 门

石斛夜光丸　　　　　　明目羊肝丸
光明眼药　　　　　　　黄连羊肝丸
杞菊地黄丸　　　　　　障眼明片
明目地黄丸　　　　　　磁朱丸

咽喉口齿门

牙痛一粒丸　　　　　　冰硼散
六神丸　　　　　　　　炎得平胶囊
牛黄益金丸　　　　　　清音丸
双料喉风散　　　　　　喉症丸
牙痛水　　　　　　　　锡类散

耳 鼻 门

耳聋左慈丸　　　　　　鼻炎糖浆
鼻渊丸　　　　　　　　藿胆丸
鼻炎片

其他

白癜风丸　　　　　　　美容祛斑药膏
肤螨灵软膏

附录 2

现代医学病症药名索引

流行性感冒

荆防败毒丸　　　　　　　通宣理肺丸
复方大青叶注射液　　　　小青龙合剂
银翘解毒片　　　　　　　藿香正气水
感冒解热冲剂

普 通 感 冒

西羚解毒片　　　　　　　六合定中丸
羚翘解毒片　　　　　　　复方柴胡注射液
桑菊感冒片　　　　　　　牛黄上清丸
风寒感冒冲剂　　　　　　紫金锭
防风通圣丸　　　　　　　玉屏风丸
感冒清热冲剂　　　　　　养阴清肺膏
九味羌活丸　　　　　　　香砂六君丸
川芎茶调散　　　　　　　罗汉果冲剂

流行性乙型脑炎

安宫牛黄丸　　　　　　　紫雪丹
局方至宝丹　　　　　　　感冒冲剂

流行性脑脊髓膜炎

安宫牛黄丸　　　　　　　复方大青叶注射液
局方至宝丹　　　　　　　板兰根干糖浆
紫雪丹

黄疸性肝炎

云芝肝太冲剂　　　　　　茵陈五苓丸
龙胆泻肝丸　　　　　　　复肝宁片
健肝片　　　　　　　　　五苓散
灵芝糖浆

慢 性 肝 炎

越鞠丸　　　　　　　　　失笑散
木香顺气丸　　　　　　　香砂养胃丸
开胸顺气丸　　　　　　　九气拈痛丸
良附丸　　　　　　　　　沉香化滞丸
舒肝丸　　　　　　　　　黄芪建中丸
逍遥丸　　　　　　　　　小建中合剂
舒肝和胃丸　　　　　　　补中益气丸
鸡骨草丸　　　　　　　　参杞冲剂
五仁醇胶囊　　　　　　　七厘散
健肝片　　　　　　　　　脑灵素片
益肝灵片

细菌性痢疾

痢必灵　　　　　　　　　葛根芩连片
香连丸　　　　　　　　　木香槟榔丸
黄芩素铝胶囊　　　　　　枳实导滞丸

左金丸　　　　　　　　　　　银黄片

戊己丸　　　　　　　　　　　千里光片

附子理中丸　　　　　　　　　炎得平胶囊

蛔 虫 病

乌梅丸　　　　　　　　　　　驱虫片

乌梅安胃丸　　　　　　　　　使君子丸

川楝素片　　　　　　　　　　化虫丸

咽 喉 炎

六神丸　　　　　　　　　　　牛黄解毒片

喉症丸　　　　　　　　　　　栀子金花丸

双料喉风散　　　　　　　　　黄连上清丸

牛黄益金片　　　　　　　　　川贝枇杷止咳冲剂

梅花点舌丹　　　　　　　　　杏仁止咳糖浆

冰硼散　　　　　　　　　　　二冬膏

牛黄消炎丸　　　　　　　　　痰咳净

清音丸　　　　　　　　　　　罗汉果冲剂

炎得平胶囊　　　　　　　　　养阴清肺膏

百合固金丸

扁 桃 体 炎

喉症丸　　　　　　　　　　　牛黄解毒丸

冰硼散　　　　　　　　　　　四季青片

双料喉风散　　　　　　　　　养阴清肺膏

梅花点舌丹

阑 尾 炎

阑尾消炎片　　　　　　　　　千里光片

荨 麻 疹

麻杏止咳糖浆　　　　　　首乌丸
防风通圣丸

胆 道 结 石

利胆片　　　　　　　　　消炎利胆片
利胆排石片

腮 腺 炎

夏枯草膏　　　　　　　　牛黄解毒丸
紫金锭　　　　　　　　　银翘解毒片
六神丸　　　　　　　　　黄连上清丸
梅花点舌丹　　　　　　　如意金黄散
腮腺炎片　　　　　　　　板兰根干糖浆

乳 腺 炎

醒消丸　　　　　　　　　西黄丸
荆防败毒丸　　　　　　　一粒珠
小金丸

视 神 经 炎

石斛夜光丸　　　　　　　黄连羊肝丸
杞菊地黄丸　　　　　　　障眼明片
明目地黄丸

鼻 炎

藿胆丸　　　　　　　　　鼻渊丸
鼻炎片　　　　　　　　　鼻炎糖浆

清眩丸　　　　　　　　　芎菊上清丸
六神丸　　　　　　　　　川芎茶调散
双料喉风散　　　　　　　小建中合剂

肾　　炎

茵陈五苓丸　　　　　　　参苓白术散
舟车丸　　　　　　　　　六味地黄丸
五苓散　　　　　　　　　五子衍宗丸
三仁合剂　　　　　　　　海马补肾丸
八正合剂　　　　　　　　补肾宁
二妙丸　　　　　　　　　锁阳固精丸
分清五淋丸　　　　　　　补肾强身片
石淋通片　　　　　　　　青娥丸
三金片　　　　　　　　　全鹿丸
健脑补肾丸　　　　　　　六一散
妇科分清丸　　　　　　　脑灵素

甲状腺功能亢进

海藻丸　　　　　　　　　大补阴丸
夏枯草膏　　　　　　　　天王补心丹
六味地黄丸

糖　尿　病

消渴丸　　　　　　　　　大补阴丸
消渴平片　　　　　　　　全鹿丸
六味地黄丸　　　　　　　鹿胎膏
玉泉丸　　　　　　　　　脑灵素
缩泉丸　　　　　　　　　人参精

再生障碍性贫血

阿胶
人参归脾丸

小建中合剂

一般性贫血

阿胶
新阿胶
黄明胶
复方阿胶浆
升血膏
健脑补肾丸
当归补血精

鸡血藤片
补中益气丸
八珍丸
青春宝
双宝素
人参精
山东阿胶膏

肺 结 核

蛤蚧定喘丸
百合固金丸
清肺抑火丸

炙甘草合剂
生脉饮口服液

高 血 压

牛黄降压片
牛黄清脑片
舒心降压片
杜仲降压片
复方罗布麻片
罗布麻降压片
降压平片
脑立清

清脑丸
芎菊上清丸
愈风宁心片
灵芝糖浆
再造丸
防风通圣丸
六味地黄丸

动 脉 硬 化

脉乐通
活心丸
参杞冲剂

首乌丸
万氏牛黄清心丸

高 脂 血 症

降脂灵胶丸
消栓再造丸
清栓通络片

脉安冲剂
益肝灵片

冠 心 病

活心丸
益心丸
环心丹
苏冰滴丸
复方丹参片
复方丹参注射液
保心丸
速效救心丸
心可舒片

解心痛片
冠心苏合丸
舒心降压片
红花注射液
脉乐通
愈风宁心片
华佗再造丸
冠心通脉灵片

脑血管意外

安宫牛黄丸
人参再造丸
大活络丸
天麻丸

再造丸
牛黄降压片
局方牛黄清心丸

癫　痫

礞石滚痰丸	磁朱丸
医痫丸	局方至宝丹
羊痫风丸	局方牛黄清心丸
白金丸	朱砂安神丸

脑　血　栓

消栓再造丸	脉络通
消栓通络片	冠心通脉灵片

急性胃肠炎

痢必灵片	清胃保安丸
银黄片	炎得平胶囊
葛根芩连片	千里光片
四消丸	痧药
枳实导滞丸	益元散
四君子丸	行军散
保和丸	戊己丸
六合定中丸	小半夏合剂

慢　性　胃　炎

木香顺气丸	良附丸
平胃丸	开胸顺气丸
人参健脾丸	九气拈痛丸
香砂养胃丸	烂积丸
启脾丸	元胡止痛片
保和丸	三仁合剂
安胃片	

胃及十二指肠溃疡

参苓白术散　　　　　　　　左金丸
香砂六君丸　　　　　　　　舒肝丸
附子理中丸

神经官能症

安神补心丸　　　　　　　　健脑补肾丸

神 经 衰 弱

天王补心丹　　　　　　　　五味子冲剂
朱砂安神丸　　　　　　　　香砂六君丸
枕中丹　　　　　　　　　　小建中合剂
柏子养心丸　　　　　　　　黄芪建中丸
安神补心丸　　　　　　　　逍遥丸
脑灵素　　　　　　　　　　鹿胎膏
健脑补肾丸　　　　　　　　补中益气丸
健脑丸　　　　　　　　　　当归补血精
炙甘草合剂　　　　　　　　青春宝
人参归脾丸　　　　　　　　双宝素
磁朱丸　　　　　　　　　　人参精
灵芝糖浆　　　　　　　　　人参蜂王浆

高 温 中 暑

藿香正气水　　　　　　　　暑湿正气丸
祛暑丸　　　　　　　　　　清凉丹
清暑益气丸　　　　　　　　金银花露
暑症丸　　　　　　　　　　生脉饮口服液
仁丹　　　　　　　　　　　十滴水

风湿性肌纤维炎

大活络丸	武力拔寒散
小活络丸	豨莶丸
镇江膏药	九分散
风湿祛痛膏	复方当归注射液
风湿止痛膏	祛风舒筋丸
阳和解凝膏	坎离砂

风湿性关节炎

国公酒	风湿止痛膏
消络痛	阳和解凝膏
小活络丸	金不换膏药
天麻丸	冯了性药酒
独活寄生丸	舒筋活络酒
木瓜丸	祛风舒筋丸
镇江膏药	复方当归注射液
伤湿宝珍膏	九分散
伤湿止痛膏	坎离砂

骨 质 增 生

骨刺片	骨刺消痛液
骨质增生丸	大活络丸
骨刺丸	小活络丸
骨仙丸	豨莶丸

化脓性感染

抗菌消炎片	千里光片
紫草膏	牛黄解毒片

一粒珠　　　　　　　　　　　拔毒膏
蟾酥丸

骨　　折

跌打丸　　　　　　　　　　　正骨水
中华跌打丸　　　　　　　　　沈阳红药
七厘散　　　　　　　　　　　接骨散
骨折挫伤散　　　　　　　　　伸筋丹

外 伤 出 血

云南白药　　　　　　　　　　槐角丸
三七片

蜂窝组织炎

小金丸　　　　　　　　　　　蟾酥丸
栀子金花丸　　　　　　　　　拔毒膏

湿　　疹

二妙丸　　　　　　　　　　　荆防败毒丸
如意金黄散　　　　　　　　　金鸡冲剂

肿　　瘤

西黄丸　　　　　　　　　　　醒消丸
片仔癀　　　　　　　　　　　鸦胆子乳注射液
新癀片　　　　　　　　　　　宫颈癌片
核葵注射液　　　　　　　　　猴菇菌片

月 经 失 调

鸡血藤片　　　　　　　　　　乌鸡白凤丸

益母丸
逍遥丸
八宝坤顺丸
七制香附丸
妇科调经片
艾附暖宫丸
女金丹
当归养血丸
八珍益母丸

当归浸膏片
妇康宁片
千金止带丸
产后身痛片
少腹逐瘀丸
调经至宝丸
金鸡冲剂
失笑散

闭　　经

当归养血丸
妇科通经丸

大黄䗪虫丸

白　　带

白带丸
女金丹
千金止带丸
乌鸡白凤丸

艾附暖宫丸
温经丸
固经丸

痛　　经

越鞠丸
良附丸
痛经丸
温经丸
九气拈痛丸
元胡止痛片
七制香附丸
当归浸膏片

益母丸
益母草膏
失笑散
八珍益母丸
调经至宝丸
少腹逐瘀丸
金鸡冲剂

不 孕 症

鹿胎膏　　　　　　　　　　雏凤精
鹿角胶　　　　　　　　　　阿胶

习惯性流产

安胎丸　　　　　　　　　　山东阿胶膏
保胎丸

功能性子宫出血

人参归脾丸　　　　　　　　乌鸡白凤丸
阿胶　　　　　　　　　　　十灰散
女金丹　　　　　　　　　　荷叶丸

·便　　秘

麻仁丸　　　　　　　　　　枳实导滞丸
五仁润肠丸　　　　　　　　四消丸

青　光　眼

石斛夜光丸　　　　　　　　杞菊地黄丸
黄连羊肝丸

白　内　障

障眼明片　　　　　　　　　石斛夜光丸
黄连羊肝丸　　　　　　　　杞菊地黄丸

肺　　炎

百合固金丸　　　　　　　　麻杏止咳糖浆
止嗽定喘丸　　　　　　　　风寒感冒冲剂

西羚解毒片　　　　　　　三仁合剂

银翘解毒片　　　　　　　银黄片

羚翘解毒片　　　　　　　千里光片

抗菌消炎片　　　　　　　控涎丹

复方大青叶注射液

支气管哮喘

止嗽青果丸　　　　　　　鲜竹沥口服液

清肺抑火丸　　　　　　　定喘丸

止嗽定喘丸　　　　　　　痰喘丸

茯苓丸　　　　　　　　　喘舒片

小青龙合剂　　　　　　　海龙蛤蚧精

止咳喘热参片　　　　　　艾叶油气雾剂

百花定喘丸　　　　　　　苏子降气丸

慢性气管炎

二母宁嗽丸　　　　　　　半夏露

二陈丸　　　　　　　　　玉屏风丸

橘红丸　　　　　　　　　清瘟解毒丸

罗汉果冲剂　　　　　　　莱阳梨止咳糖浆

川贝枇杷止咳冲剂　　　　苏子降气丸

复方川贝精片　　　　　　止嗽定喘丸

痰咳净　　　　　　　　　喘舒片

消咳喘　　　　　　　　　礞石滚痰丸

百　日　咳

百日咳片　　　　　　　　蛇胆川贝末

蛇胆陈皮末

性神经衰弱

至宝三鞭丸

龟龄集

海龙蛤蚧精

还少丹

全鹿丸

男宝

三肾丸

海马补肾丸

补肾宁片

锁阳固精丸

海龙胶

二仙膏

鹿角胶

雏凤精

鹿胎膏

人参精

THE ENGLISH–CHINESE ENCYCLOPEDIA OF PRACTICAL TCM

(Booklist)

英汉实用中医药大全

（书目）

VOLUME	TITLE	书名
1	ESSENTIALS OF TRADITIONAL CHINESE MEDICINE	中医学基础
2	THE CHINESE MATERIA MEDICA	中药学
3	PHARMACOLOGY OF TRADITIONAL CHINESE MEDICAL FORMULAE	方剂学
4	SIMPLE AND PROVED PECIPES	单验方
5	COMMONLY USED CHINESE PATENT MEDICINES	常用中成药
6	THERAPEUTICS OF ACUPUNCTURE AND MOXIBUSTION	针灸治疗学
7	*TUINA* THERAPEUTICS	推拿治疗学
8	MEDICAL *QIGONG*	医学气功
9	MAINTAINING YOUR HEALTH	自我保健
10	INTERNAL MEDICINE	内科学

Special Thanks To
鸣　谢

The Education Commission of Shandong Province
山东省教育委员会
TCM Administrative Bureau of Shandong Province
山东省中医管理局
Jinan Factory of Traditional Chinese Drugs
济南中药厂
Shandong Donge Factory for Making Ejiao (Donkey-hide Gelatin)
山东东阿阿胶厂
Shandong Pingyin Factory for Making Ejiao (Donkey-hide Gelatin)
山东平阴阿胶厂
Medicinal General Corporation of Zhejiang Province
浙江省医药总公司
Weifang Factory of Traditional Chinese Drugs
潍坊中药厂
Shandong Zibo People's Pharmaceutical Factory
山东淄博人民制药厂
Jinan Factory of Chemicals For Daily Use
济南日化厂
Jining City Factory of Traditional Chinese Drugs
济宁市中药厂
Zhejiang Ningbo Pharmaceutical Factory
浙江宁波制药厂

Zhejiang Jinhua Shuanglong Pharmaceutical Factory

浙江金华双龙制药厂

Zhejiang Lanxi Pharmaceutical Factory

浙江兰溪制药厂

Shandong Yantai Factory of Traditional Chinese Drugs

山东烟台中药厂

Shandong Linqing Factory of Traditional Chinese Drugs

山东临清中药厂